13250173    3-25-85    46/0

**Lift Your Way to Youthful Fitness**

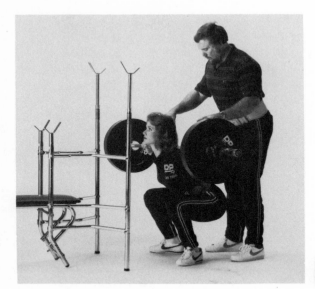

**Lift You**

# Way to Youthful Fitness

*The Comprehensive Guide to Weight Training*

**Jan Todd and Terry Todd, Ph.D.**

 A *Sports Illustrated* Book

**Little, Brown and Company • Boston • Toronto**

FIRST EDITION

*Photograph credits appear on page 341*

*Before embarking on any strenuous exercise program, including this one, everyone, particularly anyone over thirty-five or anyone with any known heart or blood-pressure problem, should be examined by a physician.*

*Library of Congress Cataloging in Publication Data*

Todd, Jan.
    Lift your way to youthful fitness.

    Bibliography: p. 323
    Includes index.
    1. Weight lifting.   2. Physical fitness.   I. Todd, Terry.   II. Title.
GV546.3.T63   1985       613.7'1       85-7
ISBN 0-316-85061-6

*Sports Illustrated* books
are published by
Little, Brown and Company
in association with
*Sports Illustrated* magazine

MV
*Published simultaneously in Canada
by Little, Brown & Company (Canada) Limited*

PRINTED IN THE UNITED STATES OF AMERICA

A few years ago, Floyd Burdette was one of the subjects in a research study conducted at Auburn University, where we then taught. The purpose of the research project, which is described in some detail in Chapter 10, was to compare the physiological effects of two programs of exercise, weight training and jogging, on two groups of middle-aged sedentary men. Floyd was in our weight-training group, and it would be fair to say that he was the least-fit subject tested. He was overweight, weak, inflexible, and in poor cardiovascular condition. He had never been active in athletics, but he was a crackerjack corporate executive, having served as the vice-president of finance at Diversified Products Corporation for fourteen years.

The lifting was tough on Floyd, both physically and emotionally, surrounded as he was by larger and stronger men, many of whom had been varsity athletes in college. But he stuck it out. He never missed a training session when he was in town, and soon his hard work began to show. His waist got smaller and his shoulders grew, while his strength seemed almost to double. The change in his spirits was no less dramatic. He was the talk of the office. Overjoyed by his newfound vigor, he trained even harder, continued to gain, and by the end of the project, he was almost literally a new man. He was leaner, stronger, more flexible, more enduring, and so enthralled by these changes that he continued his exercises faithfully once the project ended. Three days a week, Floyd, smiling, would stroll into our weight room at Auburn, gym bag in hand, and greet each young lifter by name.

On Sunday, July 17, 1983, Floyd drowned in heavy surf at Gulf Shores, Alabama. He was fifty-one years old. He was our friend, and we dedicate this book to his memory.

## Note to Readers

We researched, argued about, and finally wrote this book together, and so it seemed inappropriate to use any other pronoun than what the grammar books refer to as first person plural. Hence the "we." From time to time throughout the book, however, each of us will relate some anecdote or make some point from our own individual perspective. When we do that, we'll preface that passage with the name — in bold letters — of whichever of us is speaking, e.g., **Jan:** or **Terry:**, and we'll place the passage within quotation marks.

# Contents

# Acknowledgments

THANKS.

First, to our parents, who passed along whatever vigor and strength we have.

Second, to Bill Pearl, Doris Barrilleaux, Judy Gedney, and the Curry Family, who were kind enough to share with us their time and photographs.

Third, to the many people in the field of strength and fitness who have inspired us with their robust youthfulness, including — but not limited to — Sam Loprinzi, Milo Steinborn, Sig Klein, Bob Hoffman, John Grimek, Vic Tanny, Vic Boff, Joe Weider, Al Treloar, Ottley Coulter, David P. Willoughby, Charles A. Smith, Peary and Mabel Rader, Bill Good, Kate Sandwina, Mac Bachelor, Al Turner, Bernarr MacFadden, Roy J. McLean, Al Thomas, Pudgy Stockton, Otto Arco, Stanislaus Zbyszko, Warren Lincoln Travis, Eugen Sandow, Albert Beckles, Black Jack Woodson, Norbert Schemansky, Karl Norberg, W. A. Pullum, David Webster, Jim Witt, Precious McKenzie, Joe Greenstein, and George Hackenschmidt.

Fourth, to Dr. Mike Stone, whose research efforts in the field of resistance training have helped validate many of the physical benefits of this form of exercise.

Fifth, to the hardworking men and women who participated in the research projects we described in chapters 10 and 11.

Sixth, to Joe Hood and Dr. Waneen Spirduso of the Physical Education Department at the University of Texas at Austin, both of whom read portions of the manuscript and enlightened us with their comments.

Finally, our Seventh Seal of Approval goes to Bill Phillips of Little, Brown for his editorial guidance and constant support.

Jan and Terry Todd
Austin, Texas

PART ONE

# How This All Began

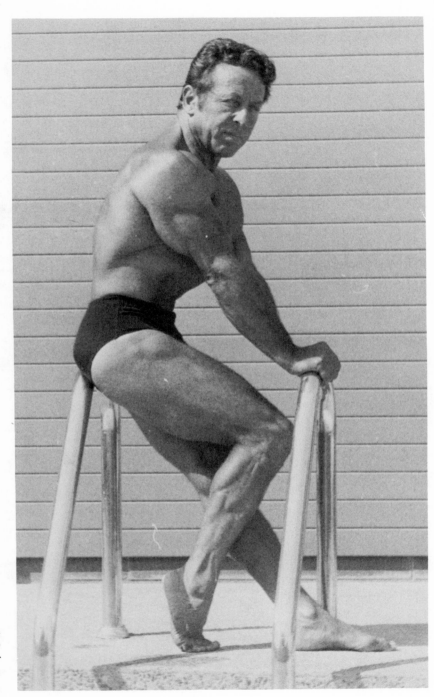

*It was this shot of Sam Loprinzi, taken when he was sixty-two, that caused us to begin wondering why so many of our weightlifting friends looked so much younger than their peers.*

I N the summer of 1978, we traveled to Portland, Oregon, to appear in a series of exhibitions at the Multnomah County Fair. The shows had been organized by a division of the Guinness Corporation, which, besides publishing the *Guinness Book of World Records,* owns several museums around the world.

One of the reasons we wanted to make the trip was to look up an old friend, Sam Loprinzi, who ran a gym in Portland, and who had been famous during the thirties, forties, and fifties for his strength and physique. Shortly after we arrived in Portland we headed for his gym to take a workout and visit.

We got there a little before Sam did, so we had time to look around a bit. On the walls of the immaculate, well-equipped gym were dozens of photos of the top bodybuilders from the past and the present, and among the faces in the frames, we saw photos of Sam himself, posed in trunks. It was interesting, because the quality of the photographs and the staging of the shots gave more evidence of the relative age of the various photos than did the body itself. On the back wall was a large color shot, obviously newer, with Sam leaning against a swimming-pool ladder, stomach flat, shoulders squared back to show the depth of his chest, the muscles of his arms and legs standing out in relief. Tanned, skin glowing, his hair dark and shiny, he looked in the photo as he always had before. He came into the room then, saw us, and as we began to catch up on days and people gone by, neither of us could resist glancing at the color photo from time to time as we talked. Finally, not able to stand the curiosity any longer, one of us asked Sam how old he was when the color shot was taken. He smiled then, turning toward the photo, and replied, "Still look pretty good for an old man, don't I? It was taken last summer. I was sixty-two." **Jan:** "I almost choked before I managed to sputter, 'You *can't* be that old. Terry told me you were a friend of his from the old days, but I thought he meant you were roughly the same age. I can't believe you're sixty-two.' Thinking back on it now and remembering how Sam looked, standing in his knit shirt and khaki slacks, I still remember my disbelief. And later, after we left, Terry commented on how amazed *he* had been, despite his knowledge of Sam's approximate age."

It's always difficult to say what it is that makes a person "look forty" or "look fifty," let alone sixty or seventy or eighty. The physical attributes of aging are so diverse and come upon us so slowly that it's hard to pinpoint when you or someone you see often starts "looking old," or even older. The two major changes that occur in both men and women and give external clues to age are the increase in the wrinkling of the skin that occurs as the skin dries and thins out, and the loss of muscular size and shape. At age twenty, most men and women are at their hereditary peak of muscularity. In untrained, average men, for instance, the output of male hormones will be at its highest level, producing in those twenty-year-old bodies the greatest density of muscle tissue. Hence the average, untrained male at age twenty will look fit, his stomach will be flat, his body erect, and the muscles in his arms and shoulders will be slightly evident. He'll have a body-fat ratio of somewhere around 15 percent (fat tissue to total body weight), which he'll be able to maintain until he's thirty-five or so if he gets some regular exercise. But around age thirty-five, things begin to get a little harder, or shall we say *softer.*

Studies at the National Institute on Aging have shown that between the ages of thirty and seventy an "average" male (one who exercises a little, doesn't smoke or drink to excess, and has a typical office work situation) will lose an inch and an eighth in height, will go from 15 percent body fat at 165 pounds of weight to 30 percent body fat at 178 pounds of weight, will find his pulse rate slowing from 200 beats per minute during vigorous exercise to only 150 beats per minute, and will notice his shoulders narrowing by at least an inch as he loses muscle tissue and the remaining muscle tissue becomes weaker and stringier. A number of other indignities occur as well, including not only a decrease in the number of erections he has but also a decrease in the angle of the erections. Lord help us.

Women go through a very similar process. The "average" woman reaches her full height by age fourteen, by which time she will have started her menstrual cycle and begun "filling out." Part of that filling-out process is the acquisition of extra adipose tissue, or fat, on her buttocks, thighs, and bustline. Unlike her male counterpart, the average woman will carry a body-fat ratio of 22 to 25 percent during her college years, which will increase to 30 percent by the time she is thirty-five, and will continue to increase with the years unless something is done to slow, halt, or reverse this process. The other area of the body where fat is stored through genetic design is what physiologists call the "ventral apron," or *tela adiposa* — your belly. Knowing that nature has preordained these deposits, however, doesn't make it any easier for most women to like them, and unless a woman is very careful in her eating habits and exercise, she'll soon find that more and more of her body is soft. Women, because they mature more quickly than men and because of differing hormonal outputs, are also left with a smaller average bone structure, hence narrower shoulders than men, a smaller thoracic cavity, shorter legs, a slightly broader pelvic structure, and, with that, a larger relative abdominal cavity. Muscularly, she is also shortchanged, and the girths and lengths of the muscles of women are smaller on the average than those in the male.

Women were also given the short end of the stick when it comes to their skin. According to dermatologists, women's skin, because it is thinner in construction and less oily, is far more prone to wrinkling than that of men. It begins to wrinkle at a much younger age, the wrinkling being due to a breakdown of collagen in the skin that is believed to be caused by repeated exposure to sunlight, heat, harsh soaps, and other environmental factors. According to Dr. Albert Klingman of the University of Pennsylvania Medical School, unexposed skin doesn't show any real age-related changes, performing pretty much the same from age fifteen to age fifty, in terms of sweating, blood supply, cell production, elasticity, and so forth. The environment produces what we think of as aging — the blemishes, blotches, dry spots, and benign tumors. Apart from looseness, every skin change that you see with your eyes and feel with your hands is the result of an environmental insult. It is not a natural thing.

Natural or not, despite the high sales figure for skin lotions and beauty creams, all women and most men find themselves heading into the fearful forties with furrows in their brows. Sartre's observation that by fifty each person deserves his own face has been corroborated recently by science. According to Dr. Klingman, wrinkles are simply the products of gravity and repeated facial expressions. As we frown, or squint, or smile, the face is set into patterns of expression again and again. In our youth the collagen and elastin (fibers in our skin that cause the skin to snap back in place) are healthy and strong. As the skin is exposed to light and heat, these fibers break down so that the folds never completely smooth back as they did in our youth. The youngest-looking skin on a man will be on his buttocks, which are rarely exposed to the sun. Dr. Klingman says, "I always show women the underside of their breast or upper arm. That's the way the skin on their face should look until age ninety. It ought to be smooth and soft and absolutely without a blemish. The only reason it isn't is that it's not protected from the environment the way the underside of the breast is. (Obviously, no one can stay indoors all the time — nor should they try — since we need some sunlight to maintain our vitamin D levels. If you're going to be outdoors for an extended period, however, wear a hat and put on some sunscreen to shield your skin as much as possible.)

The only advantage women seem to have over men in terms of appearance is in the hair of their heads. Both sexes will have a diminution in both the number of hairs on their heads and in the thickness of the hair, but women are far less prone to balding than their male counterparts.

So when we try to assess someone's age, we generally look first at the

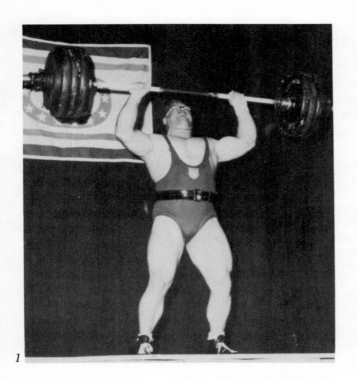

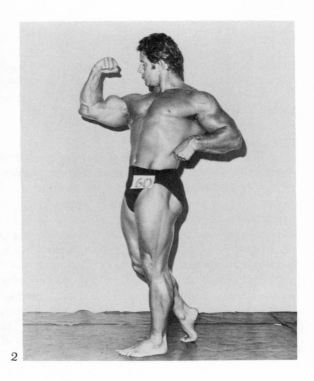

1. Nobert Schemansky, four-time Olympic medalist, shown here in his early forties. 2. Englishman Reg Park, here in his middle forties. 3. Doris Barrilleaux at fifty-one shows the results of almost thirty years of weight training. 4. Great Britain's Ron Collins, shown here at forty-two, is a seven-time world champion powerlifter.

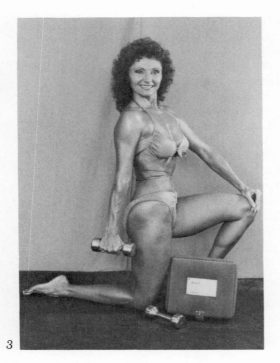

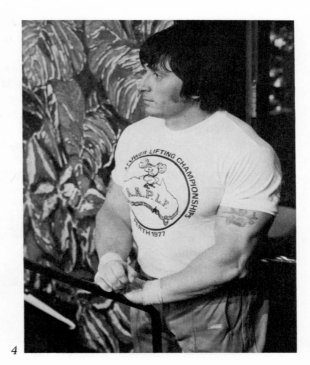

6  3

4

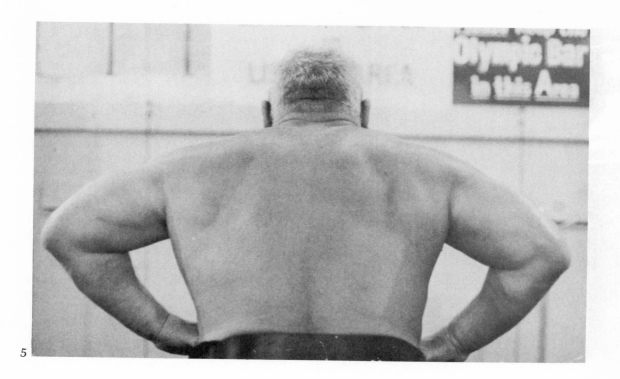

5. *Karl Norberg began training at age sixty-five. His record for bench pressing 460 pounds in his seventies is unsurpassed. 6. John Grimek dominated bodybuilding through the 1930s, 1940s, and into the 1950s. 7. Otto Arco, here in his late fifties, demonstrates an abdominal muscle control called the "rope." 8. Russian George Hackenschmidt, lifelong weightlifter, here in his eighties, hopping over a rope stretched between two chairs.*

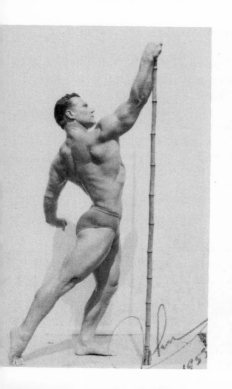

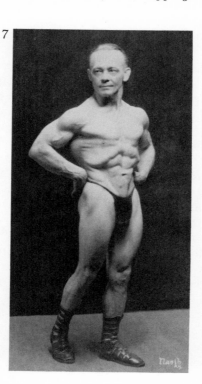

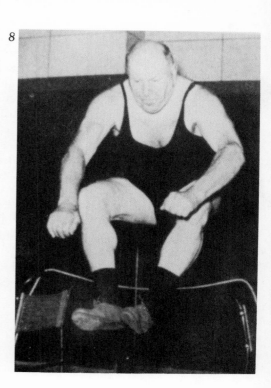

face, then at the posture and "condition" of the body. What causes posture to worsen over time, of course, is that gravity is always at work trying to cause us to stoop or slump. Only our muscles maintain the erect posture of youth. When we saw Sam Loprinzi in Portland, he defied the rules in both categories, but especially in the latter. Though his face was not that of a twenty-year-old, he certainly didn't "look sixty" either. The color in his cheeks was ruddy, his wrinkles were minimal, his skin glowed. His posture was excellent. But the most amazing thing about Sam was the fullness of his muscles and the way those muscles moved him around his gym. His step was quick and cat-sure; there was a bounce in his walk. There was none of the hesitant, short-stepped shuffling one associates with the aged. It was clear to both of us that something Sam had done along the way had helped him to maintain his remarkably youthful appearance.

Part of what made Sam different, of course, was his attitude. "I never liked the idea of losing the look and strength of a young man, and so I decided I'd fight it every way I could, with a careful diet, adequate rest, and lots of good, regular work in the weight room. I'm still fighting."

This attitude was stated best forty years ago by the Welsh poet Dylan Thomas when he advised his father:

> Do not go gentle into that good night.
> Rage, rage against the dying of the light.

That couplet is one we admire. We hold with it. The simple fact is that just as Sam has been able to ward off many of the less pleasant physical aspects of aging, so can we all. Just as we insulate our homes in the warm weather against the sharp winds of wintertime, and just as we invest in such things as IRA accounts for our retirement, we can fortify ourselves with exercise against the guerrilla warfare waged on our bodies by the passing years.

Seeing Sam that day in Portland inspired us to remember other men we'd known who'd been lifelong weight trainers and who shared many of the same characteristics of youth so evident in Sam. John Grimek, the great bodybuilding champion who is now in his seventies, came immediately to mind, as did Milo Steinborn, Otto Arco, Sig Klein, and a number of others, both living and dead. We also remembered the remarkable physical development that Doris Barrilleaux still maintained, though she was now in her fifties. Was there something in the lifting of weights that helped to create this look of youth? What happened to people who trained with weights? Why were there so many who looked ten to twenty years younger than their peers? Was the answer fitness in general, or was there something about weightlifting in particular?

We looked at photos of older athletes in other sports, and the more we looked, the wider the difference seemed between the weightlifters and their age peers from other sports — joggers, racquetball players, golfers, and so on. There had to be something going on here beyond genetic predisposition. We decided to find out what this something was, and our search was endlessly fascinating, revealing a wealth of information and several central, critical truths. We've tried to present these truths and a good deal of the information throughout this book.

We hope this will help people begin to take control of their lives in such a way that they can offset the unpleasant effects of aging. We're confident that what we have to say can benefit the average man or woman more than they could easily imagine. Perhaps we would overstate our case if we said weightlifting could produce miracles, but our own lives have at times truly *seemed* miraculous. We'd like to tell you now a bit about our lives so you can judge for yourselves.

# 1 / Terry's Story

IN the early sixties, John F. Kennedy created the President's Council on Physical Fitness, and Americans in increasingly large numbers began jogging, playing handball and tennis, spreading by word of mouth how much their new exercise program had improved the way they looked and felt. But even before those early years, I was involved in what almost everyone then considered a waste of time. I was a weightlifter. But my first athletic love was tennis.

From the time I was about thirteen until I was a sophomore in college, I spent the major part of my springs, summers, and falls on the courts. Throughout my high-school years I played on the tennis team, playing well enough to go to the state tournament, and upon graduation I went to the University of Texas in Austin and managed to earn the number-one spot on the freshman team. During my senior year in high school, I'd reached my full 6 feet 2 inches in height, and I starved myself so that I stayed around 185 pounds. I wanted to look just like a tennis player was supposed to look, and though my big frame was pretty spare back then, I had an image to maintain. The summer before I entered the University of Texas, however, I took a break from tennis and decided to begin doing a bit of dumbbell training for my left arm, which, to me, was embarrassingly small in size compared to my right. One of my friends trained with me that summer, and what had started as work for one arm gradually became a full routine as I found both the increased strength and the increased size interesting. I gained 30 to 35 pounds that summer but during my freshman year I played better tennis than ever, finding the additional strength and quickness that the weights produced an asset to my game, not a hindrance. I lettered my sophomore year and continued to lift and get bigger, reaching 230 or so that spring. In the fall of my junior year I won the team tournament at a weight of 245 pounds, and though my game was still improving, I looked like anything but a tennis player.

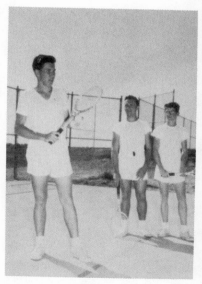

At 6'2'' and 185 pounds, eighteen-year-old Terry Todd was a sapling ready to become an oak.

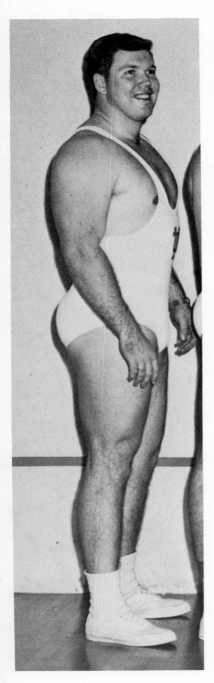

That was the late fifties, remember, before weight training became a part of the football conditioning programs, and in my junior year, I was larger than all but two of the linemen at UT, and, naturally, my new tennis coach took some ribbing about my size. However, my first college coach, Dr. Daniel Penick, actually seemed to like my size. He was eighty-seven years old when he retired and his eyesight was failing him a bit, but I remember him calling me over one day to the bench, where he sat in the sun watching the team. "Todd," he said, "you're my favorite player." I was shocked, and I managed to mumble my thanks before he went on to say, "Yes, you're my favorite. I can't tell the other men apart very well now if they're very far away, but *you*, Todd, you have a very distinctive silhouette." But my new coach liked neither my size nor the ribbing. Finally, he gave me an ultimatum — lose weight or lose your scholarship — despite the way I was playing. The implication was also clear — stop lifting weights. The unfairness of this rankled, and so I just quit, spending my last year and a half as an undergraduate concentrating on the barbells.

When I was no longer putting in the hours of regular practice on the sunny Texas courts, I not only had more time but more energy for the lifting. My strength increased dramatically, as did my size. For the next several years, as I finished up undergraduate work and began my graduate work on the history of sports, I lived the ideal athlete's life. I ate at my mother's bounteous table, and though I was, of course, interested in my research and course work, I was able to focus a major part of each day on my training, spending long hours in the gym. In three years' time, I weighed over 300 pounds and I won my first National Championship, in Olympic lifting. At about the same time, a new sort of lifting competition was being organized, called powerlifting, and I fell in love with it.

Unlike the Olympic lifts, which require great speed, flexibility, and considerable technique, the powerlifts (squat, bench press, and deadlift, all defined on pages 149–153) require mainly brute strength. The people at the York Barbell Club decided to hold a national-level meet — the first ever, in the summer of 1964 — and I began to train with renewed interest, for though I enjoyed Olympic lifting I began it too late to develop the flexibility in my hips and shoulders needed to reach the highest levels internationally.

Powerlifting came along at a convenient time, and I participated in the superheavyweight division of that first big meet, winning and outdistancing the man in the weight class below by 375 pounds. I "totalled" (squat plus bench plus deadlift) over 1600 pounds in the three lifts that year and went on to become the first man to break the barriers at 1700, 1800, and 1900 pounds officially over the next few years of my competitive career. At my peak I weighed 340 pounds and I measured 61 inches around my chest, 36¼ inches around my thighs, 22¾ inches around my biceps, 46 inches around the waist, and 17 inches in the forearm. My personal bests in the powerlifts, although they are well behind the best of today, were 800 in the squat, 525 in the bench press, and 800 in the deadlift. I was a big, strong lad.

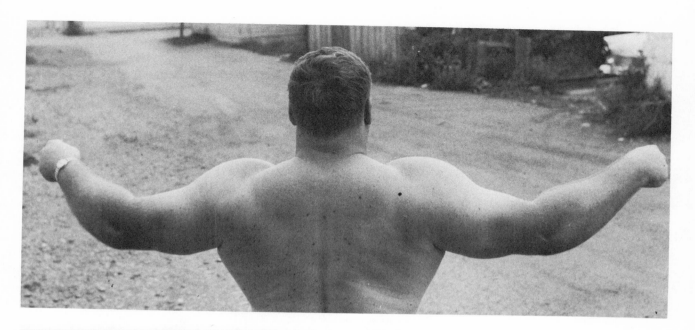

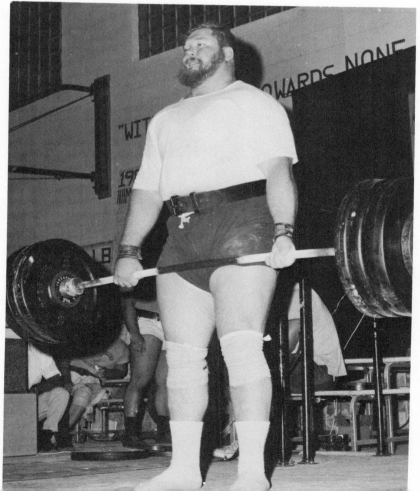

ABOVE: *By the age of twenty-six, Terry's weight had reached 300 pounds and he was having more and more trouble buying clothes.*

LEFT: *Bearded and twenty-seven, Terry had grown to his full size — 340 pounds. He's shown here winning a national championship and setting one of his many records in powerlifting.*

OPPOSITE PAGE: *At twenty-one, Terry was still 6'2'', but his weight had increased to 255 pounds.*

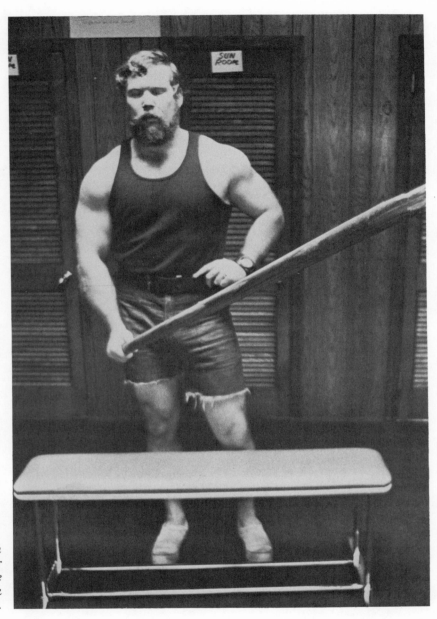

*At the age of thirty-one, Terry had been retired from competitive lifting for four years and had kept his weight within five pounds of 250. He's doing a leverage trick here with a long wooden pole.*

But the critical thing here is not how large or strong I was but how unbelievably *different* I was from the bony high-school senior who was unable to chin himself even once. The photographs on page 13 tell part of the story but only part; they don't explain the fact that even though I had gained 150 pounds, I could leap higher into the air than I could before I began lifting, or the fact that at 340 pounds, I could chin myself fifteen times. To me, and to many who saw the changes, the transformation did seem almost miraculous. And the trip back down was no less exciting.

In 1967, having been at or near the top for four years, and having set fifteen records in powerlifting, I finally finished my Ph.D. and took a job teaching at Auburn University in Alabama. I decided then to concentrate my energies on teaching and academic work — not on barbells and beefsteak — and so I began to cut back on both my training and my eating. No more bent-forward rowing with 500 pounds, no more size 60 suits and two pounds of steak at a sitting. Within a year I dropped 90 pounds, down to 250, through a combination of diet, tennis, and a reduced and radically altered weight-training program.

Since that time, almost twenty years ago, I have continued to train regularly for fitness and health purposes. Rather than being the means to the end of competition, weights have become the means to another end — fitness and the maintenance of strength and vigor.

I left Auburn in 1969 and moved to Mercer University in Macon, Georgia, where Jan and I married in 1973, and during those years in Macon, I played tennis regularly but I still managed to get to the gym a couple of times each week for thirty to forty-five minutes. I found even during the winters, when I would go for months without playing tennis, that as long as I trained, my weight stayed roughly at 250, and the quickness and flexibility of my body remained fairly constant. My routine takes very little time from the rest of my life, yet still allows me to continue to retain the musculature and power of a much younger man, to eat almost as much as I wish, to sleep well, and to have excellent health and energy. For the past eighteen years I have spent an average of no more than an hour or so a week lifting weights, yet this hour, along with a little seasonal tennis or squash and the odd day of wood splitting, has allowed me to feel terrific and to maintain, at forty-seven, the physical characteristics of a twenty-year-old athlete and the health of your average horse. I could train harder, I know. Jan often rags me about it — but I'll be satisfied to hold my own for a while yet and not have to become a slave to the gym or the running track to do it.

Through the years, I've been able to use weight training to produce a variety of effects on, *and to exercise control over,* my body. As a teenager I used the weights to gain weight and to improve my performance in tennis; in grad school I used them to gain more mass and size and so became a competitive lifter; after retiring, I used them to *lose* that great body weight, and for the past eighteen years I've used them to maintain my health, fitness, and appearance. Properly done, weights can work magic. I know.

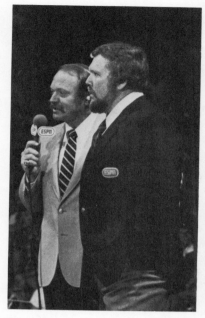

*Through the many years since his retirement, Terry has remained close to the center of the world of strength, serving more than any other person as a color commentator on national television, coaching, and writing about the strength sports for* Sports Illustrated. *Here he and Paul Maguire cover the "Strongest Man in Football" competition for ESPN.*

# 2 / Jan's Story

THE main thing I remember about growing up is that I always had a weight problem. Looking back, I realize that although part of the problem was real, part was only in my mind. I remember always looking so strange compared to the other girls my age. I was much larger in my bone structure, yet not very fat — more like a larger species of the same animal. In later years, when we were farming in Canada and worked our farm with draft horses, it struck me that the analogy I'd always looked for in regard to me and other girls was that I was more like a Percheron or a Clydesdale than a thoroughbred. Percherons aren't much taller than average horses, but their width and heft of bone is such that they *are* heavier. It was a comforting analogy.

Sadly, our culture didn't have much sympathy for girls like me who didn't fit the conventional Madison Avenue mold as we grew to womanhood.

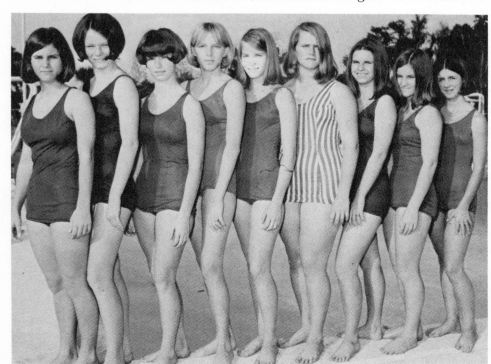

*Only fifteen and already showing the heavy bone structure that would help her break dozens of world records in the years to come, Jan Todd stands out in this photo for reasons other than just her different suit.*

It still doesn't, for that matter, though thank God that's changing a bit. During my years at college I seemed to look different every few months. I was either dieting because I was depressed about how I looked, or binging for the same reason. My personal nadir — my low point — came when a friend and I, during the spring of my sophomore year, decided to go on a diet together. We placed a bet to see who'd lose the most weight, so we had to take our "before" measurements and weigh in. I was horrified to find that I weighed 187 pounds and that my hips were 49 inches around. I was nineteen.

But I began running a mile or so in the afternoon, and since money was short, I rode to a new job on my bicycle and it all helped. I also found that by cooking for myself or by *not* cooking and getting by on a salad of some sort, I began to really lose weight. A year later I was down to about 140 pounds but even though I was 5 feet 7 inches tall, I still wasn't satisfied. I still felt too "big," even though I now looked positively cadaverous. I was nervous and didn't sleep well and my complexion wasn't good. I was eating not only too little but poorly. I was so caught in the notion of what women are "supposed" to weigh that I couldn't see clearly what I was doing to myself. I never gave a moment's thought to *what* I was eating when I dieted, only to eating less. And I still didn't look the way women were "supposed" to look: tiny and delicate with long legs and ample breasts. What's important to understand is the magnitude and yet the ordinariness of the problem I've dealt with through the years. Like the lines from the Allman Brothers' song:

> Just another lonely love song ringing;
> The only difference is this one is mine.

When I finally started my weight training after Terry and I married in the fall of 1973, the only thing I brought to the weights was a legacy of chronic weight problems. Plus round-shoulderedness. As it turned out, however, my Percheron bones were built for strength — I'd been a good swimmer and a fast runner in high school — but neither Terry nor I expected me to ever actually become a competitive lifter. There were no such things back then.

In 1973, you couldn't go to your neighborhood bookstore and find shelves of books on weight training or magazines filled with photos of our newest type of athlete — the female bodybuilder. Women simply didn't train with weights, except for a few isolated cases here and there. And so, when Terry first encouraged me to come with him to the gym for his twice-weekly workouts, I felt more than a little reluctance. No matter what he told me about muscle weighing more than fat and that you could weigh more but *be* smaller, I didn't really want to begin an activity that I was afraid would make me even bigger and heavier. But I did begin to go, and we worked on simple things, using light weights, concentrating on exercises to correct my round-shoulderedness, sit-ups for my waistline, and some light lunges for my legs. I kept waiting for unsightly bulges to appear but none did.

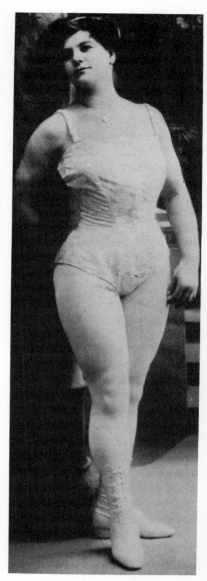

*One woman who inspired Jan to continue her lifting was the famous, 5'11", 210-pound Kate Sandwina, a center-ring attraction with the Ringling Brothers Circus in the early part of this century.*

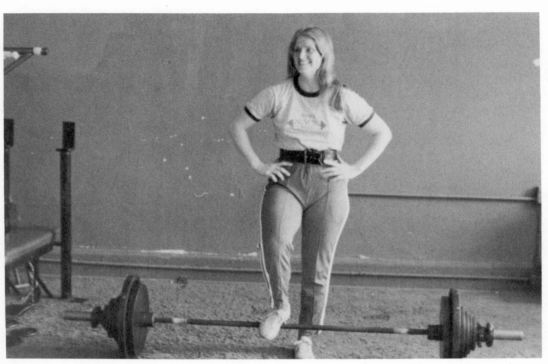

*Jan had been training hard for less than three months when this snapshot was taken. She weighed about 165 pounds.*

We spent Christmas that year in Texas and took our workout at the Texas Athletic Club, Terry's old haunt. And guess what we saw there? — another woman training, *with heavy weights*. She weighed about 115 very svelte pounds and she had worked up in the deadlift to 225 pounds. I was flabbergasted and fascinated by the combination of grace and physical power the young woman had. Later I asked Terry about using heavier weights. I had begun to find the unchanging light weights a bit boring, even though I could see a difference already in my posture and waistline, and I liked the idea of the challenge the bigger weights represented. Terry told me about some of the women at the turn of the century who earned their livings as professional strongwomen in circuses and sideshows. We poked through Terry's big collection of lifting books and came across a passage from the *Guinness Book of World Records* listing a record of 392 pounds in the "Two Hands Deadlift." It was the only lifting record listed for women, and it had been set back in 1926. I asked Terry if he thought I could break that record if I trained for it. He answered simply, yes.

So, when we got back to Macon, Terry designed a different routine for me, and I set my sights for a meet in Chattanooga, Tennessee, five months down the road. However, when we left for Chattanooga I'd only lifted 385 pounds in training, almost 10 pounds less than the record. But when the time came, I pulled 394.5 pounds and I was delighted by it. Breaking the record opened a new world for me because I realized that almost all of the fears we have and the barriers we set for ourselves as women are in our minds. I felt so free. All things seemed possible. Never before had I felt such confidence.

After we left Macon and moved to Canada I taught at the rural high school near our home. During my tenure at the school we had the most active women's powerlifting team in Canada — made up altogether of high-school girls, and me.

By then, I'd begun to do all three of the powerlifts and my goal was to be the first woman to reach 1000 pounds in the total (squat plus bench press plus deadlift), a goal I achieved in June 4, 1977, in Newfoundland, in what was probably the best meet in my life. Everything went right, and I squatted 424.4, bench pressed 176.4 and deadlifted 441 pounds for a 1042-pound total and the honor of being the first woman to total 1000 pounds. By that time I had increased my body weight — *on purpose* — to almost 200 pounds. I knew Terry had gained a great deal of weight to help his lifting and then had easily lost it, and I figured I could too. He agreed that if I didn't mind the extra flesh for a while it would definitely make me stronger, and I really wanted to be the first to make that 1000. How ironic that I, who had always felt too big and who had been so worried that weightlifting would make me even bigger, had actually *tried* to gain weight? And succeeded? And what fun it was. I love to cook as well as eat — so does Terry — and we really indulged ourselves during my heavy years.

Over the next several years I jockeyed my body weight up and down, though I was careful not to gain or lose too quickly. The lifting routine I used and the diet I followed always allowed me to maintain complete control over my gains and losses.

During this period, I made several world records, but something new was happening in the sport. The media began to focus more and more attention on powerlifting, and as the number of competitors increased and more and more distinction went along with the holding of world records, it quickly became rather clear that some women were willing to pay almost any price to win. At the Women's Nationals in 1979, the first time that NBC televised the event, there were several women entered in the competition who looked completely different from the way they had looked the year before. And they *sounded* so different. I remember standing in the warm-up area at the Nationals that year getting ready for an attempt and hearing a stream of curses that would have shocked a sailor. I turned around, thinking it fairly rude of some guy with a loud baritone voice to be talking so roughly in front of the young women, many of whom were still in high school, only to learn that the voice came from one of the lifters, a person I had known for several years and whose voice was unrecognizably changed. She was also much more masculine in her appearance, and the whispers of steroid use began to circulate as soon as the audience saw her on the platform. Because the vast majority of women in powerlifting have never taken anabolic steroids, competition is not fair, since the steroids give the users a definite advantage. What this all meant to me, personally, was that whereas I'd been able to dominate my class weighing 196 to 198 pounds, I could no longer count on coming out on top so easily. It was frustrating to know that in open competition I might well be facing someone who was willing to take whatever steroid-related risks were necessary to win, risks I was unwilling to take. So, once again I decided to try and gain a little more weight. My only hope was to fight the drug store with the food store.

And, as my weight increased, so did my poundages. My rising expectations gave me a new goal — 500 pounds in the squat. Finally, at the first Women's World Championships in May of 1979, I squatted with 507 pounds and had the highest total in the competition. I weighed 225. But though I was stronger than ever, the disadvantages of weighing 225 pounds began to wear on me, and I began to think of retiring. I was tired of having to buy my clothes in the "Lots of Love" shop and I didn't want to be thirty years old and still weigh 225 pounds. But I wanted to go out with a bang. I was helped in this aim by a call from a promoter who wanted to know if I would consider lifting in his meet, along with Bill Kazmaier, who was then considered by some to be the strongest man in the world. I became intrigued with the no-

*Jan had increased her body weight to 181 pounds by the time she was twenty-five. This 450-pound deadlift was a "world record" when it was made.*

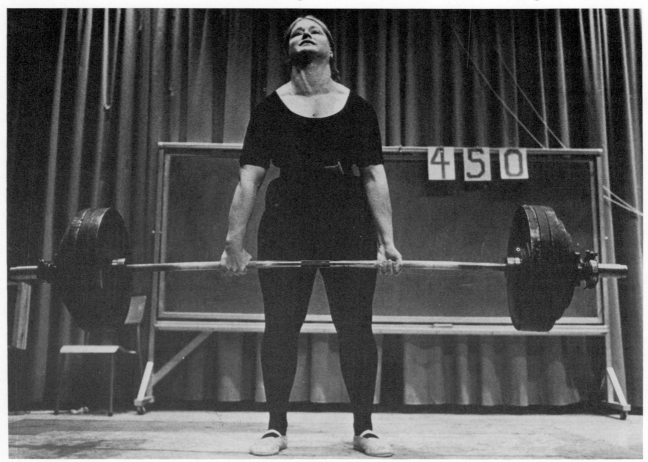

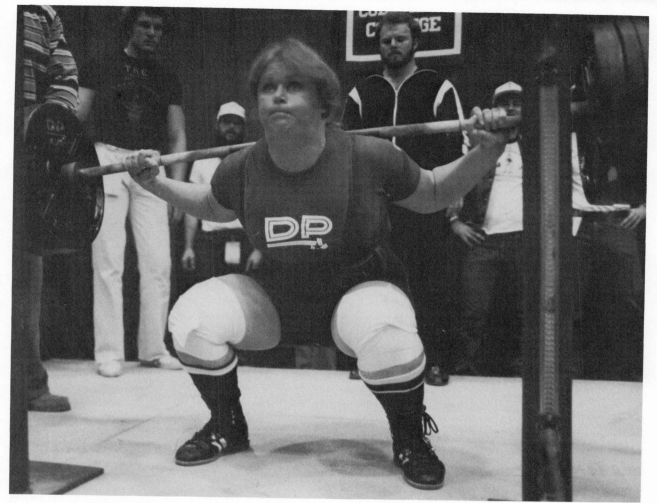

tion; never before had the "strongest man" and the "strongest woman" lifted in the same competition. So we went for it. At the meet I made world records in the squat (545 pounds), in the deadlift (480 pounds), and in the total (1230), a performance that made my retirement as a "heavy" much easier to bear.

Through the years, I'd gained over 65 pounds to increase my lifting — going from 164 pounds at Chattanooga to a smooth (and I do mean smooth) 230. At twenty-eight years of age, I knew that the longer I held the extra weight the more difficult it would be to lose, and so when I returned home I created a new routine and diet designed to burn away the extra flesh. And there was a lot to burn. At 230 pounds, my measurements were: bust: 44¼ inches; waist: 38½ inches; hips: 50½ inches; thighs (measured at the fullest part, standing straight) right: 31½ inches, left: 31 inches; calves: 17½ inches; neck: 16½ inches; biceps (measured with arm relaxed, straight down): 15½ inches; forearm: 11¾ inches; ankle: 9¼ inches; wrist: 7¼ inches.

*Jan's heaviest body weight was reached in 1981, when she weighed in at 225 pounds and set the world-record squat of 545 pounds, a record that has yet to be closely approached.*

It's pleasant today, many months later, to see the changes that have occurred, but it wasn't all fun and games getting here. I'd be lying if I said it didn't take a lot of hard work and willpower. Don't believe those people who try to say losing weight safely is a simple process. The very idea of losing weight by being jiggled by a vibrating belt, taking a steam bath, and eating the usually boring and unsafe diet of the week is ridiculous. It takes a combination of work and will but it *can* be done. Check the photos.

I knew when I started to lose, just as Terry had known, that *the barbells could be used to help me drop my weight.* Going up helped us both understand how to go down. What I really love about this whole experience — these past ten years in which I've used weights to increase, decrease, reshape, strengthen, and tone my body — is that I now have this great confidence in the fact that the weights will let me create any sort of look I want.

After I decided to reduce, my training program included weight workouts six days a week, cycling three to four days per week, and even a bit of rapid walking. Bear in mind that this is a very advanced program — I could never have done this much without considerable previous training. For the first several weeks I recorded everything I ate in my training log, and the cal-

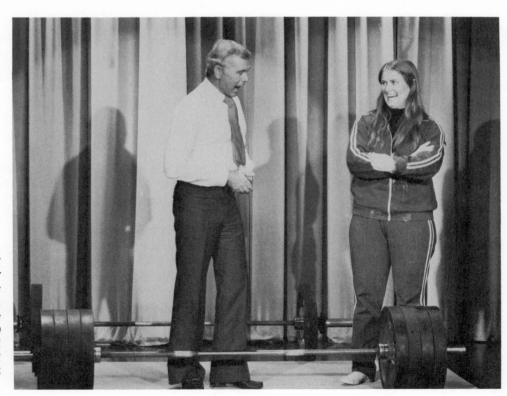

*Leading the vanguard of the growth of weight training for women, Jan has received more mainstream media attention than any other competitive lifter. Here, weighing about 200 pounds, she laughs both at and with Johnny Carson, who had just failed to budge the 415 pounds she lifted five times.*

orie totals for those first days were all in the 2500- to 3000-calorie range, which is hardly starving. However, as the days went by and my body became more satisfied with smaller amounts I dropped my caloric intake to between 1500 and 2000. By the sixteenth of November — nine months later — I weighed 171 pounds and the measurements by then had fallen to: bust: 40½ inches; waist: 30½ inches; hips: 41 inches; and thighs: 25½ inches. I looked like a completely different person. And I felt wonderful.

William Glasser has written of what he terms a "positive addiction" to exercise that often develops among marathon runners who train for several hours a day, several times per week. Research has shown that actual changes in blood chemistry occur that produce this "runners' high," as it has been called, and some very recent research suggests that the same thing happens with people who train regularly and vigorously with weights.

As the new program progressed and my body adapted to the increased workload, I became interested once again in the notion of training for strength; I hadn't lost as much power as I feared I might with the big weight loss. So, I began looking for a contest, having decided that I wanted to lift in a "drug free" meet where testing of some sort would be done to detect the use of anabolic steroids.

I started my contest training weighing around 160 pounds. Three days before the meet (I planned to lift in the 148-pound class) I took my measurements again; my bust was 39 inches, my hips were 38½ inches, my waist, 28½ inches, and my thighs, 23½ inches. I also discovered, to my extreme pleasure, that my smallest clothes from college all fit fine.

The day before the meet I took a polygraph test. I was asked if I had ever taken steroids and I said no. I passed. I weighed exactly 148½ and I managed to make the highest total in the world in that class for the year as well as a new world record deadlift with 446 pounds. What I'm proudest of in my whole career is having been the first person, man or woman, to create an official world record in a drug-free meet. I lifted twice more before I retired, and my last lift was a new world-record deadlift, which still stands, of 474 pounds. I weighed 146½. I was also tested for steroids that day, this time via urinalysis, by the International Powerlifting Federation, and I passed again.

Some time after that last meet, an old friend of ours, Bruce Randall, who won the Mr. Universe title back in 1959, came to town and stopped by to visit. He had seen me at 230, and he was shocked by the transformation. But he could relate. Bruce was himself once far larger. As in LARGE. When he entered the service in the mid-fifties he decided to take up weight training to gain a little bulk for football. As he trained, his size and strength increased, until he found himself at 250 and too hooked to play ball. He kept pumping and kept eating, and when he got out he weighed 370 pounds! Upon his discharge he found that buying his own groceries rather than getting them at the mess hall were two very different things, and after reaching his "goal" of 400 pounds, he dropped all the way back to 187 pounds. He actually went from 200 to 400 to 187 in only twenty-eight months. Unbelievable! He later trained back up to 225, at which weight he won the Mr. Universe title, and he still looks great today. In an even more dramatic fashion than Terry or I, Bruce proved you can use the weights to sculpt almost any sort of body you want — using weights and willpower to reshape the raw material of your body. And once you've gotten your body more or less where you want it, you can keep it that way for years and years.

It seems to me that this is wonderful news for adults with an interest in maintaining as many of the physical characteristics of youth as possible. No longer do we have to feel helpless as the late summer and fall of our lives approach. *We* can be in control, not the calendar.

The purpose of this book is to help those with the will to train learn *how* to train. We know that only a handful of even marginally sane people would

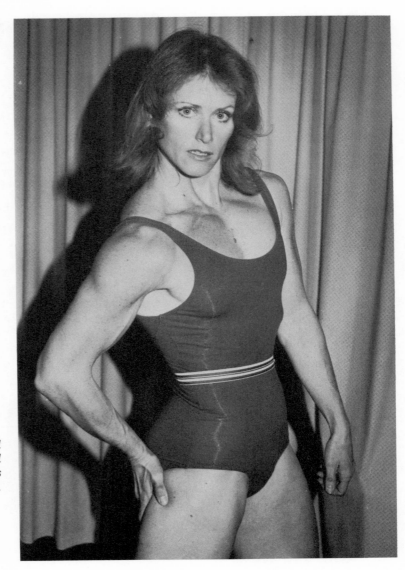

*In 1983, Jan set another world record by deadlifting 474 pounds, but instead of 226, she weighed only 146. This photo was taken the following day.*

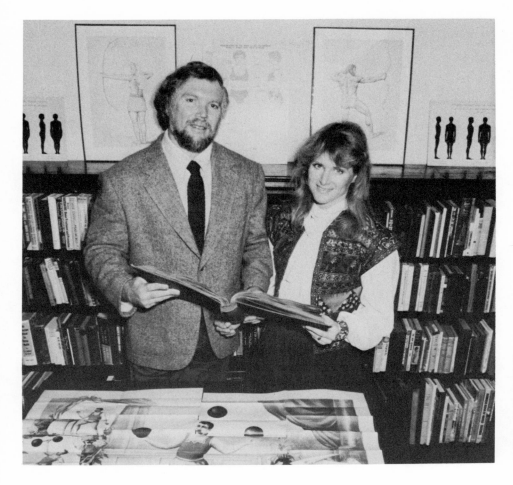

*Over the years, Jan and Terry have put together the world's largest collection of books, magazines, and other materials on weight training. They are donating the collection to the University of Texas in Austin, where they both work and teach.*

want to go through the rigors of weight gain and loss we went through in order to create lifting records, but we also know that because of our efforts in the gym and in the library we have both the experience and the knowledge to give you the guidance you need to train with safety and efficiency. We know this sounds more than a little like puffery, but we hope you understand that we want you to feel some confidence in our ability and desire to help you.

Terry is a faculty member in physical education at the University of Texas in Austin, and I work with him at UT on many research projects. Through the years we have assembled the largest and most comprehensive collection in the world on the subject of strength training, and we have tried hard to bring what we know about lifting to life in this book. If you read it carefully and use it with intelligence and commitment, it can change your life.

# PART TWO

# How Exercise Affects Aging

THERE are five major components that physiologists measure when assessing fitness — strength, muscular endurance, cardiovascular health, flexibility, and psychological fitness — and many people are surprised to discover that an older person of good health can make just as much progress toward fitness in these areas as a young person can. The older person may not be able to reach the same maximum level of performance the young person can — he or she may never get as strong in the bench press, for instance, or be able to run as fast — but a number of studies now indicate that very similar *percentages of increase* can occur using similar training methods. Because sedentary middle-aged (and older) people are generally in worse shape than a younger person who decides to start an exercise program, they will start at a lower level. Yet over time, they can improve on a percentage basis just as much as the young person can. In fact, some research has suggested that older people probably require *less* training stimulus to bring about increased fitness. All this means that it is fair to say that the effects of physical conditioning upon middle-aged and older individuals can be *life-changing,* in that they are opposite in direction to those commonly associated with the aging process. In other words, vigorous exercise will, for all practical purposes, make a middle-aged or older person "younger."

Good news indeed. And don't for a minute think we're talking only of men. For both men and women, the single greatest deterrent to vigor and health in our later years seems to be our sedentary life-style. Did you know that the muscles of the body that show no appreciable loss of size, or atrophy with the passage of years, are those such as the heart and diaphragm, which are constantly contracting, constantly working? Most of us have seen the way someone's arm looks when it has been kept in a cast for six weeks. It not only *looks* weaker, it *is* weaker, because the muscles have not been used. Living a sedentary life is like putting your entire body in a cast. Without engaging the muscles of the body in regular exercise they waste away — even in the young. Dr. John E. Dietrich, a professor at Cornell University Medical College, decided to test this notion and immobilized a group of healthy young people by placing their bodies in plaster casts from the waist down. At the end of eight weeks he found, just as Dr. Ancel Keys of the University of Minnesota had found earlier, generalized weakness and marked atrophy of the muscles. The subjects suffered significant loss of blood volume and their bones lost from 9 to 24 grams of calcium. Furthermore, their muscles lost significant amounts of nitrogen, vitamins, phosphorus, sulphur, sodium and potassium.

Dietrich's study found that muscular atrophy began within five to six *days* of immobilization. The group averaged a loss of nine pounds of muscle over the eight weeks, yet, when they were weighed on the scale after the removal of the casts, their body weights were almost exactly what they had been at the start of the experiment. Their *body-fat* levels, however, were nine pounds higher than they had been prior to the immobilization. Another important finding was that the mineral loss, particularly of calcium, was an indication that osteoporosis (weakening of the bones) was taking place as a direct result of inactivity.

In short, sitting around on your duff is increasingly bad for you as you age, and vigorous physical exercise — particularly lifting weights — is increasingly important if you want to live a robust, full life. In the chapters that follow, we'll explain in some detail just how beneficial regular weight training can be in promoting strength, muscular endurance, cardiovascular health, flexibility, and psychological fitness.

One thing we do want to stress, however, before you read further, is that some of the material in the next several chapters is rather complicated. Accordingly, some of you may want to only skim it and hit the high points. Others of you, though, may want even more thorough and technical information than we provide. Our intent is to be as clear and understandable as we can and still give you a considerable amount of research-based information to support our recommendations. We know you wouldn't have read this far had you not been motivated, and the last thing we want to do is to baby you in case you want to really dig what's left of your teeth into some of the scientific meat behind our arguments. So, for those of you with only a small hunger, we suggest you just snack along through these sections. And for the rest, bon appétit.

# 3 / Strength and Muscular Endurance

By chase our long-lived fathers earned their food,
Toil strung the nerves and purified the blood:
But we, their sons, a pampered race of men,
Are dwindled down to three score years and ten.
Better to hunt in fields for health unbought
Than fee the doctor for a nauseous draught.
The wise, for cure, on exercise depend;
God never made his work for man to mend.

(John Dryden)

ROBERT MAYNARD HUTCHINS, the former president of the University of Chicago, is supposed to have once said, "The secret of my abundant health is that whenever the impulse to exercise comes over me, I lie down until it passes." The sentiment so cleverly expressed in this frequently quoted expression is common to a great many people who don't see much reason or need for exercise, and particularly for strength, in our twentieth-century society. We, obviously, feel differently; even though our jobs are not primarily physical and our home is full of the usual labor-saving devices, we still want to feel fit, vigorous, and strong.

Strength has traditionally been synonymous with maleness. Young boys yearn to possess it not just for the advantages it provides among their peers but for what they think its effect will be on the female population. And the Boy is father to the Man. Men in their prime, even nonathletes, are often quick to test themselves at feats of strength such as arm wrestling, or wielding the sledge at the local fair to see if they can make the bell ring, or by physically outworking their fellows. And older men see the waning of their strength as a sign of age — a loss of manhood and a matter of much sadness.

And as for women, it's increasingly acceptable these days for *them* to treasure their strength. **Jan:** "As far as ultimate strength is concerned, nobody really knows yet how strong women are capable of becoming. When I began training back in 1973, the rule of thumb was that women were 60 percent as strong as men, yet women's strength and performance levels are much closer now than that to those of men. And the gap is still narrowing.

The primary reason is that it is now culturally copacetic for women to want to be stronger and to be willing to work to build lean, fit bodies. It has also become okay, since the late sixties, for growing girls to *try*. Most women now in the thirty-and-over group weren't taught to really try, as their male counterparts were, in PE classes. We had different rules for basketball so we wouldn't get tired, we were readily excused from gym class during the days of our menstrual period, we did girls' push-ups and girls' chins, and one thing you *never* did, at least where I grew up, was to beat your boyfriend in a race of some sort. The more I see, the more I believe the differences are primarily psychological rather than physiological."

In any case, to have denied women the opportunity to live not only in their bodies but through them, as men at their best have always lived, seems, in retrospect, like restricting Emily Dickinson to prose. Actually, when you take into account the amount of fat normally carried by women and compare only the *relative muscular weight* of men and women, strength differences among untrained men and untrained women are not as great as most people suppose. Recent studies have suggested, in fact, that in the lower body, when muscle weight is equal, untrained women are at least as strong as untrained men. A number of years ago, few college football teams had more than an occasional player who was as strong in the legs and hips as several of the top women lifters are today.

Clearly, though, men are demonstrably stronger than women in their upper bodies, the area in which the sexual differences between men and women becomes most apparent. Women are not as broad in the shoulders as men, they have lighter bones in their upper bodies, and, correspondingly, smaller muscles. No matter how hard a woman trains, even if she takes artificial male hormones, she's not going to change these factors. But, clearly, women can become far stronger than they ever thought they could, and this strength will make them not only healthier but more beautiful as well.

Unarguably, the bodies of both men *and* women respond to the rigors of exercise by becoming stronger, and women no less than men can be ennobled by exercise. It is not necessary to believe that men and women are the same to understand that in many respects they are similar. For instance, part of what makes a man or woman "attractive" is the grace, shape, and coherence of his or her particular body. It's possible to be both physically attractive *and* strong. The bottom line is that strength plays a vital role in *all* our lives, because it determines so much about how we look and how we feel about ourselves and because it allows us to do so much more with our lives.

**Jan:** "I'd never really thought much about my 'strength' until after I'd trained for several years and noticed how different my life had become. Before, there were so many things that I'd always said I couldn't do — not because I couldn't, but because I wasn't confident enough to try them. My strength gains radically changed my opinion of myself and of what was *possible*. They also made my days so much easier. The work on our farm took less out of me, I enjoyed my gardening more, I found groceries weren't really that heavy, and I learned that being strong didn't make me any less of a woman. All it did was make me healthier, leaner, and more confident."

In physiological terms, "strength," or "static strength," is the maximum amount of force that a muscle or group of muscles can exert in an isolated movement, and "power" is a measure not only of the force-generating properties (contraction) of the muscle but also of speed at which the muscle contracts. For instance, if two men can each lift 200 pounds in the squat, and the two men are of equal height and limb lengths, yet one can do the lift twice as fast as the other, the faster man is said to have generated more power. Most physiologists who specialize in strength believe that a person should do weight-training exercises rapidly, not slowly, so that significantly greater "power" will be developed as the central nervous system is "trained" by the quick, explosive movements.

Strength and power, however, like flexibility, are specific to individual areas and muscles within the body. It's possible, for instance, to have good leg strength yet poor upper-body strength. And it's also possible to have good biceps strength in the upper arm yet poor triceps strength. The strength of individual muscles depends on the amount and type of exercise they receive, and it has always been generally assumed that, if all other factors were equal, the larger muscle would be the stronger muscle. But besides the differences in their size and composition, difference in limb lengths, central nervous system efficiency, psychological motivations, and hormone levels also affect the ability of the muscles to contract forcefully and exhibit strength. For example, in testing situations, if a gun is fired at the exact moment a subject has been asked to contract a muscle, the unexpected gunshot acts as a stimulus that will cause the muscles to contract more forcefully than they would under normal circumstances. Shouting also has a similar effect, which is one reason you'll see lifters screaming when they're doing limit lifts in competition.

So, while muscle girths are important, they don't explain everything about strength. In fact, when a group of "young" (early twenties) weight trainers who'd been doing the same eight-week training program that an "old" group (fifty to sixty year olds) had been doing were compared, both groups made the same percentage of improvement in their *strength*, though the younger group gained more in muscular size. The researchers found that the older group's gains in strength came from their greater ability to activate the muscle fibers. The older trainers were apparently able to make more muscle fibers work at the same time, which resulted in a more powerful muscle contraction.

For many reasons, it's difficult to get a fix on precisely why any person or any muscle is as strong as he, or it, is. It's long been recognized that one of the largest roadblocks to attempts to measure absolute strength has been the inhibiting factor of the brain. Without extreme motivation, the signals sent to the muscles by the brain require the muscles to work well below their full capacity, whatever that might be. Cases such as that cited in the

*Guinness Book of World Records* of Mrs. Maxwell Rogers, who lifted the end of a 3600-pound car off her son following a traffic accident, lead one to speculate on the possibilities of increasing human strength by increasing disinhibitions. This is why attitude is so critical in weight training. It's quite possible that truly strong people derive part of their strength from being relatively fearless about trying heavier weights. One of the advantages of the type of training we recommend in this book is that the gradual, failure-free increase of poundage from week to week allows the brain and central nervous system time to adapt to heavier weights and thus become disinhibited and able to lift the heavier weights.

While it's important to work on attitude and central nervous system training by concentrating on the technique and speed of the lifts you're doing, however, the best method to increase strength still seems to be hypertrophy, or muscular enlargement. Basically, hypertrophy is the result of increased protein levels within the muscle cells that make them enlarge. For this reason it's important that anyone participating in a weight program have an adequate protein intake.

Another, still largely mysterious, aspect of muscle-tissue development is "hyperplasia," or the splitting of muscle fibers. In a famous study done on cats, whose muscle fibers are similar in structure to humans', Dr. W. J. Gonyea found that when the cats were exercised using both high speed and "high tension" (heavy weights) their muscle fibers would split. Interestingly, the muscle cells produced by these splits are smaller and seem to have a less than normal ability to undergo further hypertrophy. As for humans, we have evidence of hyperplasia in a study done on the deltoids (shoulder muscles) of a group of champion swimmers. The swimmers, who were believed to have hypertrophied because their muscles were larger than average, apparently underwent hyperplasia; biopsies showed them to have smaller but more numerous cells — which may translate into greater potential for power — characteristic of the latter condition. Far more inquiry needs to be made into this new area, however, before the scientific community will reverse its position on the ability of the human body to produce new muscle cells, which has heretofore been considered impossible. Nonetheless, it's interesting to speculate on how training methods may change if athletes begin to train to increase muscle size and strength not simply by hypertrophy but also through hyperplasia. In fact, the Bulgarians (see Chapter 10) think they already are producing hyperplasia by their training methods, which involve lifting weights not two or three times a week but five or six times a day.

Bodybuilders with their hypertrophied muscle fibers are, of course, far stronger than average individuals, yet in comparison to a trained weightlifter they come up second-best in strength even though their muscle girths are often greater. The strength of bodybuilders also depends on how they train. Those who consistently handle heavy weights in their training programs become stronger, while those who stay with lighter poundages build less strength, though they *do* significantly increase size and what we call "muscular endurance," or the ability to repeat a movement under stress for an extended period of time.

Like strength, muscular endurance is specific to certain muscles in the body, and those muscles used repeatedly will have greater muscular endurance than those used minimally. An illustration of this principle would be the ability of a normal, fairly sedentary individual to run to exhaustion compared to his ability to do sit-ups. Since our leg muscles retain some strength and endurance from our daily walking, the sedentary person should be able to run slowly for several minutes before he could go no further, but he would find it difficult to do many sit-ups because his abdominal muscles would lack endurance.

Again, one of the reasons we're so sold on the method of training we call Periodization — which we describe in Chapter 13 — is because of its ability to produce endurance as well as strength. In general, one advantage weight training has over such forms of exercise as jogging or cycling is that it allows you to create muscular endurance in all parts of your body, not just your legs and hips.

There's a fine but distinct line between muscular endurance and strength that is difficult to discuss without delving into the labyrinthian intricacies of muscle-fiber types and the way those fibers are fueled. Though there is a relationship between strength and endurance, the strongest weight trainer is not necessarily the most enduring. For instance, two weightlifters, both capable of a maximum squat of 400 pounds, might be vastly different in their ability to do repetitions with 200 pounds. Likewise, if one person could deadlift 200 pounds and another person 400, and both were tested with half their maximum for a check on endurance, it's quite possible that the weaker athlete would be able to do more repetitions with 100 pounds than the stronger could with 200.

At one time, physiologists thought that the differences between a marathon runner with a high level of endurance and a shot putter who had more explosive strength but low endurance levels could be completely explained by the two basic types of muscle fibers found in skeletal muscles — white "fast-twitch" fibers and red "slow-twitch" fibers. It is true that athletes participating in sports with high demands for endurance have a greater slow-twitch fiber concentration in their muscles, whereas shot putters and other athletes with little need for endurance primarily possess fast-twitch fibers. And it has long been believed that fast-twitch fibers were fast twitch, slow-twitch fibers were slow twitch, and neither one was capable of becoming other than what it was. Apparently, however, this belief was in error.

A good friend of ours recently made the analogy that muscle fibers were a lot like people. They're all basically made up of the same stuff, and they all work in basically the same ways, yet they produce quite different results. Some folks are fast workers, some are slow and steady, and some fall midway between. Some give their all quickly and are exhausted; some seem to keep plugging along forever, and some hold the middle ground.

As we learn more and more about the functioning of muscle fibers, other observations are beginning to be made by sports scientists who have lately defined an intermediate fiber type called FOG (fast twitch, oxidative, glycolitic). Several recent research studies have demonstrated that muscle-fiber types *do* have the capacity to change one into the other. Slow-twitch fibers can become intermediate FOG fibers, FOG fibers can become fast-twitch fibers, or vice versa. The reason for these changes is the body's adaptation to the demands of exercise, although apparently only a small percentage of the body's total muscle fibers can change in this manner, and even that change can't happen overnight.

Each of us receives as part of our genetic heritage a certain percentage of fast-twitch fibers and a certain percentage of slow-twitch fibers. No matter how hard someone like the football star Herschel Walker trained he could never change all his fast-twitch fibers to slow-twitch fibers and become a marathoner of any particular skill; his sprinting ability, his leaps into the end zone, and his strength going through the line are partly the result of his naturally high level of fast-twitch fibers. However, the intensive training he's done for years has, no doubt, contributed to his power by switching some of his FOG fibers to fast-twitch fibers and by switching some of his slow-twitch fibers to FOG fibers. But even if he started running ten to twenty miles a day tomorrow and continued doing so for the next five years he could never change all his fast-twitch fibers to slow-twitch ones. Similarly, Bill Rodgers, the great marathoner, would have trouble gaining a high level of strength and power since so much of his body is apparently composed of slow-twitch fibers. With free weight training, which mainly uses fast-twitch fibers, he could no doubt change a certain percentage of his fibers — but not all of them.

All muscle fiber types — fast twitch, slow twitch or FOG — function by the burning of a fuel called ATP (adenosine triphosphate), which is stored in small amounts within the cells. When the brain sends a message to the muscles to contract, and if the order calls for a quick reaction such as the lifting of a barbell or the running of a sprint, the fibers begin to simultaneously break down the ATP that's already stored in the muscles (which fuels the contraction) and build new ATP so the fibers can continue functioning. This new ATP is formed in fast-twitch fibers by the breakdown of a substance called creatine phosphate, which requires no oxygen for its transformation to ATP. This allows the fast-twitch fibers to respond immediately to the orders of the nervous system, to react quickly and strongly, and to keep contracting until some other form of ATP production can take over. However, the creatine phosphate reserves in the muscles are small and after five to eight seconds of vigorous activity such as a sprint requires, they are used up and must be replenished before the muscle will again be capable of fast contractions.

At this point, if the brain continues to send orders to the muscle to contract, the fast-twitch fibers shift to a second method of energy production called anaerobic glycolysis. Glycolysis is the breakdown of the stored sugar or glucose that exists in the muscle fibers. Glycolysis works rapidly, using enzymes to convert the glucose to ATP and a byproduct, pyruvic acid. ATP, of course, keeps the muscle functioning, but the price paid is that pyruvic acid becomes changed to lactic acid, which, at high levels, interferes with the process of glycolysis unless the body's *third* ATP production system, aerobic glycolysis, takes over. The buildup of lactic acid makes the cells too acidic to continue breaking down glucose, and so fatigue sets in within several minutes of vigorous exercise. Also, besides shutting down anaerobic glycolysis, the high lactic acid levels produce the "burning sensation" we associate with exercising vigorously.

Though this exercise pain diminishes almost as soon as the exercise is stopped, some researchers think the high levels of lactic acid produced through anaerobic glycolysis also bear a relationship to the muscular soreness that normally hits us twenty-four to forty-eight hours *after* we've exercised. This latter form of muscle soreness is poorly understood, and minute muscle and tendon tears, as well as lactic acid and several other "culprits," are currently under investigation. However, since weightlifting is done primarily with anaerobic ATP production, it will leave higher levels of lactic acid in your body than if you had gone out and simply jogged two miles at a moderate pace. Jogging and other forms of repetitive movement such as cycling and fast walking are primarily powered by the aerobic production of ATP and by aerobic glycolysis once lactic acid is converted back to pyruvic acid. This means that aerobic activity leaves you with lower levels of lactic acid in your muscles and in your bloodstream.

Aerobic glycolysis is the most efficient method of producing ATP since it can continue for the greatest length of time, but it is also the slowest method. The muscle cells have to have time to prepare themselves for the aerobic method, which is why a quick movement will always be fired by anaerobic means. Most of the body's movements are powered by an aerobic glycolysis, including our "muscle tone," which is actually a state of mild contraction. Just remember as you plan your workout that the *rate* of the exercise will determine which system you are stimulating — and training — in your muscles.

The byproducts of aerobic glycolysis are water and carbon dioxide, both harmless to the cell's ATP production; they leave the cell without interfering. This means that the cells could theoretically continue functioning until all their stored glycogen (glycogen is the body's form of carbohydrate that is converted to glucose for energy) is depleted or until the central nervous system can no longer function efficiently. The oxygen for aerobic glycolysis is provided by a substance within the muscle cells called myoglobin, which acts as an oxygen carrier just as hemoglobin does in the bloodstream. Slow-twitch fibers appear red because they have much higher myoglobin levels, which results in a greater capacity to store oxygen. When a runner participates in a marathon his efficient cardiovascular system will allow him to continue exercising for a long time because his blood can supply oxygen at an adequate rate to the muscle cells. However, as his muscles' demands for oxygen exceed the ability of his lungs to supply it, an "oxygen debt" develops, and the myoglobin must release its oxygen to keep the muscles functioning. (The oxygen debt is actually the result of lactic acid buildup within the muscle tissues. Without oxygen, lactic acid can't be converted back to pyruvic acid, and so the high acidity levels once again inhibit ATP production. In case you're wondering why there's *any* lactic acid present, we should explain that, for one thing, not all the lactic acid produced by anaerobic ATP production can be converted back to pyruvic acid during aerobic training and, secondly, that at the same time that the body is using aerobic glycolysis, there will still be other fibers using anaerobic glycolysis, and if you speed up or slow down, you can switch back and forth during the same exercise.)

The labored breathing of runners near the finish line and weightlifters who just finished that final set of 10 repetitions is the body's way of repaying the oxygen debt to the myoglobin molecules that have released their oxygen in order to keep us moving. The heavy breathing also allows the muscle cells to rebuild creatine phosphate so that when and if a sudden, explosive movement is needed, the muscles will be ready.

This isn't as simple as it sounds. You may be tempted to think that sprints involve *only* fast-twitch fibers and marathons involve *only* slow-twitch fibers, but we now know that these fibers work in concert and that their specialization is determined by the speed with which they can respond to the nerve's orders. When a muscle contracts, all the muscle fibers do not fire at once. Some respond immediately, others are involved only when those in the first round are exhausted. High strength levels, as we noted earlier, are partly the result of being able to fire large numbers of muscle fibers at the same time. Slow-twitch fibers take longer to tire because they have higher myoglobin levels and because they have more (and larger) mitochondria in them. This means that they can carry out aerobic ATP production for far longer than the fast-twitch fibers — with fewer mitochondria and less myoglobin — can. Yet studies have shown that fast-twitch as well as slow-twitch fibers are involved in distance races, just as slow-twitch fibers are involved in high repetition weight training, though not necessarily competitive weightlifting.

The reason we've included all this technical information is to show you that it is possible for the body to change and adapt *dramatically* with exercise, whether in the direction of strength, endurance, or both. By doing endurance training, you can actually increase the number and size of the mitochondria, which means you will have a greater ability to manufacture

ATP through aerobic glycolysis. Similarly, vigorous resistance training with weights will allow you to enlarge the size of your muscle cells (hypertrophy), possibly increase the *nunber* of cells (if you credit the new theories of hyperplasia), and it will increase the rate at which your cells can utilize ATP by anaerobic methods, which means your muscles can contract more rapidly and more strongly. Furthermore, by concentrating your training in one direction or the other (endurance or strength), those intermediate FOG fibers will likely be pulled in one direction or the other, creating even more endurance or an even greater capacity for strength.

## The Decline of Strength in Middle Age and Beyond

Only recently has very much attention been paid by science to the relationship of age and the decline in human strength. Though weakness and the loss of muscle size that accompany aging are all too observable, we are still not completely clear about why this occurs. There was a little work done on the subject during the nineteenth century and the earliest study, done in 1835, spread the rather depressing word that there was a 40 percent loss of strength by the time a man reached the age of sixty-five. But more recently it's been estimated that the *potential* strength differentiation between untrained subjects who are "young" and those who are sixty-five is more in the 10 to 20 percent range, and most of the recent research, in fact, indicates that very little change in potential occurs until well after the age of fifty. Of special interest is a project done on 100 men who worked in a machine shop. The men varied from twenty-two to sixty-two years in age and all worked at roughly the same sorts of hard manual labor. The researchers found no difference in either grip strength or in muscular endurance among the men despite the forty-year age span. Obviously, their everyday work had produced what physiologists call a "training effect" upon their strength.

There does still seem to be some disagreement regarding the rate at which average, untrained women lose strength. While some experts contend that women lose strength more rapidly than men, others say that the peak values attained and the subsequent rate of decline depends upon the demands of occupation and leisure. This may explain why many researchers have found a *slower* strength loss in women than in men, since women have primarily worked at home and not "retired" as men have. Even so, many of today's older women are still far too sedentary for their own good, but at least they get up and putter around while their husbands all too often just vegetate in their easy chairs. Unfortunately, there have been no longitudinal studies (studies conducted over a period of years) done on the specific effects of weight training on strength over a period of twenty to thirty years, though it's encouraging to observe that recent research studies take note of the relative ease with which muscles, once gained, can be maintained.

**Jan:** "It always amuses me when people see Terry train because they'll invariably ask, 'Aren't you going to do anything else? Don't you do curls for your biceps or wrist work for your forearms?' The fact is that physically he *does* look as if he works his muscles harder than he does. He's living proof that even a somewhat lazy person can maintain musculature once it's been built in the first place." **Terry:** "I prefer to think of what I do not as a lazy man's workout, but as 'quality' time."

## Hormones

One of the things that are critical to the maintenance of strength and muscle tone is hormones, which are produced by the various glands in our bodies. Hormones are fascinating: Besides their effect on muscle building, they moderate such activities as blood pressure, reproduction, glucose tolerance (related to diabetes), and even certain types of behavior. Of particular interest are the hormones testosterone (and other male hormones called androgens) and the human growth hormone, because of the role they play in "anabolism" — the building of body tissue.

## Testosterone and Related Androgens

In males, testosterone is produced in both the testes and the adrenal cortex, which sits astride the kidneys, and almost all researchers have found that an appreciable decrease occurs in testosterone levels with increased age. And since testosterone and other androgens are directly linked to anabolism, or protein synthesis (tissue building), researchers have concluded that its deficiency has been largely responsible for the general weakness and muscular atrophy that is so common among older individuals. Decreased levels of testosterone, however, can adversely affect two other cellular functions — the storage of glycogen (the energy food needed for ATP production in the cells during exercise) and the retention of water within the cells that promotes fuller-looking cells as well as better cellular function. The testicular production of testosterone is believed to begin to decrease around age twenty-five, although the related (androgen) hormones produced in the adrenal cortex seem to remain relatively constant throughout life among men and women of good health. The primary androgen produced by the adrenal glands is called androstenedione.

According to David Lamb, a leading researcher in the field of androgens and exercise, 5 to 10 milligrams per day of testosterone and 1 to 2 mg/day of androstenedione are secreted by men, while women normally produce 0.1 mg/day of testosterone (in the ovaries) and 2 to 4 mg/day of androstenedione. Testosterone is considered to be five times more powerful than androstenedione, so that, when looking at the visible changes that occur with age-related androgenic hormone decreases, most research has been done in regard to the testicular production of testosterone. In women, however, Lamb and others believe that the role of androstenedione may be more important to the problems of aging.

With the development of synthetic male hormones, the medical community has been able to determine that testosterone is essential to the proper functioning of human beings. When exogenous testosterone (testosterone from outside the body) has been given to aging patients, weakness has been lessened, feelings of well-being have been reported, calcium and other mineral loss in the bones has been turned around, and the skin has shown less evidence of aging. And an evaluation of men between the ages of sixty and seventy-nine in a longitudinal study in Baltimore led by Dr. P. D. Tsitouras noted that higher endogenous (natural) testosterone levels were linked to a higher incidence of sexual activity. Masters and Johnson are also in agreement with this position, and in their studies the use of exogenous testosterone was found to increase the sexual function of their male patients. Simple common sense would indicate that such a relationship exists, but the Baltimore study went on to speculate that higher testosterone levels were also responsible for increased sensitivity in the sex organs and other "target" tissues, which allowed for more enjoyment of the sex act and for the maintenance of an erection.

Another area that needs further investigation is the relationship between the amount of sexual activity in men and the amount of testosterone in the body. We're aware of only one such study done on humans and it's a case study of a single human being. It found that sexual activity sharply increased the secretion of testosterone, although how long such high levels lasted was not determined. Studies on primates have corroborated this hypothesis. Still another incompletely understood area is the relationship of body fat and testosterone production. In the Baltimore study, those subjects with high body-fat percentages were found to have lower testosterone levels than their "leaner" counterparts, and similar studies have found similar relationships. The question, of course, is whether the extra testosterone makes one leaner or whether the extra leanness (and likely higher activity level) makes extra testosterone.

We do know that we are sexual beings and our twentieth-century society has put the pressure on men to keep "performing" sexually much longer than have previous cultures. And we know that such pressures have in many cases led to stress and increased impotence because of the fear of failure. They have also led some individuals to experiment with synthetic hormones to increase their sexual prowess, experiments often done without a doctor's supervision, which, of course, increases the likelihood of potentially harmful side effects. The endocrine system is an extremely delicate arrangement of checks and balances, and much as we understand a man's desire to enjoy greater sexual power, no one should undertake such hormonal experimentation without the supervision of an expert endocrinologist, if then. Durk Pearson's and Sandy Shaw's *Life Extension* is an entertaining tome, but their recommendations that human growth hormone and synthetic testosterone be used by *average* (nonill) aging individuals who simply want to promote longevity and greater sexual pleasure leave us with Brave New World apprehensions. Not only are such drugs costly but there could be serious side effects to consider — which should not be lightly dismissed in the search for youth. This is especially true, in our minds, *since there is solid scientific evidence that certain types of exercise will produce natural increases in testosterone and in human growth hormone.* There is still room for further study in this area, but it certainly appears that when *vigorous* activity such as weight training is done, testosterone levels within the bloodstream will increase, along with the advantages conferred by extra testosterone.

J. R. Sutton was one of the first researchers to measure increased androgen levels following exercise. In one study, done on world-class swimmers and rowers, he found that all twenty-nine subjects in the study had increased the testosterone level within their bloodstreams following a vigorous workout. When these same subjects were asked to exercise only moderately, however (doing what we call submaximal exercise), he did *not* find any increase in androgens within the bloodstream. In another study, Sutton found that military recruits — after undergoing their six weeks of vigorous boot camp — had substantially increased levels of androgens. And a recent study done in France found increased testosterone secretion following a rigorous treadmill test. Even more important, in a study done at Louisiana State University, physiologists Mike Stone and Ronald Bird found some rather interesting androgen changes among the middle-aged men who participated in their weight-training study. The researchers used three groups of men with an average age of forty-two years. One group was placed on a twelve-week weight-training program, one group who had already been on a regular jogging program (roughly six miles per week) was asked to continue with that level of activity, and the third group served as a control, meaning that they continued doing no regular exercise. The serum testosterone levels *increased significantly* at the end of the program for the weight trainers while the joggers showed *no* change in the levels at which they started the project. The control group also showed a small increase, though not nearly as high as that of the weight-training group.

Stone and Bird point out that all males undergo certain seasonal changes in hormonal levels and that since the testosterone levels of the joggers did not show the increase seen in the other two groups, this may well mean that jogging suppresses testosterone levels. Stone and Bird further support this hypothesis by noting that aerobic training has been shown to suppress testosterone production in several animal studies. But while there is clearly a growing body of evidence that such androgen increases do occur following heavy, rigorous training, the correlation of these higher levels with increased strength and changes in body composition still needs much exploration. Simply *having* a somewhat higher testosterone level apparently won't make major differences in your appearance *unless you exercise regularly.*

The human-performance laboratory at De Anza College in California is another place where the relationships between androgens and exercise are being investigated. In an interesting study done there recently, a group of college-age males, college-age females, and high-school males were tested before and after a single bout of near-maximal weight training. The college males were further divided into two groups — experienced weight trainers and nonexperienced. The college men made significant increases in their serum testosterone levels, and the skilled group increased their levels more than the nonweight-trained males, though both groups showed significant increases. However, the high-school boys and the college-aged women showed no significant increases, a fact that might reflect the ability or willingness of the test subjects to exert a maximal effort. Perhaps inexperience and lack of aggressiveness by the female subjects and lack of motivation by the high-school students resulted in less than vigorous weight-training sessions. The college male group was well motivated and trained maximally, so the expected androgen increases occurred. The college groups were all members of the varsity football team, and, even though some had no previous weight-training experience, they were used to hard, rigorous exercising and "giving their all," a fact that helps prove how critical attitude is in exercise.

In short, there's not much doubt in our minds that different types of training will elicit different hormonal responses, but it also seems fairly safe to say that regular, vigorous exercise with weights to near-maximal levels will increase the natural levels of male hormones in your body, and if you continue to exercise vigorously and regularly, you should be able to maintain a significantly higher than normal level of testosterone for as long as you follow your training programs.

As we age, there are a number of desirable reasons to have a higher level of testosterone for a longer period of time. We know that it is associated with increased muscularity, strength, feelings of well-being, decrease in bone loss, and the proper operation of a number of body functions, not the least of which are our sexual activities.

Our personal theory is that the reason so many of the men we know who've been regular weight trainers look and act so much younger than their age mates is because the regular weight work they've done has caused them to maintain a higher level of hypertrophy than is "normal" for their age and that this hypertrophy is related to an increased androgen production. The basic principle around which all weight-training exercises work is called the "overload principle." This means that you progressively increase the weights as you exercise so that you reach near your maximum in strength with each workout. And if maximal exercise increases the body's production of androgens, then it may be that the longer a person trains the greater his ability to synthesize testosterone becomes, so that the training not only affects the growth of muscles but the actual speed at which muscles *can* be grown. Inevitably, of course, no matter how much we exercise, aging will occur. But the more active you remain, the higher your testosterone level will be for longer periods of time, and this offers *big* advantages, used intelligently.

One advantage is that there is apparently a relationship between testosterone production and success in other forms of "competition." The way it works is that testosterone acts as both the incentive to *and the payoff for* a successful competition. A study was done that revealed the fact that pulling off a successful business deal resulted in an upswing in a man's testosterone production. This upswing, of course, should create even greater feelings of confidence and competitiveness and would then give the man an extra edge in his next business deal. And, conversely, the "loser" would have a corresponding decrease in testosterone level, making him less sure of himself, less confident, less competitive, and at a disadvantage when he next began to deal. Many animal studies support the fact that those males with higher testosterone levels seem to dominate, and that this domination produces extra testosterone that makes future dominance likely.

As fascinating as this information is, it shouldn't make you so concerned with your testosterone level that you resort to the risky step of taking exogenous testosterone with all its capacity for producing severe side effects. You should, however, be encouraged by this data to train regularly and vigorously so that your *own* testosterone level will increase and remain that of a normal, healthy young man as you go into and beyond middle age. It's important to remember that in the various research projects, the effects of exercise have not increased testosterone levels enough to create a problem, as too much testosterone can be. With all its potential benefits, exogenous testosterone is closely linked to hypertension, liver disorders, atherosclerosis, and manic depression. When athletes take large amounts of testosterone there is often a great increase in blood pressure, and the larger the dosage that is taken the higher the pressure seems to rise. Unbelievable as it may seem, some athletes are now regularly taking up to a *hundred* times as much testosterone as the body normally produces. Though absolute proof of a direct connection is difficult to establish, several world-class athletes in "good shape" have suffered life-threatening heart disease in their thirties while using large amounts of testosterone. There is also growing evidence of severe personality changes accompanying these high dosages. Sadly, the use of such drugs by athletes is growing and we look with great apprehension to the future of sports.

There is, however, absolutely no reason to believe that undertaking a weight program such as we recommend will do anything but increase your health and potency as long as you follow the instructions and use common sense.

Human growth hormone's proper name is somatotrophin, often abbreviated in scientific literature (and, more recently, in bodybuilding magazines because of the recent rise in its use) as STH. It is an extremely powerful hormone. For example, administering STH to aging rats prevented the weight losses that are normally a part of aging and gave the animals a more youthful appearance. Growth hormone is a highly "anabolic" (tissue building) substance, and it is STH that helps determine how tall a person will become by its influence on the long bones of the body. When STH levels drop at the end of adolescence, the growth plates at the ends of the bones close, and even though your body will continue to produce growth hormone you will no longer get any taller. If you have abnormally high levels of growth hormone in your system or if the mechanism to reduce STH levels doesn't work, then such conditions as acromegaly or gigantism occur. Taller than normal, most acromegalics also have excessively thick hands, prominent brows, long jaws, and enlarged joints and internal organs.

Besides its obvious relationship to the bones, STH is also responsible for stimulating muscular growth, maintaining the immune system, and, of special importance to many of us, burning fat. STH is released by the pituitary in response to exercise, fasting, hypoglycemia, sleep, and trauma. A few "experts" have recommended that either exogenous STH be taken or that STH "releasors" be used to mobilize more STH into the bloodstream. Most STH releasors and STH itself are prescription drugs, although considerable press has been given recently to the amino acids arginine, ornithine and lysine, which some health-food experts contend are "natural" STH releasors. Discussions we've had with some sources suggest there may be something to the amino acid theory, though most endocrinologists give little weight to such claims. Even so, empirical evidence is increasing that suggests that some solid research needs to be done to determine if the claims for amino acid use have any substance. But some writers, even physicians such as Dr. Robert Kerr of California, persist in recommending the injection of actual growth hormone. That would *not* be our recommendation. In light of the potential side effects of STH — rapid growth and coarsening of the skin so that it becomes noticeably thicker, possible enlargement of the joints and facial bones (acromegaly), deepening of the voice due to growth of the larynx, growth of many of the internal organs, and so on — it seems too risky, even if the rather suspicious matter of the possible relationship of excess growth hormone and cancer isn't considered. There appears to be experimental evidence on both sides of the cancer question, admittedly, but why take such a chance? Our recommendation is to eat well, get plenty of sleep (since we know that additional STH is released during sleep), and use exercise to create whatever additional increases mother nature, not the local pharmacist, will allow. We know this is a conservative — some would say old-fashioned — position. But we're both still very healthy, very strong, and we have normal bones, normal joints, and good cardiovascular condition, as do many of our lifting friends, who, like us, use no prescription hormones. Do it through exercise.

Closely examined, the relationship between growth-hormone response and exercise is very interesting. Like testosterone, STH is primarily released during maximal sorts of exercise. However, if the intense effort continues for too long a period of time — as in, say, an extended run — growth-hormone levels have been found to actually decrease.

Of particular importance here is the fact that somatotrophin's potential apparently diminishes very little in our bodies as we age, and research shows that even elderly patients are able to release growth hormone when they exercise vigorously. It does seem that men achieve higher levels than women, though substantial increases did occur in subjects of both sexes. On the other hand, if older individuals become more sedentary, their bodies will release less STH. Even though the basal (normal) levels of STH among sedentary older people may be comparable to those of an average young person — the levels would be comparable only to those of an average sedentary young person.

The normal function of growth hormone is to serve as a "biochemical amplifier," enhancing the work-induced synthesis of muscle protein. And the larger quantities of growth hormone available through exercise are especially important for this purpose in an older person. STH helps in other ways as well, such as in assisting the release of fat within the body, so that when your body is exercising, more fat than lean tissue is called up to provide the energy for the cells. This means, of course, that lean body mass can be maintained while body fat is lost.

## What About Women?

Before all you women reading this join an aerobic dance class, listen to a few words about the effect of weight training on *your* hormones. We mentioned earlier that the relative levels of testosterone output are much lower in women than in men; in fact, there may be twenty to thirty times more testosterone in the "average" male than in the "average" female. This fact should never be forgotten by women who contemplate a weight-training program, because the knowledge of that one fact should dispel the fears of those who just "know" that weightlifting will turn them into an Arnold Schwarzenegger look-alike. Remember, any testosterone increase in women — and we do believe there is some — caused by training will still be within normal levels for women, not for men. Quite a few studies have been done regarding hypertrophy and women's response to weight training, and even though significant strength gains were made by women trainers, no significant changes in the girths of the muscles occurred.

**Jan:** "In the past ten years I've probably trained harder, used heavier weights, and focused more of my energies on being 'strong' than any woman anywhere. Though there are a few women who've trained longer than I, those few trained for shape, whereas I wanted to be strong and to build a body that would help that strength. During all my years of heavy training I never once missed a menstrual period, and I found no change in my basic orientation toward life as a woman — I've certainly felt no desire to be other than what I am. Many people seeing me for the first time comment that I look so 'female.' How could I look otherwise? I'm leaner now than I was in my teens, my posture is better, my skin is vastly improved, and though I wouldn't mind having slightly longer legs, I'm relatively content that I've done as much as I could with what I was given. The average man my age who has trained as hard as I have would be literally *covered* with huge muscles. In short, women don't need to be afraid of what weight training will do. What they need to be afraid of, especially as they age, is what will happen if they don't train.''

There is a sense in which it is incorrect to call testosterone a ''male'' hormone and estrogen a ''female'' hormone since they are both present in each sex. Their ability to determine and differentiate the sexes is based on their volume in the body — not their mere presence. Testosterone in women, by the way, has gotten a bad rap by folks who want to argue that strong women — or women with less than *Playboy*-type builds — are predisposed in that way because of their higher testosterone levels. While common sense would certainly indicate that this is at least *partly* true, testosterone is involved in only a part of the process of protein synthesis, and other factors may be of equal or greater importance in explaining such muscular differences.

As we mentioned earlier, women are actually harder hit by aging than men are. Menopause, the cessation of ovulation and the resultant end of the menstrual cycle, is caused by decreasing levels of the hormone estrogen. When estrogen levels become low, not only do the ovaries cease functioning but also the entire aging process is rapidly accelerated. Women's skin becomes less elastic and more wrinkled. The sexual organs shrink and intercourse can become painful because of excessive dryness. Bone brittleness also increases as do cholesterol levels and several sorts of cardiovascular disease. Muscular atrophy also occurs because estrogen is an anabolic hormone that helps with the synthesis of new body tissues.

A few doctors have recently begun prescribing small amounts of testosterone (usually used in combination with certain ''female'' hormones) to postmenopausal women and those who have had hysterectomies, and we've even read of people advocating the use of STH in healthy women. But, as we've said, why not get your hormones *naturally*? Clearly, the best antiaging program a woman can undertake would be a regular weight-training program combined with a reasonable diet and cardiovascular exercise. Rather than swallowing and injecting small amounts of growth hormone and other prescription hormones in an attempt to achieve similar ends, it certainly seems to us to make far more sense to do your best to make those changes naturally, without the risk of endocrine-system damage and with no extra cost beyond your initial investment in the barbells and benches.

# 4 / Bill Pearl –The Ageless Wonder

Fᴏʀ years bodybuilding was considered a sport for young dazzling men in their early twenties, men whose competitive careers would be little more than a memory by the time they turned forty. This, of course, was all before the second coming of Bill Pearl. Not to mention the third, when, at age forty-seven, *twenty-five years after his victory in the Mr. America competition,* he stepped back onstage for an exhibition at the 1978 Mr. America show in such amazing muscular condition that many bodybuilding authorities felt that he would have won the event had repeat winners in Mr. America competition been allowed. In any case, it is no exaggeration to say that Bill Pearl played a leading role and perhaps *the* leading role in revolutionizing the sport of bodybuilding. Perhaps more than any other individual he has demonstrated the limitlessness of human physical potential and the absurdity of setting chronological barriers regarding the condition of the body. *For almost thirty years* Bill has been able to maintain a physique that remains equal to that of the very best men in the sport. Even *he* has been surprised.

Following his 1953 Mr. America victory, Bill continued to train, and upon his release from the Navy in 1954, he opened a gym in Sacramento. He continued to compete as well, winning the Mr. USA title in 1956 and the Professional Mr. Universe title in 1961. His regular habits made him a success in his business, and soon he went from the one lone gym in Sacramento to a string of eight. But he didn't care for all the travel, and he sold out in 1962 and moved down to Los Angeles, bought a new gym, and decided to concentrate on his own training and the coaching of other bodybuilders. Gradually, as the years passed, Bill discovered that one of the "principles" of bodybuilding was definitely wrong. Even though well into his thirties, he was not slipping back, he was continuing to get better. He was able to add even more muscle mass and gain more strength and symmetry, and so, in 1967, he began preparing once more for the Professional Mr. Universe title. Bill was thirty-seven years old the night the posing lights came on in London, England, highlighting the peaks and contours of his body, and when the judges turned in their final tally he had won every judge's first-place vote. Every one.

He returned to his gym business and continued training, and he said he'd retired. But four years later, several younger bodybuilders wanted to take a crack at beating the legend, and the word began to circulate that Bill was afraid to face the current crop of competitors. Rising to the bait, Pearl sent word back through the iron grapevine that he feared no man — nor age — and that he'd meet all comers on the platform at the 1971 event. He came, they saw, he conquered. Then he said farewell forever to actual competiton. "My main reason for entering the 1971 Pro Mr. Universe was to prove a point," he explained, "and I did. The trophy or title meant very little to me. I actually felt strange on stage, and felt I should have been there as a counselor or a judge rather than a competitor. I felt I had had my day. Enough was enough."

But while *he'd* had enough, the bodybuilding world certainly hadn't; they clamored for him to guest pose and make appearances in the years that followed. Bill, however, returned to his gym business, continued his regular workouts, and worked once again at the coaching of other bodybuilders. He put to good use all the vast information he'd gleaned through his years of experimentation and training by writing a 638-page book on weight training, *Keys to the Inner Universe,* whose main strength is its listing of every known variation of every known weightlifting exercise.

"Following the 1971 Mr. Universe victory," Bill recalls, "I'd really had my fill of bodybuilding politics, and I decided to do something else for awhile. I'd always done some cycling for my cardiovascular conditioning so I decided to drop my body weight down and concentrate on that. I went from my normal weight of 230 to 185 and I competed in bicycle races until 1975, but I didn't get the satisfaction from it that I'd hoped to find. I still did weight training during those years, but I wasn't very crazy about the way I looked or the way I felt, so I decided to switch back to my old training methods. Within a year my body weight was back up to 225, and I could see that I hadn't really 'lost' anything. I was intrigued to see what sort of condition I could get into and so I agreed in 1978 to make a guest appearance at the Mr. America. I'm really glad now that I did it. I was naturally proud of the way I looked, but what I guess I'm even more proud of is that so many people have come up to me since then and said how it had opened their eyes to see me pose that night. To see me onstage, after all those years, was a revelation to a lot of people, including me. Now, I don't have *any* set ideas about what an appropriate appearance is for a person of a certain age. I just take every day as it comes and try to make the most of it. I'm going to live and train for as long as God gives me the strength and the health to do it."

While modesty often causes Bill to sound as if his immunity to aging has been an accidental blessing, he and the rest of the bodybuilding world know that the primary reason for his continued condition — he gave his last posing exhibition at age fifty-one — has been his absolute dedication to reg-

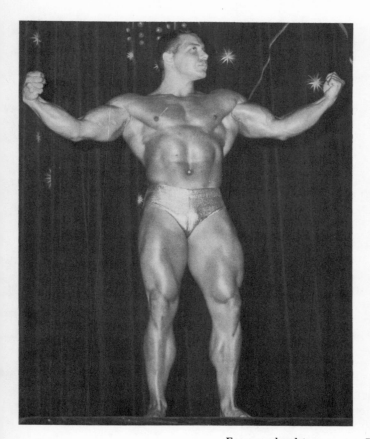
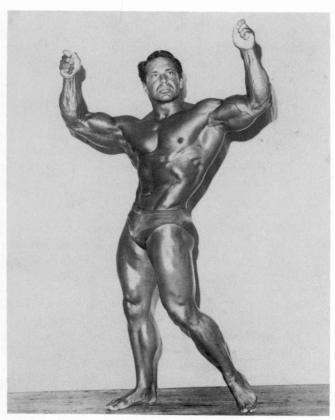

*For nearly thirty years, Bill Pearl has been a dominant force in bodybuilding. Can you believe that one of these shots was taken nearly twenty years before the other? Bill's forty-two in the photo on the right.*

ular training. His days begin with a 4:00 A.M. workout, usually shared by his wife, Judy, and several local bodybuilders. Says Bill, "I realize that 4:00 would not suit a lot of people's tastes, but if you're going to be serious about something you have to find time to do it properly. In those early morning hours I can concentrate all my attention on my training. It's like a hobby to me, a habitual hobby. No one comes in to distract me and so I can train really hard. By training in the mornings, I never have the tendency to put it off. It suits me." Each of the early morning sessions begins with a fifteen- to twenty-minute stationary bicycle ride before he begins his weight work. "I guess my one concession to aging has been the cycling warm-ups I now do," he explains. "I find it really gets me going, especially here at the farm, since the barn we train in is unheated. Sometimes in January and February I have to pedal quite a while before I feel like moving on to the barbells. But I like the coolness; it makes me move quickly through my workouts, something I should do anyway." Following the cycling, Bill moves through his scheduled exercises for the day, his routine split between upper-body days and lower-body days.

Bill is quick to say that he credits a large part of his health and appearance to his wife's careful attention to his diet. Both Pearls decided to become lacto-ovo vegetarians in 1967, meaning that they eat vegetables, fruits, grains, eggs, and dairy products. "We eat eggs and milk, and Judy knows as much about nutrition as most trained dieticians," Bill said recently, "so I've never really worried about maintaining my size without meat. But you've got to be careful, especially if you also shun eggs and milk as some vegetarians do. The fact is that people don't need nearly as much protein as they think they do. Even the bodybuilders are learning this. Very few of them eat only red meat anymore — and I can remember the days when steak was king. Now they eat mostly fish, chicken, and turkey and have greater musculature than ever before in history. Judy and I eat a well-balanced diet, lots of fresh fruits and vegetables and we take vitamin supplements as well. We both feel better without the meat, we know we're eating a lot less fat, and we have all the energy we'd want, so I guess we'll go on eating this way."

Looking at Bill today, the massive shoulders still square, the hips trim, the waistline flat, the glowing skin unwrinkled, it is indeed hard to imagine him as much more than thirty-five. And that's a drop-dead thirty-five — *not* your average. His goals now are modest. He recently told us, "I used to think, years ago, that one day I might quit training, but now I know I never will."

# 5 / Cardiovascular Fitness

Roughly 50 percent of all deaths in the United States are related to some form of cardiovascular disease. Yet cigarette sales are still high, obesity is all too common, and even though there are now millions of Americans participating in regular exercise programs, there are millions more sitting at home in front of the tube. One reason, we feel, that many folks have found it hard to stick with such activities as jogging or swimming is that, to many, they are basically boring. Further complications are access to a pool where one can actually swim laps, and the now widely documented incidence of various joint injuries (particularly in the back, knees, and ankles) that is associated with the relentless pounding of jogging. Well, there's some good news on the research front for those of you who've been bored — and for those who, like us, have always preferred weight training; it now looks as if weight training, especially when done relatively rapidly, *will* produce improvements in cardiovascular condition. This is not to say that *only* weight training should be done, but to make the point that whereas in the past most fitness experts thought lifting weights was of no cardiovascular value whatever, recent research has shown that lifting *does* produce cardiovascular improvement.

Before we talk about the latest research findings, however, let's look at the problems that accompany the aging of the cardiovascular system. The structural changes within the aging heart include a gradual loss of muscle fibers and an increasing accumulation of fat, connective tissues, and the potentially harmful pigment lipofuscin, which, by age eighty, may occupy as much as 10 percent of the total volume of the heart. The ability of the heart to pump blood is also directly affected by age, and in untrained individuals, the difference between a man of twenty and a man of ninety may be as much as 50 percent. This means that not only are the contractions weaker, but the volume of blood pumped per beat decreases, meaning that less total circulation takes place. The blood vessels, as we've noted, also change, becoming less elastic and in some cases thicker, as cross-links form in the collagen molecules.

Atherosclerosis — the accumulation of fatty deposits on the inside of the blood vessels — can begin even in adolescence, but in almost all humans it is well established by the time middle age is reached if a normal "American" diet is followed, thus increasing the blood pressure and requiring the heart to "labor" more. Obesity, as well, is directly linked to cardiovascular failure. Atherosclerosis can also reduce the amount of blood that reaches the brain at a surprisingly young age. During the Korean War, for instance, doctors doing autopsies on American servicemen often found atherosclerosis even in those under twenty years of age. These were men in the prime of life, with no visible signs of poor health. In Vietnam, the same incidence of cardiovascular disease was found. Many people are unaware that atherosclerosis begins so early in life and that by age fifty-nine there is roughly a 50 percent decrease in blood flow to the brain among inactive people. This has dramatic implications for both memory and intelligence, since both decline more rapidly among those who have cardiovascular disease and subsequent hypertension (high blood pressure). Individuals with high blood pressures (diastolic pressures), in fact, have been found to score lower on intelligence tests than individuals with low or "normal" pressures.

In another area of related research, Dr. Mike Stone of Auburn University has conducted several studies relating cardiovascular fitness and weight training. His first project, done at LSU, and described in part in Chapter 3, found changes in the blood among the middle-aged men who made up the training group. Stone and the other researchers measured three parameters of cardiovascular health in the men at LSU: (1) the "serum lipids" — the fats within the bloodstream, (2) the amount of time it took the men to reach their "target" heart rates for cardiovascular fitness (85 percent of 220 minus their age), and (3) body composition (the relationships between lean body weight and cardiovascular health are clearly established). In all three measures, the weight-training group made more positive changes than did the control group and the jogging group. It should be noted that since the joggers had already been jogging and were simply continuing with an exercise program already in progress, they were not expected to create the percentage of improvement that a new trainer shows during the start of a training program. By the end of six weeks, however, the weight-training group reached their target heart rate more slowly than the jogging group, which indicates that they had increased their aerobic condition. An important point is that these men were not training with a special emphasis on speed. As Stone says, "This supports the contention that cardiovascular effects can be derived from anaerobic work." (As we discussed, "aerobic exercise" refers to exercise in which oxygen use plays a central role *during exercise,* whereas "anaerobic exercise" refers to exercise — such as sprinting or standard weight training — in which oxygen does not play such a role. Different physiological mechanisms support the work done in these two forms of exercise.)

Research has shown that aerobic exercise alters blood lipid levels, increasing the percentage of High Density Lipoprotein (HDL), a beneficial lipid that helps to keep the arteries and veins clean while decreasing the concentration of harmful Low Density Lipoproteins (LDL), which clog the veins, creating hypertension and atherosclerosis. Such changes have been documented even among older, formerly sedentary men. Until the LSU study, however, little was known about the effect of *anaerobic* training on blood lipid levels. In fact, only one study closely approximates what Stone tried to do at LSU and that was a study done on longshoremen, whose work is very similar in nature to weight training. In an analysis made of the longshoremen's work patterns, it was found that those men who had the highest energy output had less cardiovascular disease than their peers who worked less hard, "lifted less," and had a more sedentary life-style. Even though the active longshoremen were only more active on their jobs, it was still enough to make a difference in their health.

What Stone found when he analyzed the blood samples from his previously sedentary middle-aged volunteers was that there were lowered levels of blood lipids when a vigorous program of weight training was used. As Stone says in his discussion of the changes, "The mechanisms by which exercise causes the changes in serum lipids are unclear. The positive changes in serum lipids occurring with aerobic training may be related to fat mobilization and metabolism during the exercise. However, the exercise associated with resistive training (weight training) in this study is supported primarily with anaerobic mechanisms and should not affect fat metabolism significantly. Weight training produces a very large oxygen debt relative to the amount of time spent training. The total oxygen debt may exceed fifteen liters. Much of the oxygen debt would be paid back using an elevated metabolism during recovery, thus serum lipids may be affected at this time rather than in the actual exercise."

In other words, in aerobic exercises such as jogging and running, blood lipid (fats) are "burned away" by the demands of aerobic process. Weight training, on the other hand, uses anaerobic energy sources, yet it also apparently alters blood lipid levels, partly because of the time it takes to recover one's breath following a set of exercise. Even though you're not continually moving during your weight-training sessions, if you train relatively rapidly, and with significantly heavy weights — as the men did in the study — you can create an oxygen debt that will, along with other mechanisms still not clearly understood, improve your cardiovascular fitness. Whatever the mechanism, it works, and in a subsequent analysis of the serum lipid levels done on the middle-aged weight trainers in the LSU study, lipids again decreased following a regular weight-training program, as did the percentage of body fat of the men who trained with weights.

# 6 / Flexibility

ONE of the least pleasant changes that comes with age is the loss of joint flexibility. Is it not with a mixture of joy and sadness that we observe the remarkable flexibility of babies who can — *and do* — put their toes effortlessly in their mouths? Tried it lately? Have you even touched your toes lately? Can you *see* your toes? All of us well past our majority realize all too well that after our bones harden and muscles become fully developed our ability to stretch out, to bend, and to reach is slowly but surely diminished by the passage of time. Very old sedentary people have joints with little range of motion and a shuffling, short-gaited walk — two of the telltale signs of decrepitude. This gradual loss of flexibility not only contributes to poor posture and leaves us more subject to injury, it also stops us from doing the things we previously could do. It narrows our life. It diminishes us. And, to a large degree, it can be counteracted by the sensible program of stretching we outline for you in Chapter 16. You can *definitely* reverse the process of joint stiffening and, for a very long time, maintain excellent flexibility and ease the various aches and pains we all associate with advancing age.

Basically, there are two main factors that limit flexibility. The first is individual bone structure and the second is the structure of the soft tissues (muscles, tendons, etc.) of the body. Your bone structure, of course, remains virtually unchanged throughout life once the growth plates (epiphyseal processes) on your bones have hardened, so you must concentrate your efforts on the body's soft tissues in order to combat the stiffness of old age. Flexibility, simply stated, is the capacity of your joints and muscles to move through a full range of motion. The relative lengths of your muscles, your tendons, and your ligaments will determine the amount of movement possible at each joint. (Ligaments are the connective tissues that attach bones to bones at the joints. Tendons connect muscles to bones.) The degree to which you're able to maintain the body's potential flexibility is determined by stretching the joints.

As our bodies move us through our daily activities, many of the body's joints are stretched and worked without our being conscious of "stretching." But these are rarely full-range stretches, and as our activity level decreases with advancing years, the unconscious stretching that occurs during an average day also declines. For this reason, it is very important that flexibility work be included in your routines and, furthermore, that you stretch each of the joints of the body through a full range of motion as often as possible. Many people don't understand that flexibility is a characteristic specific to each joint. A person can be very flexible in the hips and legs, as many dancers are, yet not be flexible at all through the shoulder girdle. One of the old myths about weight training is that it makes you "muscle bound" or inflexible — tight and clumsy — but actually the converse is true. Flexibility studies done on subjects who'd been on weight-training programs for a set period of time found that in every case joint flexibility *increased* by the end of the program. And in those studies in which standard stretching exercises were included as a warm-up and/or cool-down procedure for the routine, the flexibility gains were even better. But the myth of muscle binding has died hard. The superior flexibility of Olympic lifters, shot putters, and a host of other athletes who use weights was ignored for years by coaches who, largely because of ignorance, urged their athletes to stay away from the weights.

One of the less well-known effects of exercise is that it helps to strengthen and thicken the cartilage found in joints, where it serves as "padding" between the ends of the bones. Cartilage is primarily composed of a substance called collagen, and with aging, collagen loses elasticity through the formation of cross-links and becomes thinner. (If you'd like to know more about this, read the section called Theories of Aging on page 307.) These changes in cartilage begin early in adulthood and progressively worsen as we age. This means we not only lose some of the flexibility we enjoyed in our joints during our youth, but the shrinking of the cartilage makes the joints less stable and so joint injuries become more prevalent. Exercising helps prevent this loss of flexibility and stability both by increasing the volume of the cartilage and by making the musculature around the joints stronger so that less slippage can take place.

Tendons and ligaments also lose elasticity with age, leading to a higher incidence of tears and pulls. Tendons and ligaments, like other connective tissues, contain high levels of collagen, and, as happens elsewhere, the formation of cross-links inhibits its elastic properties. The fact that there is a decreased blood flow in older, especially inactive, individuals is also thought to predispose them to connective-tissue injuries. Tendon tears, for instance, are usually found in those spots on the tendon where there is the least blood supply. Fortunately, this loss of elasticity can be moderated by exercise and stretching.

There are two kinds of arthritic conditions that attack the joints as we age, osteoarthritis and rheumatoid arthritis. Osteoarthritis, found in more than 80 percent of people over sixty years of age, primarily attacks the joints in the knee, hip, and spine, where it causes stiffness and pain. Far more serious, however, is rheumatoid arthritis, in which the joints also swell and, in some cases, actually "lock up" so they can't even be used.

The three best corrective medicines for both conditions appear to be (1) flexibility work to stretch the joints and keep them limber, (2) keeping the body weight within normal limits so as not to place extra stress on the joints, and (3) exercising to strengthen the surrounding muscles of the joints involved. Pain killing and anti-inflammatory drugs are sometimes necessary in the early stages of rheumatoid arthritis, but we all know that since they have rather long-term side effects they should be avoided, if possible. When arthritis of either type strikes an individual, the normal response is to reduce the activity level and wait for the pain to go away. Many arthritis specialists, however, now feel that in the long run this exacerbates the problem by allowing the joints to lose flexibility and become less stable through muscle shrinkage and weakness. One further thing you should know is that many people have osteoarthritic conditions without having any accompanying pain. Quite often osteoarthritis will begin to develop during early middle age, but since there is no pain or swelling, you may not even be aware that it's there. So, just because you're not at all conscious of the slow loss of your flexibility doesn't mean you shouldn't do anything to fight it, because, by the time the pain manifests itself, you've got a much more serious problem on your hands. Arthritis, even in the early stages, is a serious medical condition, however, and no one who suffers from it should attempt any of the stretching or weight-training exercises in this text without prior medical approval.

Some people won't let arthritis rob their lives of joy, however, and they develop the patience and the intestinal fortitude to continue stretching the joints, even after the onset of the pain. One such person is Milo Steinborn, one of the greatest weightlifters and pro wrestlers of all time. Milo recently turned ninety, but he only retired a few years ago from his work as a wrestling promoter. He lives by himself, has a sharpness of mind and a memory a man of thirty would envy, and still does regular weight training as well as some wrestling with his son, Henry. Over fifty years ago Milo was stricken with rheumatoid arthritis in his hands, but he decided to keep using them even though the pain was at times almost unbearable. He kept stretching them back into a normal shape, yet his arthritis became even more acute and his fingers began to curve inward. So, along with his daily finger exercises and stretching, every night he strapped his hands, palms down, to two boards, so that the fingers were straight. He's done it for fifty years and *he still does it*. His hands are far from perfect, and he still has considerable swelling in the knuckles and, from time to time, pain. But the tough old German uses his hands to drive his car, fix his own meals, handle his business and office affairs, hold his dumbbells, and even to grab his son, Henry, when they wrestle. We've talked with him about his condition on several occasions and about how courageous we feel he's been to keep fighting such a crippling condition — which most older people would have given up on long ago. He merely smiles. "What should I have done," he asked us once, "give up? Never."

## Osteoporosis

Osteoporosis (weakening of the bones) is a major problem in later years, as this bone weakening makes older people more subject to debilitating fractures and breaks. It also often inhibits people from walking or participating in an exercise program because they fear they'll fall and break something. For some reason, the loss of bone calcium is higher in women than men, and though it begins prior to the start of menopause (usually around age thirty-five, whereas menopause is generally cited as occurring in the forty-seven to fifty-two age range), some researchers speculate that the loss of estrogen accelerates the process. Others, however, are looking at other hormones as the culprit, though much more data needs to be collected before anyone can say for certain why it happens.

What we *do* know for certain is that *exercise will slow down and in some cases reverse this process — even among the elderly*. A study done on extremely elderly women subjects (the average age of the group was eighty-two) showed that they gained 4.2 percent in bone minerals as a result of exercising for an extended period compared to a control (nonexercise) group who, during the same period of time, lost 2.5 percent. When this information is considered in light of the estimated 20 percent average bone mineral loss for men and *30 percent* loss for women by age ninety, a 6.7 percent average gain (which is how much better off those women were than the ones who didn't exercise at all) is highly significant.

A further problem with osteoporosis is that the released calcium goes into the bloodstream, where it then misbehaves in all sorts of ways. Much of the calcium is thought to attach itself to the walls of the blood vessels, depriving them of elasticity, but it also impairs the functions of other body tissues as well.

Senile osteoporosis (osteoporosis among the elderly) is characterized by an increased vulnerability to fracture, as well as degeneration in the vertebrae of the spine. We mentioned earlier that we all shrink in height because of the compression of the discs between the vertebrae, but senile osteoporosis causes the vertebrae themselves to become more fragile and porous as calcium is leached away; they can actually "crumble" if severe calcium deficiency levels are reached. Chronic backache is another problem that has been associated with osteoporosis, though in all fairness we should note that weakened back muscles as well as weakened bones are responsible for both the pain and the poor posture we have come to associate with old age. A related condition known as "kyphosis," characterized by rounded shoulders and "dowager's hump," is primarily caused by the weakening of the back and neck muscles.

Such poor posture, besides causing back pain and an unsightly appearance, also inhibits proper breathing. As kyphosis develops, the rib cage and diaphragm are sunk further back into the abdomen, breathing becomes more shallow, and not nearly as much oxygen is transported into the lungs. Less oxygen, of course, means less efficiency, less efficiency means poorer health, poorer health means a person is less likely to exercise, and so you have a vicious circle. But take note of the fact that kyphosis can be limited through proper exercises to strengthen the neck, shoulder, and back muscles.

Another spinal disorder frequently seen among the elderly is scoliosis, in which the spine forms a side-to-side "S." Like kyphosis, scoliosis is caused by the gradual weakening of the back muscles, the increasing osteoporosis of the vertebrae, and the loss of flexibility through lack of exercise and/or arthritic conditions. Some people are born with scoliotic or kyphotic conditions that don't manifest themselves until later in life, when a lack of exercise helps to aggravate the condition and create back pains. There is every reason to believe, however, that exercises to strengthen the back muscles might make the ultimate course of such disorders as kyphosis and scoliosis significantly different.

A case in point is a young friend of ours, Lamar Gant, who in 1984 won his tenth straight world championship in powerlifting. Lamar has severe scoliosis; in fact, one physician told him that he thought it made a five- to six-inch difference in his height. Even so, Lamar was active as a child, and in junior high school he began wrestling and weight training. He won his first national championship in powerlifting at the age of eighteen, and he has set dozens of world records in the sport. He suffers no back pain. Astonished physicians and chiropractors who've examined him have usually agreed that the heavy weight training he's done has so strengthened the muscles that it has completely eliminated the debilitating effects usually suffered by someone with such a severe case of scoliosis. They've advised him to keep it up.

*We are not, however, recommending that all people with severe or even moderate back problems become powerlifters.* What we are recommending is that if you should have such a problem (even if it does not at this time seem serious), consult your family physician and ask if he or she would recommend your doing some light weight-training work to help strengthen the adjacent muscles. Then, *if you get permission,* work to *gradually* strengthen the muscles. And don't forget to do some flexibility work while you're at it. Strength and flexibility, after all, are the keys to avoiding joint problems, poor posture, and other related indignities associated with getting older.

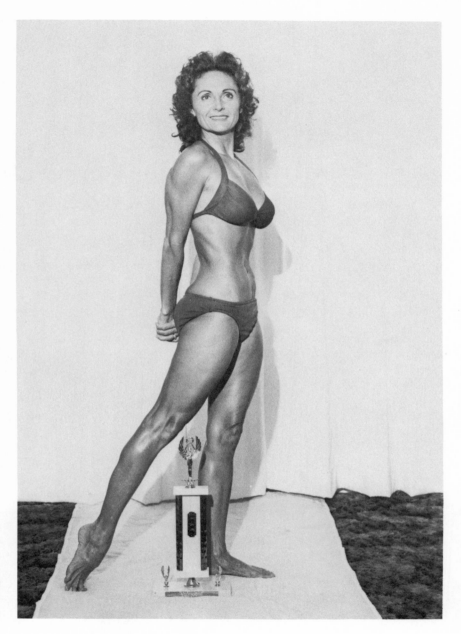

*At forty-seven years of age, Doris Barrilleaux left her Florida home to go to Canton, Ohio, and compete in the first women's bodybuilding contest ever held. This photo was taken the day following the championships in which she placed third against women half her age.*

# 7 / Doris Barrilleaux — Bodybuilding's Pioneer

THE first thing you should know about Doris Barrilleaux, if you can tear your eyes away from that show-stopping body, is that she's fifty-three years old. The second thing is that she's the mother of five children, grandmother of eight, and has a regular job as an airline stewardess. The third thing you should know is that more than any other person, Doris Barrilleaux is responsible for the rapid growth of women's bodybuilding in the United States.

Doris participated in the first modern women's bodybuilding championships at the age of forty-seven and left those championships filled with ideas and plans for a new women's sport. As Doris explains, "It was never my intention to become a bodybuilder or to become involved in the administration of the sport. I was a normal working mother who trained at home, alone for the most part, whose only aspiration as a weight trainer was to keep my body in shape and to have enough strength so that I could keep up with five growing youngsters. But, at the urging of several of my friends, I traveled to Canton, Ohio, back in 1978 to compete in what turned out to be the first modern women's physique contest. I was so upset at the way the men thought women should look that I decided someone had to head the sport in a different direction."

Doris has indeed headed the women in a different and, we think, appropriate direction. Women's bodybuilding, as a sport, had to overcome the heritage of beauty contests and the cultural antipathy toward women who took up a "masculine" sport. "At the Ohio meet, where I placed third, we all wore bikinis, of course. Some meet promoters thought we should be required to wear high heels so we wouldn't put off people in the audience who'd never seen a weight-trained woman with muscles before, let alone a woman *posing* those muscles. So, when I came home I talked to several of my friends here in Central Florida who trained with weights as I did, and we decided that if there was a future for women's bodybuilding it should not be a future in which men determined how the ideal feminine physique was supposed to look. I felt then, and feel now, that women bodybuilders should first and foremost look like women. Women who train exceptionally hard and diet with unstinting dedication can become both very muscular and very lean — but they should still look like women. I'm very much against the 'anorexic look.' Bodybuilding's a great sport, but it should *encourage* better health, not tear it down through the use of starvation diets or artificial hormones."

Doris's love affair with barbells began when she realized she was no longer able to do the things she had done when she was younger and that her body, possessed though it was of a fine bone structure and good skin, did not look as she remembered it. "I married very young, and by the time I was twenty-one, I had already had three children. I didn't 'work' at that point, though I worked plenty keeping up with the babies, and because I was young and busy I didn't give much thought to how I looked. As the years passed and we got out of diapers and into the yard, I began to think a bit more about myself, though I didn't do any exercises of any sort. But I knew from the way my clothes fit that the four babies had taken their toll, and then one day, when I had taken the kids down to the local park, I had one of those life-changing experiences people are always talking about. Mine wasn't a divine vision; it was more a matter of embarrassment. We'd been in the park for about an hour and the kids had run on to play with some friends when I got the urge to hang on the chinning bars by my knees. I used to love to climb trees when I was a kid, and I'd always been very active when I was young, so I was really shocked when, despite everything I tried, I couldn't raise my feet to the bar. I was twenty-five years old. I was also infuriated for having let myself get in that kind of shape."

But Doris used her anger to fuel a new exercise program. "I started out doing exercises at home — sit-ups, side bends, and things of that sort — but once I began to train, I wanted to do more. As I thought about it — remember, this was 1956 — I decided that I wanted to begin doing some barbell training in addition to what I was doing with calisthenics. After that first couple of weeks of training at home, I decided that I was going to join a regular men's gym and learn what to do."

The training made a difference in the look of her body, and it made a tremendous difference in her health. "I could tell that I was feeling better, had more energy, and all that, but when I had my fifth pregnancy in 1958, I discovered what a *real* change had occurred in me. Until the eighth month, I didn't really feel pregnant at all. I backed down some on the exercises during this time, though I still continued to train with light weights. Even the delivery and recovery phase of the birth were easier than those in the past, though I was considerably older. I was in labor for only an hour."

As Doris will admit, with five kids and a husband to take care of, it wasn't easy to squeeze in time for her training. "Please don't get the idea," she told us, "that I've been doing some huge, time-consuming workout day after day after day. I really don't do all that much compared to what a lot of people do, but I've always been regular about doing it."

It's been twenty-eight years now since Doris began her weight work.

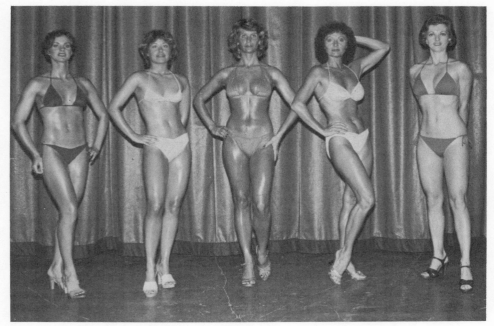

*More than any other woman, Doris is responsible for the rapid growth of women's bodybuilding. She founded the first official women's bodybuilding organization, which drew up judging guidelines for women and sponsored contests such as this 1979 Ms. Gold Coast Competition in Tampa.*

Naturally, there were times during those years when she couldn't train as she wanted, even periods when she hardly trained with weights at all. "When I couldn't get to the gym in the old days, I'd still try to do something here at home. All the kids went to Catholic schools and so every week I had twenty-five white shirts to starch and iron for them, plus five for my husband. Well, I used to save them all up and do them at once, and the whole time I was ironing or washing dishes I'd do calf raises. Other times, when I was vacuuming, I'd do lunges as I worked, just so I didn't lose all my muscle tone. The kids used to think I was pretty strange, but now they're all very proud of what I've been able to accomplish."

Today, Doris's 5 foot 5 inch, 36-25¼-36-inch body is maintained by three weekly workouts and a sensible eating program. When her schedule permits it, she trains at home, but when she's on flight duty for Aerosun International, or off in some distant corner of the world judging a bodybuilding show, she trains in her hotel room. But, wherever she is, she trains.

"A lot of people have come to me over the years and talked about weight training and a lot of them have said that they feel inspired by what I've been able to do. Nice as that is to hear, I'm also sort of amused by the fact that so many people seem to think that staying fit is so terribly difficult. I've often thought that it would be interesting to see how the Miss America contestants of 1956 look today, compared to the way I look. I don't say that out of pure vanity, though I suppose there's some there, of course. What I'm trying to say, I guess, is that the difference between the way beauty contestants

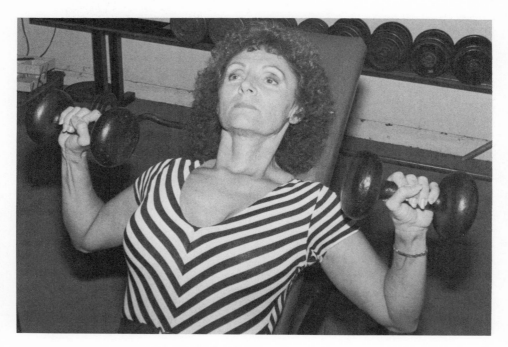

*With five children and a career as a stewardess, Doris has had to squeeze her weight workouts in when she could. She's found that training at home has made it possible for her to work out on many days when she couldn't afford the time to go all the way to the gym.*

look and the way women bodybuilders look is the difference between good genetics coupled with youth and average genetics coupled with hard work. What's interesting to me is that once youth fades, good genetics alone won't allow a woman to continue to look as she once did. Yet even a woman of average 'beauty' can continue to look fantastic for years and years through weight training. It's really pretty simple, and it doesn't even take much time, just commitment and regularity.''

# 8 / Fitness of the Mind

IF there is any aspect of aging that is even more unpleasant to contemplate than the gradual loss of the power and shape of our bodies, it would surely have to be the gradual loss of mental sharpness, memory, and reaction time.

We've all heard of the dangers of having older drivers — whose reactions in many cases aren't what they once were — on our streets and highways. And we're all also aware that older people often have more trouble remembering things (particularly those things in the recent past) when they are asked to remember quickly, in what's known as a "time press." We know as well that it's hard for many elderly people to make decisions; when confronted with several problems, older people often become confused. The reason for these changes, of course, is that the central nervous system ages in much the same way other systems in the body do — it slowly breaks down. None of this is news, but what most of you are probably unaware of is that there's a growing body of evidence that suggests the fitness of the central nervous system is connected to the fitness of the rest of your body. The old Latin goal *mens sana in corpore sano* — a sound mind in a sound body — is apparently a lot closer to the truth than many had previously thought.

Aging of the central nervous system has always been a highly individual matter, but a number of cross-sectional studies (investigations of a group of individuals) have proven that there's a direct relationship between a person's physical activity level and his neurological "fitness." Most of us have probably been in "rest" homes at one time or another and observed the high level of senility that usually is found there. Some of you with family members who have had to be institutionalized may even have had the unpleasant experience of observing the generally rapid deterioration that accompanied a move from home, where there were chores to do, to an institutional situation where there was no reason to be active. There are, of course, a number of causes other than a lack of physical activity for the onset of senility, but the fact that so many people in their later years don't even walk on a regular basis is now thought to contribute to the problem more than was previously suspected. Although much is still not known about this, one explanation of what happens when a person becomes inactive is that the lessened oxygen supply to the brain causes the brain cells to function less efficiently, which means information is processed more slowly, memory is affected, and the total number of brain cells diminishes more rapidly. One "proof" of this theory is that if an older person is given extra oxygen (which is more available to a fit young person) while asked to perform certain central nervous system tasks such as memorization, he or she will score higher than without the supplemental oxygen.

Happier news is that training has a very beneficial effect on the central nervous systems of old as well as young people. When young sedentary subjects were compared to young active subjects, for instance, the response times — the time it takes a subject to respond to a stimulus — of the sedentary group were significantly slower. In fact, when young nonathletes were compared to old *athletes,* the older athletes often turned in faster reaction times. A study that exemplifies this was done by Waneen W. Spirduso in 1975 at the University of Texas in Austin. Dr. Spirduso tested a group of older (aged fifty-nine to seventy) hand-eye-coordination-sports players (squash, tennis, and handball) who played on an average of three times a week, against a group of healthy "normal" twenty- to thirty-year-olds who were not regularly involved in exercise. She also tested a group of young players and an inactive "old" group. Her findings showed that when members of the old inactive group were tested for reaction times they had very serious central nervous system deterioration. The "active" group of comparable age, however, turned in scores that were equal to or better than those of the twenty- to thirty-year-olds who were not regularly involved in an exercise program, even though there was a thirty- to forty-year difference in their ages. Dr. Spirduso also found, in a subsequent research project, that regular exercise can postpone deterioration in some motor areas of the brain that are associated with aging. In collaboration with Drs. Richard Wilcox and Roger Farrar, she did research showing that routine exercise can curb the reduction of a substance called dopamine, a neurotransmitter closely related to motor control. This is important because the depletion of dopamine is probably the primary cause of the loss of movement control experienced in aging and in Parkinson's disease, which is characterized by severe motor dysfunction. Another interesting thing to consider is that at several Olympic Games, research measuring reaction times on representatives from all the different sports has shown weightlifters to score at the very top of this large group of elite athletes. It's believed by several leading strength sport theorists that the explosive training movements of weightlifting have a stimulating effect on the central nervous system.

Although it is common knowledge that conditions such as atherosclerosis (accumulation of fat on the inside of the blood vessels) reduce the amount of blood that reaches the brain, you may not be aware of the fact that these blood-flow reductions can begin at a young age. Many people are unaware that atherosclerosis begins so early in life, or that by age fifty-nine there is roughly a 50 percent decrease in blood flow to the brain among inactive people.

A new area of investigation has been the relationship between atherosclerosis and reaction times, and the evidence is mounting that high cholesterol levels in the blood, which minimize the oxygen that reaches the brain cells — and which can be lowered by regular exercise — also lower the speed at which a person reacts to an outside stimulus. In the past five years there has also been research into the question of intelligence levels and cardiovascular fitness that suggests that both memory and intelligence decline more rapidly among those people who have cardiovascular disease and subsequent hypertension (high blood pressure). In fact, individuals with high blood pressures (diastolic pressures) have even been found to score lower on intelligence tests than individuals with low or "normal" pressures.

Another interesting phenomenon occurs within the brain itself. Scientists have now learned that there are sections of the brain called motor centers, which control various activities. When a person exercises, not only does the blood flow increase to the *muscles* being used, it now is known that it also increases in the motor center of the brain that's sending the instructions. It's believed that inactive people, who therefore don't use all their motor centers, have lessened blood flow into these areas, which means the brain cells in those particular parts of the brain deteriorate even *more* rapidly with age. The person who engages in regular exercise maintains the blood flow to these motor centers and therefore escapes some of the brain-cell deterioration.

Apparently, through exercise, not only are the brain cells that signal the muscles to move affected, but the portions of the brain that plan the movements are also stimulated. So, exercise has a bracing effect on large portions of the brain. Weight training — which allows you to vigorously exercise a wide variety of muscles rather than just those of the legs and buttocks as is done in jogging — has an advantage in stimulating a wide variety of motor centers. Done rapidly, or in combination with a good cycling or walking program, weight training should be invaluable in providing brain stimulation.

A brand-new area of research is the effect exercise has on the nerves themselves. Nerve tissue can apparently undergo a form of hypertrophy similar in some ways to that of muscle tissue. In a 1965 study E. Retzlaff and J. Fontaine found that exercise increases the integrative action of the spinal neurons and the speed at which they can conduct messages, both of which are important factors for efficient functioning of the brain as well as the body. And, in 1981, Drs. Waneen Spirduso and Roger Farrar completed a similar study on rats and found at the conclusion of a six-month training regimen that their exercised rats were able to respond more rapidly to stimuli than the rats' untrained age-mates and, furthermore, that the fit rats exhibited other characteristics of fitness such as proper body posture and muscular strength.

One of the most amazing effects that exercise has on the central nervous system is its capacity to "tranquilize" a person who exercises. One famous study done by Dr. Herbert DeVries at the University of Southern California found that bouts of exercise were more efficient than tranquilizers at relieving tension. DeVries found that even ninety minutes after exercise, there was less tension, or electromyographically measurable activity, in the muscles of his test subjects who'd exercised than in those who'd taken tranquilizers.

Quite a few sports psychologists have found that adherence to a regular exercise program can make dramatic differences in the way people feel about themselves. "Self-concept" studies on both young and older exercisers have found significant increases in feelings of self-worth following several weeks of regular training. We assisted Dr. James Hilyer at Auburn University in several research projects concerning the relationship of weight training and self-concept among young as well as older individuals. He conducted self-concept studies as part of the weight-training studies detailed in chapters 10 and 11 and found significant improvements in middle-aged men and women. He has also done similar work on teenaged and "emotionally disturbed" subjects and found significant improvements there as well.

Much more research in this area needs to be done, of course, especially in light of the rapidly increasing average age of our population, not to mention the high sales figures for tranquilizers. Our own experiences and those of our weight-trained pals would certainly corroborate the findings of the various scientists who have researched the relationship between vigorous exercise, brain function, and psychological fitness. Apparently, weight training increases not only your neurological health but also the pride you take in your appearance, thus giving you a "younger" central nervous system, more self-confidence, and the emotional tranquility necessary to eat and rest better. Not bad.

# 9 / Fitness vs. Fatness

ONE of the factors physiologists look at when determining a person's fitness is the relative proportion of fat tissue to lean tissue, a proportion usually referred to as "percent body fat." The most accurate way to determine this percentage is to have your body ground up and then immersed in organic solvent, which burns away the fat, leaving only the lean weight — the ground-up bones, muscles, teeth, hair, etc. For those unwilling to pay the price for such scientific accuracy, we suggest two alternative methods — skin-fold calipers or hydrostatic (underwater) weighing. The caliper method is the most widely used by physiologists and coaches, but, though quicker, it is far less accurate. In this method, sections of the subject's skin are "pinched up" by the tester in places such as the back of the arm, directly under the scapula on the back, at the waistline, or on the back of the thigh. The thicknesses of these folds are then measured by the caliper, and the combination of these measurements gives a good general indication of the relative percent of fat the person is carrying.

In hydrostatic weighing, the person's "dry" weight is first taken, then he or she is lowered into a water-filled tank, completely submerged, and then weighed again, underwater, on a frame inside the tank. Because fat is lighter than muscle and bone and tends to float, the sports scientist is able to approximate, through the use of a mathematical formula based on cadaver studies, the actual percentage of fat in a subject's body.

**Jan:** "I remember the first time I was underwater-weighed. I turned out to have forty-seven pounds of fat on my frame. I was horrified. While the poundage itself was certainly enough to frighten me, what was even more offensive was the sudden thought of how all that fat, piled up in one big lump, would look. The thought was a little disturbing, despite the fact that I was at that time training primarily for strength, *not* for looks."

The importance of your percent body fat cannot be ignored by anyone with serious aspirations for fitness, especially those concerned with aging.

Weighing yourself on a regular scale as you embark on a program of weight training, however, is often not only of little or no help, but actually misleading. What can be misleading is that you may gain good, lean weight, yet, thinking you are getting fatter, cut back on your food intake, which will make it more difficult for you to recover properly from your workouts. The best way to handle this matter, if you can't make arrangements to have yourself underwater-weighed periodically, is to simply pay very little attention to your body weight. Be guided more by how you *feel* and how your pants fit. One measurement you can use to monitor body-fat changes is the difference between the diameter of your upper arm when flexed and the same arm measured straight down at your side, unflexed. The greater the difference, the less fat the arm. (This method should *not* be used to compare one person with another. It works only as a way of comparing a fatter you with a leaner you.)

One of the sad things about society's notions of appropriate body weights is that quite often people who begin an exercise program are distressed to find they've gained a few pounds after training for a few months, even if the gain was all muscle tissue. What is important here is that lean or muscle tissue is good, whereas fat is mostly bad. They even *look* different. Next time you're in a supermarket, ask your grocer for a pound of suet; if it's winter, you can feed it to the birds. When the butcher brings it out, get a good look at the actual size — the physical dimensions — of a pound of fat. Then walk down to the steaks and look at the difference. Actually, a pound of fish makes an even better contrast because even "lean" steak carries a high percentage of interstitial fat (fat within the muscle tissue). Once you've made this comparison, you can understand how it is possible to gain weight and lose inches.

All fat, however, isn't bad. Mother nature requires some for the proper functioning of the organs in the body. And not only does fat help to cushion the internal organs and keep them in place, it provides a reserve of food that the body calls upon in times of trouble. However, excess fat is the excess food we eat. The amount of food we take in beyond what we expend every day through exercise and just living determines how much fat we'll gain or maintain through the years.

Since the hydrostatic weighing method has been put into use, a number of studies have been completed that have determined the body composition of a number of different age groups. For college-age men and women, for instance, the percent body-fat averages seem to fall between 20 to 24 percent for women and 12 to 15 percent for men. These are not figures for trained athletes, mind you, but for average, fairly active students. As people age, the "averages" for percent body fat correspondingly increase. This increase in body fat is the result not only of our decrease in exercise, but our corresponding *non*decrease in calorie consumption. Furthermore, as we age, our metabolic rate slows — which means we burn fewer calories during an average day. There are several reasons for the metabolic slowdown that accompanies aging, one of which you can do something about — your "muscularity." According to physiologists, the greater the percentage of muscle tissue in a body, the higher the metabolic rate. So, one way to combat your body's natural slowing down is to stay lean; being lean and muscular you will burn more calories naturally than if your body possessed a higher percentage of fat.

In each of us, as we read, walk, sleep, run, make love, type, eat, and simply sit and think, calories are being burned to fuel the energy needs of our cells. The more vigorous the activity, such as running or weight training, the more calories are burned to continue the movement. (See chart on page 74.) A calorie, more properly called a kilocalorie, is the amount of energy needed to raise one kilogram (2.2 pounds) of water 1 degree centigrade. Almost all of us burn over 1000 calories every day simply by going through our normal activities. The average, full-grown man, for instance, normally uses between 1500 and 1800 calories per day to maintain his non-exercise activities. Women usually have a slightly slower metabolic rate than men, which, coupled with their smaller relative size, makes their caloric needs less. The exception to this, of course, is the nursing mother, who should be aware that the production of milk normally requires an additional 1000 calories per day. Naturally, larger individuals need more calories per day to maintain their weight than do smaller people. And older individuals, with their slower metabolic rates, generally need fewer calories per day to maintain their weight than do the young.

If you plan to make a concerted effort to lose body fat as you train with weights, use common sense about your dieting, and before you start cutting back, analyze your body's own particular caloric requirements. The easiest way to approximate *your* metabolic rate is to simply determine your weight in kilos by weighing on a good scale and then dividing your weight in pounds by 2.2. Then, multiply your kilo weight by 24 calories. If, for instance, you weigh 154 pounds, or 70 kilos, then you would multiply 70 × 24, which equals 1680 calories. This figure, the 1680, should then serve as a base around which you plan your diet. Naturally, this is not a hard and fast figure. You may burn more or fewer calories per day than this estimate, but you can use it as a general guide for determining how many calories per day you can eat to lose weight.

A more accurate method is to determine your *total* calorie expenditure in a day by recording all of your activities for an average day in minutes. **Jan:** "For instance, one day in September of 1982, I calculated my total caloric expenditure for the day as follows:

| | | | |
|---|---|---|---|
| 11 P.M. to 6 A.M. | Sleep | 420 minutes × 1.2 cal per minute = | 504 |
| 6 to 6:30 | Make coffee, wash face, etc. | 30 minutes × 2.6 cal per minute = | 78 |
| 6:30 to 8:00 | Typing, correspondence | 90 minutes × 2.0 cal per minute = | 180 |
| 8:00 to 8:30 | Cook and eat breakfast | 30 minutes × 1.5 cal per minute = | 45 |
| 8:30 to 8:45 | Barn chores | 15 minutes × 3.8 cal per minute = | 57 |
| 8:45 A.M. to 1:30 P.M. | Writing/typing | 285 minutes × 2.0 cal per minute = | 570 |
| 1:30 to 2:15 | Cook and eat lunch | 45 minutes × 2.6 cal per minute = | 117 |
| 2:15 to 3:30 | Pay bills/talk on telephone | 75 minutes × 2.0 cal per minute = | 150 |
| 3:30 to 4:30 | Get ready for gym/ drive to gym | 60 minutes × 2.5 cal per minute = | 150 |
| 4:30 to 6:00 | *Very* rapid weight training | 90 minutes × 8.0 cal per minute = | 720 |
| 6:00 to 6:15 | Running | 15 minutes × 8.0 cal per minute = | 120 |
| 6:15 to 7:30 | Drive home, cook supper | 75 minutes × 2.5 cal per minute = | 187.5 |
| 7:30 to 8:30 | Eat supper/talk | 60 minutes × 1.3 cal per minute = | 78 |
| 8:30 to 9:00 | Dishes/clean kitchen | 30 minutes × 2.6 cal per minute = | 78 |
| 9:00 to 9:30 | Write letter | 30 minutes × 2.0 cal per minute = | 60 |
| 9:30 to 10:30 | Bathe/wash hair | 60 minutes × 1.8 cal per minute = | 108 |
| 10:30 to 11:00 | Read | 30 minutes × 1.3 cal per minute = | 39 |
| | | Total | 3241.5 |

"Since I weighed 152 pounds on the day I recorded my activities, I had no further adjustments to make to the final total, as these figures are based on a 150-pound individual. However, for each 15 pounds *over* 150 that you weigh, you should increase the total by 15 percent. Likewise, for each 10 pounds *under* 150, subtract 10 percent from the total. This enables you to know more precisely what your individual body burns in calories in an average day and what you need to consume in order to lose weight, gain, or remain the same.

"By knowing approximately what I burned in calories for that day, I was then able to go to my food charts, where I recorded everything I ate on that same day, and determine whether or not I would gain or lose weight. On this particular day, I ate only 1629 calories (based on the estimates of calories from my USDA calorie charts), which means that I had a deficit of roughly 1600 calories. Since a pound of stored fat consists of 3500 calories, I would come close to losing a full pound in two days of such activity and diet.

"One thing I found to be instructive was to keep track of my food intake from time to time as I started dropping weight to see exactly how many calories I was consuming. In the beginning, I did it for several weeks straight until I learned more about relative caloric levels, and then I did it whenever I seemed to hit a plateau and stopped losing. Often, the reason my weight hadn't continued to drop was that I was eating more than I realized.

"I also kept a notebook for motivational reasons. Recording all my food on a daily basis — even the tastes and small bites I took while I was cooking — made me stop and think about whether or not I really wanted — or needed — to eat a certain item. More often than not, realizing it had to go in the book, I'd wait for my regular meal and skip the snack."

Recently, we've become even more convinced of the importance of recording what you eat and how you exercise as we've followed the remarkable progress of a Texas couple who came to us for advice on diet and exercise. The man, at age 40, was 5 feet 5½ inches tall and weighed 238 pounds. His wife, at 39, was 5 feet 3 inches and 177 pounds. Their body-fat percentages were 39.3 and 37.7, respectively. We started them on an exercise program that now includes weight training, cycling, and powerwalking, but their physical condition also required diet counseling and so we urged them to begin keeping records as a way for us to monitor their diet and for them to begin thinking and learning about calories and the amounts and sorts of foods they were eating.

To say the program has been a success would be a classic understatement. Our male friend, Doyle, after 5½ months, has lost 51 pounds and his wife, Margaret, has lost 30. Their cardiovascular progress has also amazed their physician. Doyle, for instance, decreased his resting pulse from 82 beats per minute to *40 per minute*. Even *we* were amazed. Part of their success, of course, came from persistence and effort, but part came from the careful and complete records they kept of their food intake, their exercise program, and their pulse rate changes.

The most complete set of calorie charts we've found are those published by the U.S. Department of Agriculture in a book called *Composition of Foods*. (See Suggestions for Further Reading for information on ordering.) The advantage it has over other similar texts is that it is far more complete, even including such wonderful entries as roast muskrat, canned turtle meat, and raw whale. And besides listing the caloric equivalents for thousands of different types of foodstuffs, it also includes breakdowns on each item's protein level, carbohydrate level, and sodium level, plus ten other minerals and vitamins *and* the fiber content. It will tell you, in other words, more than you really *care* to know about food.

**Jan:** "When I sat down in the evening to analyze my calories and my activity for the day, I also checked in *Composition of Foods* to see how much protein I ate every day, what vitamins I'd ingested from my meals, and what my carbohydrate intake had been for the day. In this way, even though I was eating less than I had in the past, I was still able to guarantee that I wasn't becoming deficient in one particular area. I think that's one reason I felt so well during my dieting. I always had energy for my training, slept well, and wasn't nervous. It took a little time, at first, but now I can finish a meal and pretty well estimate how many calories I've eaten without looking anything up."

Another matter of importance, if you're trying to lose, is the relative sodium levels in different foods, because sodium contributes to the retention of fluid in the tissues of the body. People become depressed when they see

| Activity | Cal / min | Activity | Cal / min | Activity | Cal / min |
|---|---|---|---|---|---|
| Sleeping | 1.2 | Chain-saw work | 6.2 | Handball and Squash | 10.0 |
| Resting in bed | 1.3 | Stone, masonry | 6.3 | Mountain Climbing | 10.0 |
| Sitting, normally | 1.3 | Pick-and-shovel work | 6.7 | Skipping rope | 10.0–15.0 |
| Sitting, reading | 1.3 | Farming, haying, plowing with horse | 6.7 | Judo and Karate | 13.0 |
| Lying, quietly | 1.3 | Shoveling (miners) | 6.8 | Football (while active) | 13.3 |
| Sitting, eating | 1.5 | Walking downstairs | 7.1 | Wrestling | 14.4 |
| Sitting, playing cards | 1.5 | Chopping wood | 7.5 | Skiing: | |
| Standing, normally | 1.5 | Crosscut-saw work | 7.5–10.5 | Moderate to Steep | 8.0–12.0 |
| Lecture (listening to) | 1.7 | Tree felling (ax) | 8.4–12.7 | Downhill Racing | 16.5 |
| Conversing | 1.8 | Gardening, digging | 8.6 | Cross-Country: 3–8 mph | 9.0–17.0 |
| Personal toilet | 2.0 | Walking upstairs | 10.0–18.0 | Swimming: | |
| Sitting, writing | 2.6 | Pool or billiards | 1.8 | Pleasure | 6.0 |
| Standing, light activity | 2.6 | Canoeing: 2.5–4.0 mph | 3.0–7.0 | Crawl: 25–50 yds/min | 6.0–12.5 |
| Washing and dressing | 2.6 | Volleyball: Recreational– Competitive | 3.5–8.0 | Butterfly: 50 yds/min | 14.0 |
| Washing and shaving | 2.6 | Golf: Foursome–Twosome | 3.7–5.0 | Backstroke: 25–50 yds/min | 6.0–12.5 |
| Driving a car | 2.8 | Horseshoes | 3.8 | Breaststroke: 25–50 yds/min | 6.0–12.5 |
| Washing clothes | 3.1 | Baseball (except pitcher) | 4.7 | Sidestroke: 40 yds/min | 11.0 |
| Walking indoors | 3.1 | Ping-Pong–Table Tennis | 4.9–7.0 | Dancing: | |
| Shining shoes | 3.2 | Calisthenics | 5.0 | Modern: Moderate– Vigorous | 4.2–5.7 |
| Making bed | 3.4 | Rowing: Pleasure–Vigorous | 5.0–15.0 | Ballroom: Waltz–Rumba | 5.7–7.0 |
| Dressing | 3.4 | Cycling: 5–15 mph (10 speed) | 5.0–12.0 | Square | 7.7 |
| Showering | 3.4 | Skating: Recreational– Vigorous | 5.0–15.0 | Walking: | |
| Driving motorcycle | 3.4 | Archery | 5.2 | Road–Field (3.5 mph) | 5.6–7.0 |
| Metalworking | 3.5 | Badminton: Recreational– Competitive | 5.2–10.0 | Snow: Hard–Soft (3.5–2.5 mph) | 10.0–20.0 |
| House painting | 3.5 | Basketball: Half–Full Court | 6.0–9.0 | Uphill: 5–10–15% (3.5 mph) | 8.0–11.0–15.0 |
| Cleaning windows | 3.7 | Bowling (while active) | 7.0 | Downhill: 5–10% (2.5 mph) | 3.5–3.6 |
| Carpentry | 3.8 | Tennis: Recreational– Competitive | 7.0–11.0 | 15–20% (2.5 mph) | 3.7–4.3 |
| Farming chores | 3.8 | Waterskiing | 8.0 | Hiking: 40 lb pack (3.0 mph) | 6.8 |
| Sweeping floors | 3.9 | Soccer | 9.0 | Weight Training (Rapid) (authors' estimate) | 8.0 |
| Plastering walls | 4.1 | Snowshoeing (2.5 mph) | 9.0 | Running: | |
| Truck and automobile repair | 4.2 | | | 12 min mile (5 mph) | 10.0 |
| Ironing clothes | 4.2 | | | 8 min mile (7.5 mph) | 15.0 |
| Farming, planting, hoeing, raking | 4.7 | | | 6 min mile (10 mph) | 20.0 |
| Mixing cement | 4.7 | | | 5 min mile (12 mph) | 25.0 |
| Mopping floors | 4.9 | | | | |
| Repaving roads | 5.0 | | | | |
| Gardening, weeding | 5.6 | | | | |
| Stacking lumber | 5.8 | | | | |

(Sources: Consolazio, Johnson, & Pecora, 1963; Human Performance Laboratory, University of Montana, 1964–1978; Passmore & Durnin, 1955; Roth, 1968.)

*Physiology of Fitness*, by Brian J. Sharkey, copyright 1980 by Human Kinetics Publishers Inc. Reprinted by permission of the publisher.

no real changes on the scale but it's often because they've been retaining fluid. We have both become conscious of our sodium intake for this reason and because there are direct connections between high sodium use and atherosclerosis and other cardiovascular diseases.

As we share these thoughts on diet with you, bear in mind that neither of us is an expert in the field of nutrition. Bear in mind, also, however, that the physiological basis of weight control, as we've explained it, *is fairly simple*. Any physicist will tell you that if, indeed, you eat less than your body normally expends in energy, you will lose weight because your body will have to find that energy from someplace else. So, unless you create a fuel *deficit* through either increased activity or through a decrease in the amount of calories you consume, you won't lose weight. One word of caution. For various reasons, some understood and some not, our bodies don't take *all* their energy needs from our stored fat. When energy demands are very high and intake is low, the body will also begin breaking down muscle tissue to meet its requirements. To avoid this, try not to lose weight too fast. By losing weight more slowly, not only will you lose less lean tissue but your skin will have more time to "shrink" enough to fit your new contours. So follow a slow, logical approach to weight control. Don't do it overnight. Even if you have a lot to lose, give yourself several months or even a year to lose the weight you want.

To best lose body fat, common sense suggests the following steps. Using the chart on the opposite page, determine your total caloric expenditure for several average days. Don't make your calculations when you're on a trip or vacation or when you've been walking all day while shopping. Do the figures for at least three normal days, then average the figures to see what your daily caloric expenditure is. Do this before you start your training program so you'll understand what you've been doing and why your body is in the shape it's in.

Next, for those same days, keep track of every single thing you eat or drink. Don't diet on these days — just get as accurate an idea as possible of the total number of calories you *normally* consume. **Terry:** "I remember Jan came moaning into the living room one evening because the cheese sauce she'd made to go with some low-calorie steamed broccoli contained over 1100 calories when she added up the cup of half-and-half, the cup of cheddar cheese, the three tablespoons of flour, the three tablespoons of butter, and the four tablespoons of parmesan cheese. Naturally, you shouldn't eat cheese sauce by the cup, but it *is* instructive to realize how something as simple as cheese sauce can absolutely ruin what would otherwise have been a very low-cal meal of steamed broccoli, broiled fish, and spinach salad. Don't get me wrong. We still have cheese sauce, but now Jan uses skim milk, less butter, and low-fat cheese and I can't really tell *too* much difference in the taste. But until she started her food records, neither one of us ever gave much thought to the calories in cheese sauce. So keep track of everything, because it all adds up. And *shows* up."

If your two figures — calorie consumption and calorie expenditure — are close, and if they are an accurate representation of how you've been eating and living, then you probably have not been gaining or losing too much over the past few months. If, however, you're eating 100 calories or more per day over your daily caloric expenditure, you may have discovered the reason why you've been slowly gaining weight. A hundred calories is roughly the caloric equivalent of a tablespoon of butter. Doesn't sound like much, does it? But, in terms of a month, that's a gain of roughly 3,000 calories, which, continued over twelve months, means 10 pounds or so of extra body weight. And a 10-pound weight gain in a year is enough to worry any of us, especially when, through ignorance, we go on gaining an extra 10 year after year.

Now you have to decide how much weight you wish to lose and how quickly you wish to lose it. (Please keep in mind, here, that when we talk of losing "weight" we are actually referring to losing *body fat,* so while the scale will give you *some* clues as to what changes are occurring in your body, the real test is either underwater weighing or the way your clothes fit.) We recommend that you use a combination of exercise *and* diet if you want rapid changes in your body. If you look at the activity chart, you'll see that it takes a considerable amount of time to exercise off 500 calories, while most of us can cut 500 calories from our diet rather easily.

By cutting back to a more moderate eating level and increasing your exercise level, you should find the weight slowly but surely falling away. Once you've gotten into your third week of training, recalculate your average daily calorie expenditure based on the amount of time you now spend in weight training or doing pure cardiovascular work. Then, look at your food records, which you should have been keeping during those same weeks to help regulate your diet, and see where you now stand. Are you still eating more than you burn in an average day? If so, either cut back further on your food or exercise for longer periods of time. At no point should you feel as if you're starving. Be patient; don't rush the process. Just pay attention to what you eat, how long you exercise, how vigorously you exercise, and use your head.

We don't, however, want to make it sound *too* simple, because it's not. The *formula* is simple; applying the formula is not. While it's nice to say, "eat more and you'll gain and eat less and you'll lose," there *are* other factors involved in weight control, some of which are well understood, many of which are still mysteries. The research that's been done on weight control is endless, and more dollars have been made by "experts" selling diets to the American public than can be believed. Over the past twenty years, as our fascination with leanness has deepened, books describing all-meat diets, liquid-protein diets, vegetarian diets, fasting, movie-star diets, fiber diets, juice diets, vitamin diets, etc., have become *big* best-sellers. Yet we wonder if people would want to spend the rest of their lives eating as these popular books suggest. The problem with most of these "diets" is that they are quick fixes for a lifelong problem. They capitalize — do they ever — on our ardent wish for the Easy Way. Fortunes have been made on the gullibility of otherwise intelligent, albeit somewhat chubby, people.

As might be imagined, we've had quite a few people at the university come to us over the past years asking for help with losing weight. One of them, Sally, had been using an extremely popular liquid diet plan for almost two months when we saw her one day and complimented her on her weight loss. "I'm so frustrated," she said. "I wanted to lose the weight, and I suppose I'm glad I did it, but I find I can't make the adjustment back to normal food. I've tried everything but as soon as I quit eating just the diet stuff exclusively, I start to gain again."

This is an old story to us by now, and we don't mean to single out just liquid diet plans. As we sat and talked with Sally it became clear that her main problem was in not knowing *what* to eat, or how. She would normally skip breakfast, have a hamburger, iced tea, and fries for her lunch, and then eat a large supper, generally with some sort of beef, lamb, or pork playing the starring role. She disliked chicken, she said, and only liked fried fish, so avoided it most of the time. Steak was her "diet" food. Well, in case you haven't spent any time with your calorie charts lately, a broiled T-bone steak that weighs 114 grams (about ¼ pound) contains 539 calories *if* you don't trim off every bit of fat before you broil it. Few of us actually do trim the fat before cooking — Sally surely didn't — even though she cut "most of" the fat off at her plate. But even if you *did* first cut off all the fat, which should reduce the calories by nearly one half, when was the last time you ate only a quarter pound of steak and felt satisfied?

All this is by way of urging you, at the start of this whole fitness program, to spend some time with your calorie chart and learn a little about food values. You don't need to be an expert — just take thirty minutes some morning over your coffee to look up some of your favorite foods, and then decide whether or not you can continue, as you age, to eat them all the time. Despite Sally's good intentions, her problem in maintaining her new low weight came from simple ignorance. Many who have tried to lose weight in the past may also be guilty. You may have eaten *less,* but by not understanding your own caloric needs, you were still overeating. Conversely, until you understand how many calories you burn in a day, even gaining would be difficult until you're regularly consuming more than your body expends in energy.

We mentioned earlier that you should also take note of the relative sodium or salt levels in your foods, but there's another aspect of dieting we'd like to stress as well, and that's a *regular* schedule. And the most important aspect of that schedule involves eating a good breakfast every morning. But you hate breakfast, right? And it's a lot of trouble to cook an egg, right? Listen. By not eating breakfast, many of us end up with headaches by 10:30 from low blood-sugar levels that make us overeat at lunch so that we come back to our work full and sleepy for the rest of the afternoon. So fixing breakfast *is* a little trouble. So is ill health. Try to find something good that you can either enjoy or at least tolerate for breakfast and stick with it. If you skip *any* meal, skip dinner. Eating late in the day is far more fat producing than eating in the morning. In a recent study at a Boston hospital two different groups of obese patients were fed the same meal — calorie for calorie. Both groups were fed only one meal per day, and the only difference was that one group was given their meal in the mornings and the other group was given theirs in the evenings. And even though the activity levels of the two groups and all other factors were as equal as the scientists could make them, the group fed at night did not lose weight as rapidly as the group that ate in the morning. Why? The reasons are quite complicated, but the simplest way to say it is that our digestive system makes better use of food when it is consumed during the early part of the day (breakfast and lunch), when we still have time to expend more energy *that day*. Accordingly, you should eat sparingly in the evenings if you want to become leaner.

Another factor you can't overlook is that food is a great socializer. Meals are often the only time during the day when many of us come together with our families or friends to talk and relax. And because many of us like to let these times last as long as possible, we take second and even third helpings to stay longer at the table. Try to school yourself, if you really want to lose weight, to take only one helping per meal. If you linger and talk and you feel as if you have to be doing something, drink some extra water, or some calorie-free beverage, such as iced tea, but don't continue to pick at the food just because you're still sitting at the table.

Another consideration is your food preferences. Naturally, we all have certain foods we love and are accustomed to eating. Most of us tend to like the same sorts of foods our parents liked, and there are often foods, sometimes ethnic in origin, that will always appeal to us in a deep, basic way, no matter how much we learn about calories, diet, or nutrition in general. There is, indeed, a satisfaction in these foods that cannot and, we feel, *should* not be ignored. That's why neither of us would feel confident about recommending a diet to anyone that was not based on the calorie-counting method. Single-food diets, liquid-protein diets, and so on, are almost all doomed to failure over the long haul because they deny us the sensual and emotional satisfactions we get from the foods we love.

By counting your calories and charting your food consumption, you can teach yourself how to eat sensibly, year after year. You can learn that if Aunt Gladys or Cousin Tony cooks up something so wonderful you simply can't refuse it, you know you can have some and then either cut back on your other foods the next day or exercise a little more. You learn to make trade-offs and to create an eating program that will allow you to control your weight, always. We want you to avoid the quick, 14-day diets "guaranteed" to help you lose 20 pounds. Instead, we'd like you to learn for yourself what you can and cannot eat regularly, given your level of activity, and then stick with this sensible program for the rest of your life. To help you along with this, we've provided a chart from Brian Sharkey's *Physiology of Fitness,* which will allow you to calculate your average daily calorie expenditure and which gives calorie equivalents for a variety of exercises that you might be involved in beyond your regular weight work. For your food analysis, we again recommend the USDA's *Composition of Foods,* though Barbara Kraus's *Calorie Guide to Brand Names and Basic Foods* might also be helpful if you eat a lot of processed or prepared foods. *The Natural Foods Calorie Counter* is helpful if you shop in health food stores. (See Suggestions for Further Reading for information.)

## Gaining Muscular Body Weight

There may be others — lucky others? — who feel the need to gain weight. If so, the same mathematical formulae apply to gaining weight as to losing; you simply need to eat more than you burn every day. You must exercise care and concern, however, that the weight you put on is good, lean muscle weight — not fat — and to do that you must first reconcile yourself to gaining slowly. To build muscle, you must train hard, and you must make sure that you're getting sufficient protein every day so your body can build muscles properly. **Terry:** "When Jan decided to gain weight, she took desiccated liver tablets twice a day to increase her protein supply and to make sure she was ingesting good, lean protein. In my own case, when I decided to start moving up in weight back in the late 1950s, I started drinking more milk and eating as much chicken, fish, beef, and eggs as possible, along with fresh fruits and vegetables. Both of us ate balanced diets and both of us also took some vitamin supplements from time to time throughout our weight gains as well as our weight losses, but the primary thing we *both* did was to have patience. You can't gain lean weight overnight nor can you lose fat overnight. A goodly number of my fellow superheavyweights have found out to their sorrow how debilitating and health-destroying rapid weight gain can be. Friends of mine who have gained 60 or 80 pounds in a year often suffered from severe hypertension (high blood pressure), besides being unable to walk more than 100 yards or so without puffing like steam engines. Gaining as much as Jan and I gained — *even doing it slowly* — is not without its risks, but to force the pace beyond your body's ability to adapt to it is foolish in the extreme."

If you decide instead to gain by eating everything in sight, you'll soon find yourself looking more and more like a Pillsbury doughperson. And don't forget that excess protein is stored as fat, just like excess carbohydrates and fats, when it is consumed in amounts above the energy needs of the body. If you're exercising for forty-five minutes to an hour every day, you may need to be eating only 2500 to 3000 calories per day to gain, but if you have an active job in which you're moving all day long you may need far more. Only you can decide that. Only you know how active you are during your days and how much you normally eat. So, whether or not your wish is to lose weight or to gain, a simple recording system will make it easy for you to know how to proceed.

## Vitamins

We are often asked what sort of vitamin supplements to take. Well, according to the Food and Drug Administration, no careful eater should ever need to take any sort of extra vitamin supplements. They're probably right, though we admit to some skepticism about it. We're fortunate to have usually lived on small farms where we've raised a great deal of our own food. We've kept hens for eggs, various poultry and animals for our meat, and even here in Austin, we've put in a small organic garden that produces some of our vegetables; and we get our meat from a relative's ranch. We also have several fruit and pecan trees. Naturally, we both feel better and even a bit self-righteous about doing all this, but our primary motivation has been to make sure we're eating wholesome, tasty foods that are as fresh as they can possibly be. There's really no need to go into all the various preservatives or the high sodium levels that are found in most packaged foods, nor to discuss the length of time that most "fresh" fruits and vegetables sit in cold storage before being put up for sale, nor to comment on how this storage affects the *taste* of the foods, since anyone interested enough to read this book has no doubt been exposed to these sorts of discussions before.

What we want to do is simply to remind you, and to urge you, to eat whole foods — such as an apple *plus* the peeling, whole wheat flour rather than white, the potato *and* the peeling — and to eat as many raw fruits and vegetables as you can so that you give yourself the best chance of getting the nutrients you need from your regular diet. But, if you're still concerned, then take some vitamin supplements. Hedge your bet. We usually take a few vitamins ourselves: vitamin C, vitamin E, vitamin B Complex, calcium, vitamins A and D, magnesium, potassium, lecithin, vitamin B-12, vitamin B-6, and multimineral supplements. This list is not designed to be a prescription for anyone. If you're satisfied by the FDA position and you eat a carefully balanced diet, disregard the list. We offer it only as information so that when and if you decide you may need extra supplementation you'll have some idea of what other lifters take.

# 10 / The Middle-Aged Sedentary Men's Study

**T**ERRY: "In 1980, Mike Stone joined the faculty of Auburn University as an exercise physiologist. Mike had established a reputation at LSU as one of the few physiologists in the country whose primary interest was research in heavy resistance training, and I was interested in the LSU study he had recently completed on the effect of resistance training on middle-aged men. I was *particularly* interested in the fact that resistance training seemed to stimulate the production of testosterone in those middle-aged men, as we discussed earlier. I told Mike that his research might help explain why so many older weight trainers looked so much younger than they really were, and I suggested that he repeat the experiment on a larger and more rigorous scale, a suggestion that meshed with his own plans to redesign and repeat the experiment once adequate funding could be secured.

"Hearing this, I set about to raise the $50,000 or so Mike needed for equipment and to find enough volunteers to do the weight training, both of which I was able to do. Once the money and the men were ready, Mike's new research design, in which he was aided to some extent by Danny Blessing, Dr. Dennis Wilson, and Ralph Rozenek, was put into effect. It involved three groups of middle-aged sedentary men — one group would lift weights, one would jog, and one would continue being sedentary and thereby serve as the 'control' group.

"I helped supervise most all the weight-training sessions of the men in the study, and it was interesting to watch them as they brought their middle-aged bodies back into shape. Many of the men in the weight-training group had been athletes in college and high school, so they were familiar with sweat and effort, and although many of them missed more sessions — because of their work — than would have been ideal for the purposes of the study, they really bore down when they were in the gym. And once they got over their initial soreness, they were both pleased and surprised at the progress they made in the weights they could handle and in the way their clothes began to fit. Several of the men made truly dramatic changes, both physically and psychologically.''

Raymond "Buddy" Pilgrim is a burly, ex-college lineman with a boyhood of farming behind him. He was forty-five years old when he was in the weight-training group and, as in everything he does, he was one of the hardest workers we had. A highly successful executive vice-president of a large corporation, Pilgrim was delighted with his results. Here's what he has to say:

"I'd been wanting to stop smoking for years but I kept finding reasons to put it off till the exercise program came along. That gave me something to hang my decision on and so I stopped, cold. The training gave me regularity in my life and a reason to get away from the office. And as I got into the lifting I began to notice that rather than making me tired for my work in the afternoons it actually seemed to revive me. And as I lost weight and got stronger I had more energy in all the areas of my life. I've always been a pusher, but I'd noticed that I'd been slowing down a little. I needed more rest and couldn't handle constant travel as well as I did when I was younger. But the weights turned that around. Since the study ended I've laid off several times but every time I did I began to feel 'old' again and my weight would begin to creep up. So, I've learned my lesson. I'm back on a good program now and I don't ever plan to quit."

When Floyd Burdette—to whom this book is dedicated — began training with weights he took considerable joshing from his friends and business associates. A relatively small man, Burdette was vice-president for finance of the same corporation Buddy Pilgrim serves as executive vice-president. Burdette was never very active in athletics as a youngster, and after he graduated from college in 1955, he concentrated on raising his family and making his mark in the business world. And, as is the case with many middle-aged men, his small frame became increasingly overlaid with extra flesh, rather like that of one of J. R. R. Tolkien's hobbits. But he also had the hobbitlike virtue of dogged persistence, and he fought through those tough early days and went on to become one of our stars. This is what he told us shortly before he drowned.

"I'd never done any sports and I sure wasn't very strong to begin with, and maybe that's why it all meant so much to me. I've gotten more than twice as strong and I feel better in every way a man can. I sleep better, my digestion is better, I have more get-up-and-go and I can do my chores around the house without even breathing hard. I guess I never figured I'd do anything like this, but since the study's been over I've stayed right with it. I'd never want to go back to the way I was again. They teased me a lot at first but now everyone brags on me for the way I've redistributed my weight. I feel blessed by it all. The only bad thing about it is that I've had to spend a little money to have some of my trousers taken in at the waist."

Lanier Johnson is an average-sized man who was forty-one years old when he was involved with the study. An executive in a large corporation, Lanier was an all-around athlete in high school but since that time his main recreational activity has been golf.

"I'd fooled around with the weights a time or two but never used them with much regularity, and I was curious as to what effect the training would have on my golf game. I got a little sore at first, but by the time we were near the end of our group workouts I was at least ten yards longer off the tee, and maybe a little straighter. I've played the same course for years so I'm sure I wasn't just imagining the extra distance. I was also delighted to drop almost four inches off my midsection. I tend to put weight on my waist, and I flattened out quite a bit there and put a little muscle on my upper body. Not a bad swap."

**Terry:** "Testimony such as this can be had from other members of the weight-training group as well. Watching them train and gain as they did was, quite literally, inspirational to all of us who were involved in the project.

"One of the ways they improved that really meant a lot to them was in their appearance. Although they neither gained nor lost much weight, since we stressed the importance of continuing to eat as they had been eating (so that any changes they might make by the end of the twelve-week exercise period would have resulted from the exercise itself and not a change in diet), they all lost fat and gained lean body weight. This switch from fat to muscle had in many cases a considerable effect on their measurements, which, although it wasn't part of Mike's research design, I kept on my own to let the men see what sorts of changes might occur."

The changes in inches are listed below:

## Men's Study Training Results

| NECK | | SHOULDERS | | BICEPS | | WAIST | | THIGH | |
|---|---|---|---|---|---|---|---|---|---|
| Before | After | Before | After | Before | After | Before | After | Before | After |
| 15 | 15½ | 45½ | 46½ | 12¾ | 14¼ | 39 | 37½ | 21 | 23¼ |
| 15¼ | 16 | 45¾ | 48 | 13¼ | 14 | 36 | 35¼ | 21 | 24½ |
| 16 | 16⅞ | 47 | 49½ | 15⅛ | 15¾ | 38¾ | 36¾ | 23⅞ | 25 |
| 14¾ | 16 | 46 | 47 | 13½ | 13⅞ | 36 | 37 | 23½ | 25½ |
| 15 | 16½ | 47¾ | 48½ | 13 | 14¼ | 37¼ | 36 | 22½ | 25 |
| 15⅞ | 16⅝ | 47¾ | 48⅜ | 13½ | 14 | 38⅛ | 34 | 23⅞ | 24 |
| 15⅞ | 16½ | 48¾ | 48¾ | 14⅛ | 15⅛ | 42 | 41 | 23⅞ | 26 |
| 17¾ | 19 | 53⅛ | 54¾ | 15¾ | 17 | 43½ | 40½ | 25⅝ | 29 |
| 15 | 16⅛ | 44⅝ | 47⅜ | 12⅞ | 13⅞ | 41 | 37¼ | 21½ | 24 |
| 16 | 16¾ | 51¼ | 52½ | 14⅛ | 14⅝ | 41 | 37 | 23⅜ | 24¼ |

The weight-training group became "younger" in other ways as well — they became more flexible, their strength grew wonderfully, their muscular endurance and cardiovascular fitness increased, and their pride and self-image underwent a positive change. And again, as in the LSU study, their output of testosterone increased.

## The Bulgarian Connection

**Terry:** "On a recent trip to Bulgaria to visit the training camp of the renowned Bulgarian weightlifting team and talk to the sports scientists and coaches who have helped create the team, I was privileged to spend a day with Dr. Pavel Dobrev, who is in charge of weight-training research at the National Institute of Sport and Physical Culture. Dr. Dobrev had heard of my interest in the effects of weight training on the aging process and so he invited me to make rounds with him one morning as he went from one training site to another in the capital city of Sofia.

"Our first stop was at the weight-training hall at the National Stadium, and there I was introduced to a group of thirty men ranging in age from forty-five to eighty-seven. All the men were training when we arrived, and the thing that first caught my eye was the fact that the men were lifting really substantial weights. And the more I watched, the more astonished I became as I saw how much weight these men were using in their exercises.

"Dr. Dobrev smiled when I expressed my astonishment and then suggested we visit another training hall. The next hall was much like the first, filled with middle-aged and what can only be called old men. And, as before, the men were handling heavy iron. And not only were they strong and vigorous, they *looked* strong and vigorous. I spoke to quite a few of them — to most through an interpreter, to a few in English — and they spoke glowingly of how well the weight training made them feel and how devoted to it they were.

"That afternoon, Dr. Dobrev explained in some detail how he had begun to conduct case-study experiments involving weight training and older men fifteen years ago and how his experiments had grown in scope. He now has trained literally hundreds of men from forty on up, and his results have baffled medical experts in his country. He explained with a laugh that when word got around in the university that he was training "old" men with heavy weights he came under attack from many physicians, particularly cardiologists. But he persevered, and gradually he won over his critics to such an extent that he will soon be named director of a new facility in Sofia connected with the National University and called the Institute of Juvenology.

"The institute will continue his research and attempt to better understand how some of the literally miraculous physical recoveries he has supervised have occurred. I say miraculous because Dr. Dobrev doesn't work only

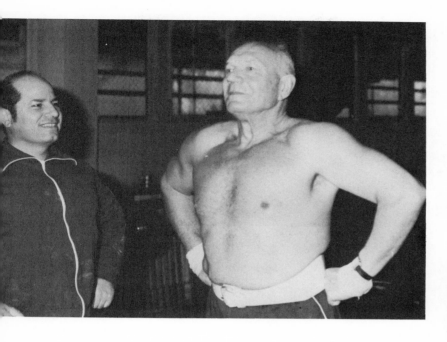

UPPER LEFT: *Dr. Dobrev, fifty-one years old and Dr. Ivanov, who at seventy-four can bench press over 350 pounds.* LOWER LEFT: *Dr. Dobrev looks on as eighty-seven-year-old Yanko Angelov deadlifts 264 pounds for five repetitions.* BELOW: *Yanko Angelov.*

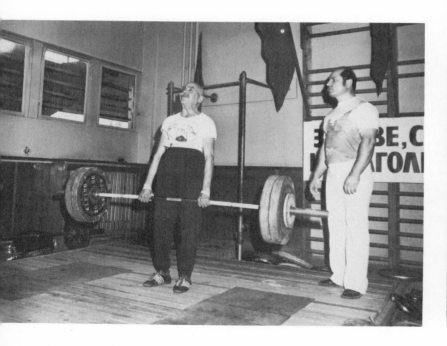

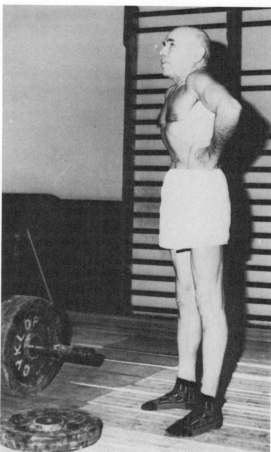

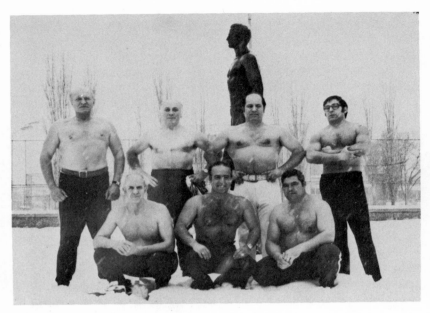

*Dr. Dobrev (second from right, back row) and a group of his fellow Bulgarian men braved the snow for a photograph outside the training hall last winter. Believe it or not, the average age of the men in the photograph is sixty-one.*

with well men; he also works with men who are decidedly unwell. I saw at least fifteen men training with heavy weights who had either undergone bypass surgery or had a stroke, and I saw one whose life was dependent on kidney dialysis. Apparently, Dr. Dobrev believes that the effects of frequent heavy workouts with weights are the single best guardian against the encroachments of age and ill health and he claims to have the research to prove it. He told me that the work he and his fellow scientists have done with these older men — most of whom had never trained before — reveals significant improvements not only in cardiovascular fitness but also in strength, flexibility, and even in the output of testosterone.

"You can imagine how excited I was to learn that such extensive work in Bulgaria bolstered what we have learned here in this country about the phenomenon of dramatic physical improvement resulting from weight training. I told him many of the things I had learned in my own reading and research, and the time flew by. But we parted with an exchange of addresses and a vow to share the results of our subsequent research. The last thing Dr. Dobrev did before I had to leave was give me some photographs of the older men with whom he has worked. It is with much pleasure that I share these photos."

# 11 / The Middle-Aged Sedentary Women's Study

THE idea of a women's study, a counterpart to the middle-aged sedentary men's study, took root at the barbecue we hosted in honor of the men completing their final testing. The men were really feeling good about themselves, and in the midst of barbecue, beer, and bravado, one of the wives asked for some advice on losing weight. Soon, several other women were gathered round and one rather loudly said, "I've been so envious of what Bill's been doing that I sure wish we could all get together and do some training ourselves." **Jan:** "One of the husbands snickered, but I rose to the bait and told them I didn't see why we couldn't set up a women's program. I told the women that, if nothing else, it would give all of them a chance to learn the exercises."

So, the women spent most of the rest of the evening talking about what they hoped to have happen, choosing rather pointedly *not* to listen to the claims of improved strength and virility being made by their husbands — claims that grew increasingly outrageous as the party progressed.

But the possibilities of such an exercise program with a group of women were fascinating. For one thing, we were unaware of any research on the effects of weight training with middle-aged women, and in talking the idea over we became enthused, and decided that, rather than simply give the women some general guidance about exercise, we would conduct a ten-week study that would be patterned after the men's study. We even arranged to have a small control group — whose members would be the baseline against which the women who lifted would be tested — but, unfortunately, some of the women in the control group "cheated" by exercising on a regular basis, which forced us to abandon that aspect of the study. Even so, the project was fascinating.

The composition of the group of exercisers was such that all the women were between the ages of thirty-five and forty-eight, and only two of them

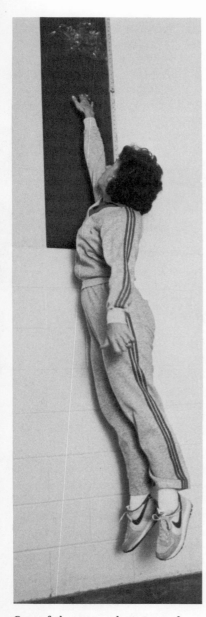

One of the tests administered to the women at the beginning and the end of the study was the vertical jump, a test of leg and hip power. Carol Davis shows good extension.

had been involved in any sort of regular exercise program over the course of the previous year or more. One woman did calisthenics from time to time and our other exerciser was a jogger, a woman of thirty-six who had been running two miles a day, several days a week, for six months. Most of the group would have been considered a bit overweight according to actuarial tables and none of them had done any weight training before. They were, in other words, exactly the sort of group we wanted — physically average American women in their early middle age.

Unfortunately, we lacked the necessary funds to do the same blood analysis on the women that we did on the men, but we used all the other tests that had been administered to the men, including a self-image profile. On our first testing day the women came to the lab, where they were weighed underwater to determine their body-fat percentages and given a standard stress test to determine their cardiovascular fitness. As with the men, the stress tests were performed on an exercise bicycle. We were able to develop two significant figures from this test: the endurance time of the women and their oxygen uptake levels (the rate at which the body is able to take in and utilize oxygen from the air).

While the stress tests were enervating for the women, more traumatic for most was the underwater weighing procedure, a procedure we felt was especially important. Prior to the testing day we had looked through the scientific journals, but were unable to find any standards for the body-fat percentages of women in their middle years. We even called the National Institute on Aging but no one there could help us. And so, although we knew what sorts of body-fat percentages women athletes of university age maintained (16 to 18 percent) and what average college women generally posessed (22 to 26 percent), we were as curious as the women themselves about what the underwater test would reveal. The high readings surprised us. Three of the women were *over 40 percent fat,* according to our calculations, and only one (the runner) was under 30 percent! Clearly, we all had some work to do. Naturally, the women themselves were dismayed to discover where they stood individually. All admitted to being larger than they'd been in high school, but the realization that so much of the firm flesh of youth had been displaced by fat came hard to many of them, though it strengthened their resolve to train hard for the next ten weeks and see what could be changed.

The other nonlifting tests administered prior to the study were the same as with the men — a self-image test, a flexibility test, and a vertical jump. Finally, after taking some standard bodily measurements with a tape, we tested the women in the same two standard weightlifting movements we had used with the men: the bench press and the partial squat. As you can see from the chart (page 92), none of the women showed exceptional strength in either exercise prior to the start of training. But what was most impressive about the strength test day was that the women really did try hard. They were beginning to be as caught up in the whole idea of the "ex-

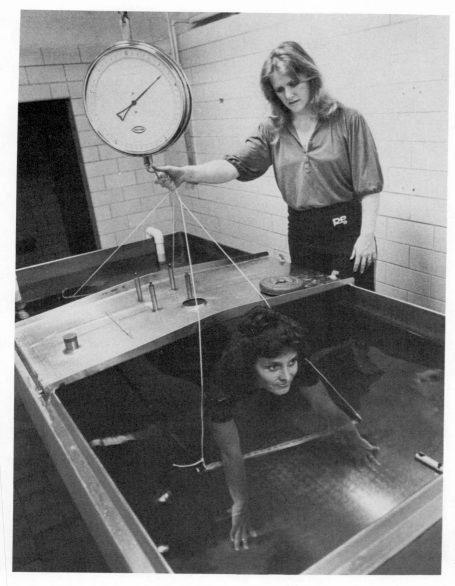

*Underwater weighing was done to determine the percent of body fat that each woman possessed at the beginning and the end of the study. Jeannie Johnson is readying herself to take the first of three plunges necessary for the calculations.*

periment" as we were, and they were determined to try with all their meager might.

Having finished with all our testing, we met the women for the first time at a local spa on July fifteenth, and divided them into two training groups in order to maximize the time each woman would have on the various pieces of equipment. We also introduced them to the eleven stretching

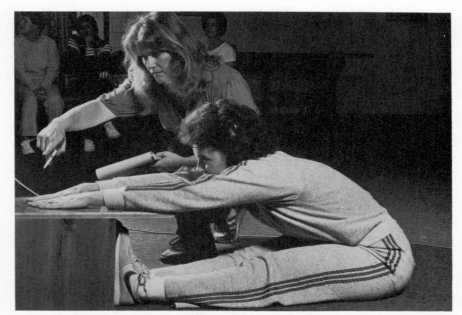

To test flexibility, the women were asked to do the "sit and reach" test. Carol, as you can see, has exceptionally good flexibility for a person her age — the result of her regular stretching program.

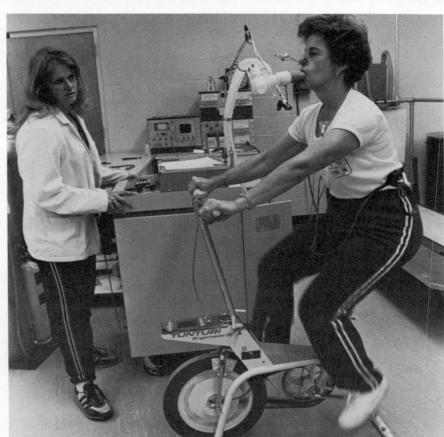

The "hardest" test was the cycle ergometer ride that tested the women for endurance. Betty Letlow is hooked up to a Beckmann Metabolic Cart, which measures her oxygen uptake level as she pedals. The clip on Betty's nose is to make sure no outside air is allowed into her lungs.

positions that would serve as a warm-up for each of the exercise sessions and that we describe in our chapter on stretching. We also brought the women along *very* slowly, because *anyone,* particularly someone who is middle-aged or older, who has not been involved in a regular exercise program should work into weight training or any other activity *gradually.* Many of the women had not been active for ten to twenty years, and they found themselves quite sore from simply the calisthenic movements and light stationary cycling we gave them at first. Had we pushed them to start in immediately with the weights, they would have not only run the risk of injury, but they would possibly have become so sore that they might have felt unable to continue with the study.

During the three weeks it took to ease the women into the full program, all of them experienced some soreness following almost every exercise session, and in order to help them understand, we explained that this was a natural part of the strengthening process. And though "pain" had not been a regular part of their lives before, they quickly adapted to the feeling of tightness and soreness that accompanies beginning workouts and began to joke about how wonderful this particular movement or that particular poundage was going to make them feel the next day.

**Jan:** "I conducted the exercise sessions and I had to remind myself that while the women were willing to work hard and do what we asked, their primary motivation for participation in the study was their desire to improve figures and their health, not get stronger. However, as they trained they began to see for themselves small but evident changes, not only in their strength levels but also in their bodies, and these changes naturally encouraged them to keep trying. And the more they worked and the more strength they gained, the more their bodies improved."

All told, the group met for ten weeks, not counting the testing days prior to the first class days at the gym. Three weeks had been spent working

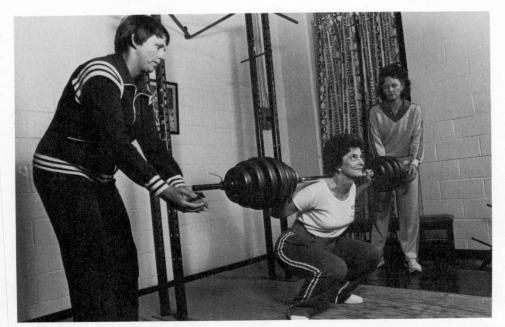

*Squats played a major part in the women's workouts. Here Betty Letlow shows exceptionally good form in the full squat.*

| Body Weight (lbs.) | | Percentage Body Fat | | Pounds of Body Fat | | Endurance Time (minutes) | | Oxygen Uptake | | Flexibility (inches) | | Vertical Jump (inches) | | Squat (lbs.) | | Bench Press (lbs.) | |
|---|---|---|---|---|---|---|---|---|---|---|---|---|---|---|---|---|---|
| PRE | POST | PRE | POST | PRE | POST | PRE | POST | PRE | POST | PRE | POST | PRE | POST | PRE | POST | PRE | POST |
| 157.9 | 158.6 | 39.2 | 34.1 | 61.8 | 55.0 | 5.40 | 6.35 | 21.6 | 24.1 | 1.25 | 4.0 | 9.5 | 11.25 | 110 | 220 | 55 | 66 |
| 157.0 | 156.7 | 41.4 | 36.9 | 65.1 | 57.9 | 4.30 | 5.30 | 16.7 | 21.2 | 2.0 | 3.25 | 6.5 | 10.0 | 110 | 303 | 60.5 | 71.5 |
| 143.7 | 139.7 | 38.2 | 32.0 | 54.8 | 44.9 | 5.0 | 5.30 | 20.8 | 22.0 | 1.5 | 3.0 | 7.5 | 11.75 | 220 | 286 | 60.5 | 71.5 |
| 139.0 | 139.3 | 28.2 | 23.1 | 39.2 | 32.1 | 7.0 | 7.0 | 28.3 | 31.3 | 10.5 | 10.75 | 12.0 | 14.0 | 198 | 303 | 60.5 | 71.5 |
| 152.2 | 157.3 | 39.6 | 33.8 | 60.3 | 52.8 | 6.0 | 6.0 | 21.5 | 27.1 | 3.0 | 4.0 | 9.5 | 13.0 | 220 | 408 | 55 | 93.5 |
| 159.3 | 159.5 | 41.0 | 33.8 | 65.3 | 53.9 | 5.0 | 5.30 | 15.9 | 18.5 | 4.75 | 5.0 | 6.5 | 8.75 | 132 | 308 | 49.5 | 71.5 |
| 152.0 | 152.2 | 42.3 | 34.3 | 64.4 | 52.2 | 5.0 | 5.0 | 22.4 | 22.8 | 5.75 | 7.25 | 6.5 | 8.5 | 110 | 275 | 55 | 71.5 |
| 144.1 | 143.2 | 35.6 | 27.34 | 51.3 | 39.2 | 6.40 | 6.30 | 26.3 | 28.7 | 3.0 | 3.5 | 8.0 | 11.75 | 132 | 286 | 60.5 | 88 |
| | | | | | | | | | Average | | | | | | | | |
| 150.6 | 150.8 | 38.18 | 32.0 | 57.8 | 48.5 | 5.36 | 5.57 | 21.69 | 24.48 | 3.96 | 5.25 | 8.25 | 11.12 | 154 | 298.6 | 56.9 | 75.6 |

into the program gradually, four weeks had been spent doing 5 sets of 10 repetitions per exercise, and three weeks were spent doing 5 sets of 5. No special instructions were given to the women regarding their diets, and they had been asked from the first not to alter their diet or their normal activities. We made this request so we could determine what effect the weight training would have — not the weight training combined with a new diet.

As for the training program itself, was there an effect? Did the lifting really change the way the women looked and felt? Perhaps some of their comments, as well as the hard data presented in the chart above, might be of interest.

**Joyce Newland:** "Where I noticed the biggest difference was in my posture. I've been round-shouldered all my life, and as I'm fairly large-busted, the problem didn't improve as I got older. It got worse. I guess I'd trained for about four weeks when someone at church commented to me about how much better I was looking. 'You know,' she said, 'looks to me like you're standing up straighter.' Until it was pointed out, I hadn't been conscious of it, but I really *had* improved. By the end of the program I stood really straight, and I've continued going to the spa on my own since then because I don't want to ever look like that again. I train by myself now, and that's harder than it was with the group, but I've just decided that I've got too much going to not take care of *me*. The training has really changed the way I feel about myself. It's not just that I'm stronger or that my body is firmer and my skin clearer than it was in the past, it has somehow changed my whole attitude to life. I feel more confident, less afraid to try new things, and I suppose that the pride in my new appearance has helped me a lot socially and with my business contacts. I don't train as hard as we did in the group but I use basically the same exercises and still do about five sets with each. I've simply decided that I'm not going to be hunchbacked and weak when I'm fifty — even if all my friends can hardly get out of their chairs. I've got too much to do, too much to see, not to try to make the most of the years I have left."

**Jeannie Johnson:** "I've always been on some sort of diet since my teens. Like many women, I've got larger hips than my upper body really needs, and so I constantly feel like I need to lose ten pounds or so. During the weight work I could tell that my body had really firmed up. Oh, it was still far from ideal, but in a pair of shorts my legs looked better than they had for a while. I was amazed at how I changed in so short a time. We got our boy an exercise machine for Christmas this year, and since I can't seem to organize my life to get to the spa, I've been working out with my son."

**Kathryn Pilgrim:** "I found the training hard when we started out. I'd been in a car accident about ten years ago that left me virtually paralyzed. I had to relearn a lot of basic motor patterns — including how to walk. This was really the first time I had tried any sort of regular exercise program since then. As we trained and I grew in confidence, I could feel the difference in my body. I suppose I'd always been afraid to push myself following the accident because I'd had to come back so far from where I was during those early days in the hospital. But with the training I found the extra strength was really an asset. I began to feel much more as I had prior to the accident, when I was also a good deal younger. It was a strange feeling, as if the years just fell away. The other thing I remember most about the program, besides the early soreness, was a comment my husband made to me one night while we were dressing to go out. We were pretty near the end of the ten weeks, when he turned and said, 'You know, Kathryn, your legs are looking better than they have in years.' I can't tell you what that meant to me. Not because it was a nice compliment from my husband — although those always mean a lot. It meant a lot to me because I knew that I had done something really physical and been successful at it. It was as if a whole portion or aspect of my life was no longer cut off from me. That, let me tell you, was a wonderful realization."

**Mary Ann Pokorny:** "At age forty-six, I was one of the oldest women in the group, and I suppose I should also have been among the most scared because of my age. But you know, from the very first I enjoyed the weight work. I've always stayed active — though I never did anything regularly — and it was really nice to get together with all the girls and push ourselves a bit. As we trained I began to get genuinely interested in my growing strength. For some reason I was never afraid, like a few of the girls were, to train hard and handle heavier weights. I guess that's one reason I made such good progress during the time. You know, I lost over 7 percent of my body fat during that time, even though I actually only lost about half a pound of weight. I could sure see a big difference in my body, though, especially in the way my clothes fit."

Actually, Mary Ann's body-fat loss was not that unusual for the group. As you can see in the chart, the group averaged a loss of 6.18 percent during the ten-week period, which we thought was remarkable. Translated into pounds of actual fat lost during the training period, the average for the group was a body-composition change of 9.3 pounds. None of the women lost weight in the traditional sense — because we told them not to change their diets — but all lost fat and inches. In fact, the only area of the retesting in which the group did not show dramatic improvement was in the stress test, in which both endurance time and oxygen uptake were measured. All of the women scored better in their ability to utilize oxygen, and they also made good gains in their endurance, but the substantial gains in these two areas only seem small because of the startling gains they made in every other test. One main factor — the relationship between the size of our group and the amount of equipment we had available — probably accounted for the less significant changes in cardiovascular conditioning. As it was, because of the size of the group and the limitations of the spa, the women were not able to go through their workouts as quickly as would have been optimal. The spa had ony one set of squat racks, only one bench, only one leg-press machine, only one leg-curl/leg-extension machine, and so on, which meant that even if the women had wanted to train more quickly than they did, they couldn't have.

In all the other areas, however, the results were far better than we had expected. As the chart reveals, most of the women made dramatic strength increases during the time. Several of them more than doubled their leg strength, and they all made at least a five-kilo increase in the bench press during the ten weeks. Five kilos (eleven pounds) may not sound like much, but it is a considerable gain in ten weeks for a woman of any age. Besides the expected strength gains, they added an average of three inches to their vertical jump and increased their flexibility by over an inch. Not bad for a bunch of middle-aged sedentary women.

The conversion the women made — changing nine pounds of fat to nine pounds of muscle — caused all of them to make some changes in their measurements. They averaged a half-inch gain in their bust, lost approximately one inch on their waist, and one and a quarter inches on their hips. Their arm and thigh measurements stayed the same because we asked them not to diet and because the fat they lost in those areas was replaced by firm flesh. The woman who made the most striking change in her physique during the study was Sandra Underwood, who lost two full inches on her hips, an inch and a half on her waist, three quarters of an inch on her thighs, and had a half-inch increase in the size of her bust. Sandra, who was not able to make every class session (she attended eighteen out of a possible twenty-six days), does not show up in the final chart because for statistical purposes we only included those women who had attended at least 75 percent of the sessions. However, even though she missed roughly a third of the training sessions, she increased her strength, her flexibility, her vertical jump ability, and she lowered her body fat of 35.16 percent to 27.34 percent. What Sandra did do was to work very hard on those days when she was there, and the effort certainly paid off.

And there were other gains besides the physical ones. One of the things we tested both before and after the ten-week training period was the self-image of the women involved. As he had been earlier with the men, Dr. James Hilyer, then of Auburn University, was in charge of determining whether or not the lifting affected the way our subjects perceived them-

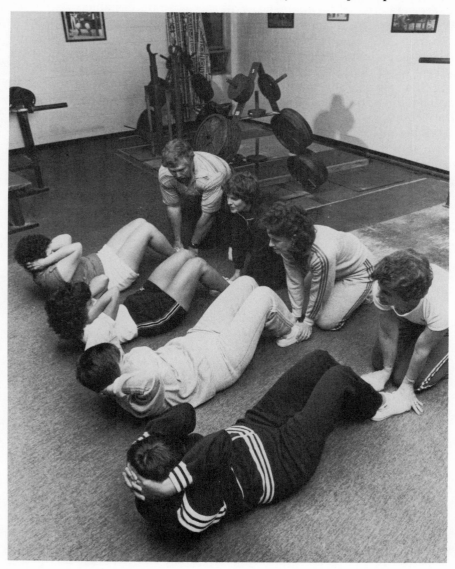

*No workout was complete until the abdominal work was done. Crunches were usually the group's first choice as a waist exercise.*

selves. What he found was that the women made an even greater increase in positive self-concept than the men had made.

Many of the women in the study were of a generation that often not only failed to encourage vigorous participation by girls and young women in sports or fitness activities but also actually discouraged it. And nowhere was this wrongheaded waste more prevalent than in the South. The image of the delicate southern belle has been slow to change. Nor has it changed completely even now for young women, which makes the gains that our middle-aged exercisers created for themselves all the more remarkable.

We want to say it straight and say it publicly — we are proud of what these women did. They made physical and psychological gains we quite honestly did not expect and they learned a considerable amount about themselves while doing so. They showed themselves and, in the process of showing themselves, they showed us just how astonishingly well the human body will adapt to graduated stress, *at any age*. And they showed themselves that they could sweat, too, and sweat intelligently. "I've never done such hard work before," Carol York said, not long after the study had ended, "but I've never done anything that opened my eyes so fast as to how little time was necessary to really look younger again."

# 12 / Judy Gedney — Petite but Powerful

J UDY GEDNEY has a grace and gentleness of spirit that would seem to some to be as appropriate in a weight room as Dick Butkus would be in a ladies' dancercize class. She has a diminutive stature — an asset during her days as a gymnast — and the sort of quiet, sunny disposition found only among the self-confident and truly happy. At 4 feet 11 inches, she has a pixielike quality to go with her charming personality, and she is a very popular college professor of physical education at Western Illinois University in Macomb, Illinois. But her gentleness and small size most certainly do not denote weakness; she has a body stronger than almost anyone else her size and sex in the world. Though she had a full life, Judy decided, at age thirty-nine, to become a powerlifter — a competitive weightlifter — and, as she'll tell you, she's loved every minute of it.

"I've been a gymnastics coach for about eighteen years now, and my husband, Roger, has trained with weights for approximately that long, which is one reason I think he still looks as wonderful as he does. But I never touched a weight until 1980, when I began to think of ways to rehabilitate one of the gymnasts who had radical knee surgery. It was Roger's idea to get her to work with weights and it sounded okay to me until he suggested that I work out along with her. I was hesitant, to say the least, because I was afraid I'd build a lot of extra muscle mass, but how glad I am that we put this plan into action; you can't imagine the changes it has made in me.

"Roger devised a workout for us, and we started in April of 1980. Within six weeks we noticed great improvements; my legs felt more solid, and the girl with the leg-strength problem was not only higher in her tumbling runs but the extra arm strength gave her more control in her other routines. All of this was more than enough to sell me on the benefits of training, but we all also noticed a big difference in the appearance of my body. I guess I'd figured that at forty nothing was going to change except for

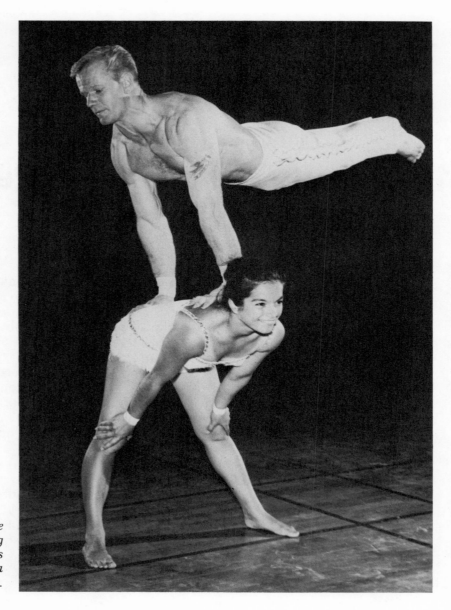

*Judy Gedney built a strength base for the world records that followed by spending years as a gymnast. Here she supports her husband, Roger, as he performs a difficult planche.*

the worse, but you could see a definite improvement in the way my legs and hips looked after just six weeks, and I lost some of the fat that I tended to carry there.''

Judy's metamorphosis led to a resurgence of the sort of competitive spirit that had fired her youth. As a teenager, growing up in Chicago, she was active in both dance and tumbling. "I entered Iowa University in 1958

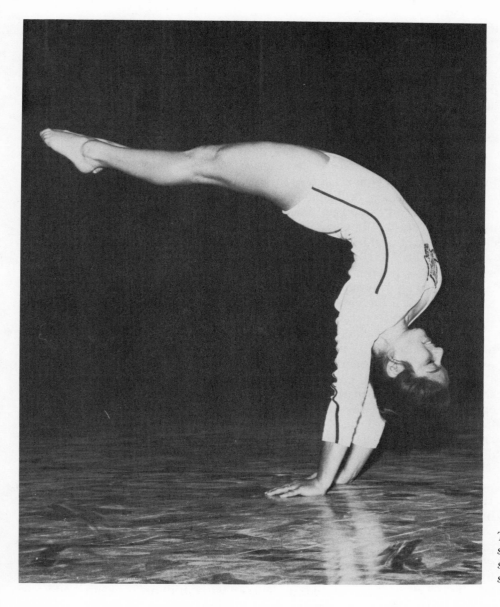

*Today, at forty-two, Judy is still limber enough to do all the stunts she did as a gymnast, such as this tricky handstand.*

and was encouraged to try out for the gymnastics team. With my natural size advantage, I did pretty well during college. I did a lot of gymnastics clinics during that time, including some in South America.

"As we trained during that first six weeks, I was pleased to see my strength go up so quickly. We've tried to find ways to account for my unusual upper-body strength and the only thing Roger and I can figure out is that my early work in gymnastics plus the years of spotting and coaching that I've done must have been giving me more of a workout than I thought. Coaching gymnastics is *hard* work. Your main job is to serve as the spotter, which means you spend 95 percent of your time catching kids who come flying at you through the air, turning them over, and then putting them down safely. When you do that for two hours a day, five days a week, and when they all weigh ten to forty pounds more than you do, you get a pretty good workout plus a lot of bruises.''

As Judy and her young friends trained, she discovered an extraordinary ability in the bench press. Masters lifting, for those over forty, was just getting organized for women at this time, and while Judy was far ahead of anyone else her age, she and Roger discovered that she was also ahead of most of the women *half* her age. "Neither of us were big followers of powerlifting," Judy recalls, "but when we realized where I stood in comparison to other women, I decided to enter a meet and see how I liked it."

So on May 25, 1980, Judy and Roger traveled to Lombard, Illinois; Judy weighed 96¼ pounds that day and after only six weeks of training she benched 115 pounds, squatted 180 pounds, and deadlifted 225. She won the first-place medal for her weight class and discovered how much she loved competing again.

Several weeks later, June 15, to be exact, Judy entered her second meet, squatting 170, benching 121, and deadlifting 236 pounds. She weighed 96¾ and again took home the first-place trophy. But this time her 121-pound bench had caused the powerlifting world to take notice. Though she didn't realize it at the time, she was within only a few pounds of the open-division world record. However, shortly after returning to Macomb, tragedy struck, and Judy had a wreck on her moped that left her with, among other injuries, a broken clavicle. While she recovered from her accident, she continued to train as much as she could, and in August took her women's team to a meet in Ames, Iowa. Did her performance suffer as one would imagine? Not much. She was successful with a 175-pound squat, a 120 bench, and a 230-pound deadlift. Her total was only 15 pounds less than her previous best.

As Judy's enthusiasm for competition grew, so did the ranks of her powerlifting team. Devout Christians, Judy and Roger decided to set up two different powerlifting teams, one to be called the Western Illinois Powerlifting Club and another, open to both students and nonstudents, called Athletes for Christ. "Roger and I have worked with students for years and know the pleasures that come from such coaching experiences. We've always wanted to find a way to combine our love of athletics with our love of God."

As coaches, one of the decisions Roger and Judy made was to take their teams to as many powerlifting meets as they could afford. In September of that same year, they traveled to Ottumwa, Iowa, to take the team to an open meet. Judy lifted in order to make sure the team scored well, then she, Roger, and several of the girls packed up, got in their cars, and traveled

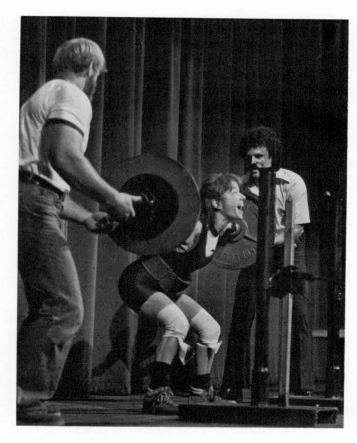

*Only 4'11" and 97 pounds, Judy
seems dwarfed by the huge weights and
the men who spot her as she drives up out
of a heavy squat.*

through the night to Purdue University, where the *very next day* she lifted
again (weighing 94.5 pounds), setting her first official world record in the
bench press with a 123.5-pound effort. Those not intimate with the psyches
and bodies of powerlifters may not understand the rarity of this. Lifting in
back-to-back powerlifting meets is akin to running the marathon or playing
college or pro football two days in a row. You just don't do it. When you push
the body to its maximum, you become not only physically exhausted but also
emotionally drained. "I can't begin to tell you the joy I felt when that bench
press left my chest and I knew I could lock it out. That world record was one
of the most exciting moments of my life."

Since Judy's early example, highlighted by her historic world record,
other Masters women (over forty) have shown that age is no barrier to the
development of strength and health. Women from forty to seventy have entered competitions both on the Masters and open levels and there's no doubt
that Judy's early example had a definite effect. More than one wife who'd
lost her husband to the iron mistress found not only togetherness but also a

greatly improved appearance by joining her man in the gym. If someone so tiny and so pretty as Judy could be *that* strong, why couldn't they? It was a good question and more than a few women answered it by heading to the weight room with their husbands.

"I'm not a political person, and I'm certainly no crusader," Judy said recently at the National Masters Championships, "but if someone wants to use me as an example of what's possible through weight training, that's fine with me. I have never gotten into the real bodybuilding-type training that so many women do nowadays. I just stick to the basics. This is probably because I'm somewhat lazy, and short on time, and since I've started competing I've decided to train to maximize my strength, rather than to maximize *me* by building a lot of muscle. Roger is very thoughtful about our training programs, and for the past couple of meets we've been following a version of the periodization method Jan recommended to me." (See Chapter 13.)

The training has, of course, altered the appearance of Judy's body. When she started, she weighed around 102, but, as we mentioned earlier, the 102 was not the same quality as the 97 pounds she carries today. "I never let myself go, and even though I wasn't involved in any sort of regular exercise program since my years as a gymnast, I still tried to do a little something every day and to watch what I ate. I tried jogging several years back but it was so boring that it almost drove me crazy. One thing I do still work on is flexibility. I can still do full splits and backbends despite my 'muscles.' I don't spend a lot of time in front of mirrors and, as I said, I'm not training to create the 'feminine ideal'; but from what I can remember of the old days, my body looks far better than it did when I was a college gymnast. I have more gray in my hair than many women my age but I'm very satisfied with what the Lord has allowed me."

At age forty-two Judy has now lifted in thirty-eight meets and has broken the open-division world record several times in the bench press and once in the deadlift, with 309 pounds. The number of Masters records she has set is staggering. Thirty-eight meets within a three-year career is amazing, and Judy will be the first to admit that it's far too many for ideal gains. Most lifters generally limit themselves to three, possibly four meets a year, as the long training cycles used today work better with only occasional peak performances. Were Judy not the sort of loving, outgoing, compassionate woman she is, she would no doubt train as all the others do. But she has a greater plan. The same selflessness that has caused her to house a score of foster children through the years has also made her put the needs of her teammates first. If there's a meet, the team goes, even if it means, as it did that day in Iowa prior to her first world record, that it may disrupt Judy's own lifting. "Lifting is not my life," she says. "It's not some philosophy that I live by. It's a sport, and I do it because it's fun and because I think it helps people. I have a lot of other things in my life that are just as important to me and several that are *more* important. Sports are for fun. Like hobbies. I have fun when I lift and the extra strength and fitness has brought me a lot of joy. But it isn't *everything* and it needs to be kept in perspective."

**Jan:** "When I recently stepped down as head of women's powerlifting in the United States, Judy took my place, and she plans to keep lifting, coaching, and serving as an administrator as long as possible. And with all the different Masters categories available now, it's possible that she could be setting records for the next thirty years. " Says Judy, "I can see a day when I might retire, but it's hard for me to imagine not lifting for the sake of my health. I suppose that may come, but I plan on doing this for a long time yet."

# PART THREE

# Approaching the Weights

W<sup>E</sup> hope you're beginning to understand the enormous difference weight training can make in your life. Without ever leaving the privacy of your home, you can change the way you look, become stronger and more flexible, find renewed energy for your daily activities, and feel better about yourself physically and mentally than you have in years. As you train with weights, you can learn a lot of things about yourself that have little to do with strength, but a lot to do with taking charge of your appearance and health. None of us can hold back the chariot of time, but you *can* make its passage far less significant. You simply need to become regular about your training and to adopt a diet and life-style that's conducive to the kind of physique and fitness level you want to maintain.

**How This Section Is Organized**

Most weight-training books place the exercises together at the end of the book with some suggestions, usually without scientific grounding, as to how those exercises should be incorporated into "routines." We thought it would be more helpful to group the exercises and our recommendations for their implementation into three divisions based on the sort of equipment available to you, since knowing that leg presses are an excellent leg exercise will do you little good if you have no leg-press machine. Therefore, we have split the exercises into three groups according to the equipment you'd have if you chose to train either at home with only a small investment of time and money, at home with a fully equipped home gym, or at a regular gym or health spa where you would have access to a greater number of machines and specialized pieces of equipment. Training at home has a number of things to recommend it, such as convenience, privacy, and the saving of gym membership fees; some people, however, find it difficult to motivate themselves at home, preferring the camaraderie and, at times, competitiveness of a gym. But regardless of your choice of location, the same training principles will apply. Your workouts should be based on the training approach we call periodization, and no matter where you train, *you should all do your first training cycle following the same basic program unless you are already a regular user of the weights.* If you are a novice at the weights, the basic program will give your body a chance to get in shape. Then, after you've done

one full training cycle on the basic program, you can try the more advanced routines we explain in the following sections.

Another reason we organized the exercises and routines into these three divisions is to help you keep from making the very common mistake of trying to do or buy too much at once. We would rather see you start out at home, with a small investment in both time and money. That way, you can find out if training really does help. Then, you can decide if it makes sense to acquire more equipment for use at home or to join a more fully equipped spa to continue your workouts. And whether you train at home or at a gym, one thing you *don't* want to do is to start out on some long, involved routine that you're not presently in shape to handle and that will make you so unbelievably sore that you'll never want to see the weights again. Before beginning to train, make sure to get a physical examination, especially if you're over thirty-five or if you have had heart or blood-pressure problems. And, start out slow. Even though the basic routine seems brief to the point of nakedness, it *will* create positive changes *if you follow the instructions carefully and begin to pay attention to your diet while you train.* You've got a lot of years ahead of you to try out the different exercises we've explained here in the book; give your body time to adjust to the new stresses of training.

Periodization allows you to take charge of your workouts and to set reachable goals for yourself each week. It will also, in time, allow you to tailor a workout to specifically meet your own particular needs. No two people are alike, so no two people should ever train exactly alike — pound for pound, exercise for exercise.

A thorough understanding of periodization will let you avoid some of the common mistakes made by those who want to test their limits every time they hit the gym or those who want to do too many exercises in one session. Just follow the instructions and be conservative at first. Keep in mind that periodization works because it lets your body *gradually* adjust to the weights. It's the safest way we know to train.

# 13 / Periodization

P ERIODIZATION'' is the scientific community's name for weight training in a cycle of increasing intensity and decreasing volume, with the cycle being made up of several distinct *periods*. It's important that you understand periodization because research has shown this method of weight work to be the most result-producing way a person can train. In other words, we're not telling you to train using the periodization model because *we* train that way but because study after research study has concluded that this method of training produces more positive physical results — more strength, more power, and more lean body weight — than any other method known. If this book can be said to have a central truth, this is it. Periodization is the best way to train.

We know, of course, that few of you are interested in really concentrating on the production of maximum strength. Neither, any longer, are we. And, while periodization can clearly be used to create great, even *incredible* strength gains, we suggest this method to you because it is also the best weight-training method to increase your level of fitness in every way. Used properly, it will make you more flexible, more enduring, more fit cardiovascularly, and — as an added plus — it is more interesting than other methods of training.

The psychological benefits of periodization training alone would sell us on it as a training method, since the worst thing that can happen to a would-be trainer is to get started on a program that's always the same. Boredom kills more fitness programs than any other villain — more than injuries, more than lack of time, more than lack of equipment. People get tired of doing the same things all the time, whether it's working on an assembly line or running laps around a small indoor track. The advantage of periodization is that no two workouts are ever the same. Every day you'll either vary the exercises, the poundage, or the number of repetitions so that you have different things to think about, different "goals." Periodization has a built-in reward system. By increasing your training poundages gradually, you condition yourself to succeed and your self-confidence will grow. In time, this will allow you to make weight training a permanent part of your life, a part that will pay dividends as long as you live.

**Terry:** "In the early sixties, when I was beginning to consider myself a 'weightlifter,' I used to read and try everything I could get my hands on about how to train. When *Strength and Health* magazine began talking about isometric contraction, my training partners and I all tried isometric contraction; when Paul Anderson said the secret to strength lay in partial movements, we all did partial movements; when someone wrote in *Iron Man* magazine that the key was high repetition work, we all did lots of high reps. We tried, in other words, *everything,* looking for the talisman that would give us strength and size and, we hoped, a national title. And while my buddies and I were training in Austin — and learning from our training — other athletes were doing the same thing. And eventually, through trial and error, we found and shared systems that seemed to work. The system we finally hit upon was a crude form of cycle training, and it involved using a variety of repetitions and weights rather than repeating a set number of repetitions day after day.

"While athletes here in the United States were using trial and error methods to achieve optimal performance, U.S. sports scientists began research studies in an effort to determine which combination of sets and repetitions created the greatest gains in strength. In 1962, Dr. Richard Berger published an article in *Research Quarterly* stating that he felt the optimal routine for developing strength was 3 sets of 6 repetitions per exercise, 3 times per week. Then, in 1966, Dr. Patrick O'Shea strengthened Berger's claims with another study that again found that 3 sets of 6 produced the greatest short-term gains. However, despite the laboratory evidence, most advanced weightlifters from the mid-sixties on didn't train year-round using 3 sets of 6 reps. What the athletes of this era had discovered was that no matter how much they *wanted* to train 'heavy' all the time, their bodies and minds wouldn't allow them to do it.

"There were some guys around who worked to their limit either on reps or singles all the time in their training, but they didn't last long. They either burned out or got an injury of.some sort. Those of us who lasted and continued to improve found that we had to start out conservatively — to use light weights for a while and then go on to the increasingly heavier poundages. Then, following a meet, we'd always take a break before coming back to begin again with light weights."

To best understand how periodization came about, we must journey to the Soviet Union — home of the world's strongest men and women and home of Dmitri Matveyev, a renowned sports scientist. For years, Matveyev studied hundreds of world-class athletes from a variety of sports to ascertain which training systems created the best gains. He looked at not just a normal eight- to ten-week precontest preparation period but at the entire year. He found that most world-class athletes trained so that they used "high volume–low intensity" training in the early part of their "cycle," then switched to "low volume–high intensity" work. He called this training method "periodization." A Russian weightlifter, for example, would do several sets of high repetitions (repetitions representing volume — in other words, the higher the repetitions the higher the volume of work) with relatively light weights (weights representing intensity — the lighter the weight in any given exercise, the lower the intensity of the work being done). This high volume (high repetitions)–low intensity (light weights) pattern would be followed during the first period of the weightlifter's training cycle. Then, in the next period of the training cycle, the trainer would switch to fewer repetitions (lower volume) and heavier weights (higher intensity) as his cycle drew to an end.

There are some who cite Matveyev's work as one of the reasons for the advances made by Soviet athletes during the 1960s, when, in sports such as weightlifting, for instance, they dramatically outdistanced their American counterparts. In any case, Matveyev's model of training didn't really enter the American sports bloodstream until the mid-1970s, and even now most American athletes who train with weights use either a rather crude form of periodization based mostly on intuition and past successes or some other method of training altogether.

Matveyev's theories of periodization, it should be noted, were based on his observation of the many, many world-class athletes who were already *using* periodization long before Matveyev "discovered" it. But his formalization of the theory was quickly applied by the Soviet sports establishment, which exerts considerable control over the training practices of their athletes. We do know that some Soviet athletes were using extremely sophisticated periodization systems well before the full explanation of Matveyev's findings had hit the United States.

Matveyev's findings corroborated in the world of sports those of the eminent Canadian scientist Dr. Hans Selye, who, through his own experiments and observations, formulated what is called the General Adaptation Syndrome. Selye feels that there are three levels, or phases, of adaptation that people undergo when they begin to exercise. The initial phase, the "alarm stage," is characterized by stiffness and muscle soreness, especially if the trainer hasn't been involved in any sort of exercise program for some time. The second phase, "resistance," is the development of a greater training capacity, or "fitness," as the body accustoms itself to the demands of the exercise and prepares itself to move on to higher levels. The third phase, "overtraining," or fatigue, is caused by training too hard or too long without adequate rest periods.

Periodization is successful because it allows the body to gradually adapt to the stress of exercise. Also, some 1978 research done by Morehouse and Miller suggests that the high volume–low intensity training that constitutes the beginning phase of periodization creates maximum muscular hypertrophy (muscular enlargement), which is important because other research has shown that larger muscles have a greater capacity to gain in strength. Morehouse and Miller's research further suggests that the best way to achieve muscular hypertrophy is to use 3 to 5 sets with between 8 and 20 repetitions per set, a suggestion that has been borne out by subsequent studies.

Within the past several years, numerous research projects have been completed that compare periodization training to the more traditional 3-sets-of-6 approach and to other popular training methods. Much of this work has been done by Dr. Mike Stone, who has consistently found that periodization trainers make better progress than those using other methods. In particular, the gains made in hip and leg strength through periodization were exceptional compared to other methods of training. Studies by Stone, and sometimes by us, have been done on Olympic weightlifters, a women's softball team, football teams, teenagers, children, middle-aged men and women, and several groups of "average" students enrolled in university weight-training classes, and *all* have shown that the periodization approach produces the greatest gains.

**Jan:** "I used a periodization approach to powerlifting almost from the beginning. And as we've come to understand more of the physiological underpinnings for periodization's success, I've adapted my workouts more closely to what research now tells us will create the greatest gains in performance. It seems to have worked." We've also encouraged the members of our powerlifting team here at UT to train according to these methods and those who've stuck with the system have made remarkable gains, often becoming national and world champions. Judy Gedney attributes much of her success to the periodization approach she has used for the past two years. Indeed, more and more of the top powerlifters and Olympic lifters now in the United States are using or switching to some form of periodization.

In short, periodization works. But those of you whose desires run more toward fitness and fun than toward competition and conquest may be wondering why you need to be concerned with such seemingly complicated planning for your workouts. Well, first of all, if you're going to invest both time and money in a new fitness program, you deserve to get something back that's really worthwhile. Naturally, doing *anything* — if you've been doing nothing — is a step in the right direction, but you deserve more than just a step for your efforts. You deserve to *arrive*. Periodization will allow you not only to start but also to arrive. The form of periodization we recommend has four basic parts:

## 1. Hypertrophy: High Volume — Low Intensity

The Hypertrophy (muscle increase) phase is designed to allow the lifter to adapt physiologically so that he or she is better able, when the time comes later in the cycle, to perform at higher levels of intensity. Three to five sets of ten repetitions are used in each exercise. Besides the increase in lean muscle weight that the Hypertrophy phase brings, another benefit is the building of short-term endurance (anaerobic capacity). This increased anaerobic activity will combat fatigue during the higher intensity work that follows.

One thing to remember about the Hypertrophy stage of training is that you should not expect to make large increases in strength at this time. The purpose of this first stage of training is to prepare you to make large gains in strength later in the cycle, *after* your body has adapted to the program through Hypertrophy and an increased anaerobic capacity. That's why when the second stage, called Basic Strength, is reached, your strength should increase more rapidly. In your Hypertrophy training, concentrate on using good speed and weights heavy enough so that you feel as if you've really worked out. But don't worry if you can't add much extra weight. Try to increase the weights slightly each week, of course, but be careful not to add so much that you can't do the required number of repetitions.

## 2. Basic Strength: Moderate Volume — Medium Intensity

The Basic Strength phase is characterized by 3 to 5 sets of 5 repetitions per exercise with increasingly heavy weights. Here, it's important that you set goal, or target, weights for yourself each week in all your exercises and that you do your best to attain those weights (see pages 116 and 117). Basic Strength is an intermediate stage between the light weights of Hypertrophy and the heavy weights of the Power phase. Basic Strength allows both the body and mind to adapt to the greater weights to come.

## 3. Power: Low Volume — High Intensity

In the Power stage, the decreased volume — 3 to 5 sets of 2 or 3 repetitions — allows the body to be even less fatigued, though heavier weights are being lifted. This means that as you concentrate more on explosive power, you'll be able to lift heavier weights. During this phase, emphasis should be placed on the technique of the lifts and the speed with which the weights are moved. If you're doing squats, for instance, control the weight on the way down but then explode upward, moving the weight as rapidly as possible without jumping off the floor at the top. (In all your exercises, move the weight as rapidly as possible while still using good form, even though you're using heavier weights.) This high-intensity training is believed to have a positive effect on the central nervous system. By concentrating on the speed of the lifts, the nerves are trained to send the right patterns of neural orders to the muscles so that they perform explosively.

It is still important in this stage of your training, however, that you not miss any of the repetitions with the heavier weights — not a single rep. While more research needs to be done in this area, it appears that you can train yourself to fail just as you can train yourself to succeed. Choosing weights that are too heavy is not only dangerous but it teaches the central nervous system to give way rather than fight through. It conditions you to fail, making subsequent failure easier. It can also create a fear of heavy poundages.

Once the Power phase is completed, a weightlifter, for instance, would enter a competition. A football player, however, facing a long season, would go on a *maintenance* program to keep as much of his strength and power for as long as possible during the season. It's generally felt that athletes with extended seasons should train with weights at least twice a week and use only 3 sets of between 3 and 5 repetitions per set in order to maintain their strength level and to avoid staleness and overtraining.

## 4. Rejuvenation: Very Low Volume — Very Low Intensity

The Rejuvenation, or Active Rest phase, is simply a time for you to let your physical and mental well fill up again. This is a time for racquetball, hiking, cycling, and trying out new exercises with the weights. Rejuvenation can last for as little as a week or up to a month depending on the physiological and emotional needs of the trainer. This phase *is* important and should not be omitted. As Dr. Stone pointed out in this regard, "The reasons for the necessity of active rest (Rejuvenation) are not completely clear but certainly it contributes to the reduction of physical and mental (especially emotional) fatigue. Thus it reduces the possibility of overtraining during the next cycle."

In order for the concept of periodization to be fully understood, we urge you now to examine the following chart outlining the way it works.

One thing you must remember about periodization is this: as the body adapts, you have to continue to stress it. And, as your level of strength grows, you have to load yourself more heavily to keep making gains. Even though the Hypertrophy phase calls for "light" weights, the target weight (See page 117 for information on how to choose your target weight) would only be light for you if you had to lift it but once or twice. Even in hypertrophy, your target weight should be heavy for you to use for 3 sets of 10 repetitions.

We recommend further, at least for the first couple of cycles, that 3 sets of repetitions, rather than 5, be done in each exercise in which you are using the target weight for the day. For instance, if you were in the Hypertrophy stage of your training, this would mean that you would want to do 3 sets of 10 repetitions with your goal weight for the day. If that goal weight was 135

## Periodization

| Period | Phase | Description | Duration | Sets and Repetitions |
|---|---|---|---|---|
| ONE | HYPERTROPHY | High volume (High repetitions)<br><br>Low intensity (Light weights) | 4 weeks | 1 set of 10 with warm-up weight<br>1 set of 10 with intermediate weight<br>3 sets of 10 with target weight |
| TWO | BASIC STRENGTH | Moderate volume (Moderate repetitions)<br><br>Medium intensity (medium weights) | 4 weeks | 1 set of 10 with warm-up weight<br>1 set of 5 with intermediate weight<br>3 sets of 5 with target weight<br>1 set of 10 with 70% of target weight* |
| THREE | POWER | Low volume (Low repetitions)<br><br>High intensity (Heavy weights) | 2 weeks | 1 set of 10 with warm-up weight<br>1 set of 3 with light intermediate weight<br>1 set of 3 with intermediate weight<br>3 sets of 3 at target weight<br>1 set of 10 with 70% of target weight* |
| FOUR | REJUVENATION (ACTIVE REST) | Very low volume (Few repetitions; light forms of other exercise)<br><br>Very low intensity (Very light weights or no weight training) | 1 to 2 weeks | Do no organized weight work. Experiment with new exercises: cycle, play racquetball, swim, etc. Do not try to keep making gains. |

* These single sets with 70% — sometimes called "down sets" — help to maintain the gains in lean body weight made during Hypertrophy.

pounds, say, you'd do a *warm-up* of 10 reps with around 95 pounds, an intermediate set of 10 reps with 115 pounds, and then you'd jump to 135 pounds for 3 sets of 10 before going on to your next exercise. So, your full workout would consist of 5 sets of 10, even though only 3 of those sets would be at your "target weight" for the day.

As for the exercises, we outline our particular recommendations in the following sections of the book. What exercises you choose will depend on the equipment available to you. Any weight-training exercise can be used in a periodization program. The only weight-training exercises that are different are abdominal exercises such as sit-ups and leg raises. We say this *not* because the muscles involved wouldn't adapt well to periodization but because it is technically difficult to attach enough weight to the legs, for instance, so that 2 or 3 reps in the leg raise would be your limit. So, just do higher reps in your waist work and work as quickly as you can.

The main thing you'll need to do with periodization is to choose weights that are close to your limit for your sets at the "target weight." What we mean by "target weight" is that if your routine calls for 3 sets of 10 repetitions in the squat, you should be able to make all 10 reps in all 3 sets with the same poundage. The tenth rep in the third set should be a tough one — even the last 3 or 4 repetitions should be. *But don't miss.* Forgive us for harping on this, but periodization is based on the body's *gradual accommodation* to the increasingly heavy loads with which you exercise. Make sure you allow your body time to adjust. Be conservative about your increases from week to week to insure that you can make all the reps for the right number of sets. *This is especially important during your first, basic training cycle,* when you will be primarily adjusting yourself to your new exercise program.

If you haven't trained with weights at all before, it might be a good idea for you to think of your first twelve-week cycle as part of a larger "macrocycle." Perhaps if you can visualize it as the foundation cycle for two or three other cycles that you will also do in the coming year, it will allow you to accept the fact that you need to be realistic and conservative in your approach to the first cycle and that you especially need to choose weights you can handle for all the desired repetitions. With one cycle under your lifting belt, you'll know your body better, and you can then afford to be a bit more adventurous and push yourself a bit harder. Just remember, you've got a lot of good, productive years ahead of you — don't rush things.

Naturally, on your first cycle, you'll need to spend some time working into the program. Remember, it took three full weeks for the members of the sedentary women's study to work in to the full routine. If you have not been involved in any sort of exercise program, please make sure to do as the women in our study did and adjust yourself gradually to the increased activity. You'll still feel some soreness and stiffness at first — what Selye calls the alarm stage — but don't take a week off because of it, or you'll have to go through the pain again. Just follow our suggestions, don't neglect your stretching and don't do more than we suggest, even though you may feel as if you can.

In the research work done on periodization, and this is crucial, it was found that the greatest strength increases occurred when a particular group of muscles was stressed really vigorously — maximally — only once a week. In our recommendations we have followed this principle, designating one day a "heavy day" and one a "light day" in the basic program, in which you train only twice a week. As you train longer, you may wish to train more days per week, but even in more complicated routines, it is still important that you vary the resistance from day to day and that a "light" and a "heavy" day be designated for each body part per week. This allows the body adequate rest, and you'll progress much faster than if you try to go heavy at each workout. The light day, however, is not a cakewalk. It is designed to be approximately 85 percent as heavy as your other training day, which, if you're doing as you should and choosing weights that really tax you on your heavy day, will still make this light day vigorous. For example, if you did 3 sets of 10 with 100 pounds on Thursday in the squat, on your light day the following Sunday, you'd use 85 pounds as your target weight for 3 sets of 10.

The final thing we need to discuss is choosing your target weights. In this, working with someone who's done some weight training is really valuable to a beginner, because what seems hard to a beginner is often not hard when viewed in light of the enormous capabilities of the human body. Even so, during the Hypertrophy stage, your target weights for the first couple of weeks should seem relatively easy. You shouldn't feel exhausted or be sopping with sweat when you finish. Remember, you are using very light weights, at first, to prevent soreness. At the end of Hypertrophy, however, you should be using a weight for your 3 sets of 10 that *will* make you perspire, that *will* make your heart pump vigorously, and that you can barely lift for the final few reps of that third set. Understandably, there's no way for us to predict what that weight will be for you. Men and women have very different natural levels of strength, as do people of different ages and activity levels. The best advice we can give is for you to choose a target weight for your heavy day that you can use for all 3 sets of 10, a weight that is, on the final set, quite hard for you to lift the required number of times. After you've gone through a couple of cycles, you'll understand a lot more about your body's limitations and will be able to judge your poundages pretty accurately.

Sometimes, despite your best intentions, you'll miss some of your repetitions on a particular day. If this happens, *do not increase the weights on your next heavy day,* but repeat the workout of the previous week and try hard to get the desired number of repetitions. Never move up in weight until you have done your 3 full sets with the right weight for the scheduled number of reps.

Naturally, sometimes you'll make an increase that is beyond you, but when this happens, simply repeat the same weight — unless the weight was obviously *far* too heavy — the next week on your heavy day. In the beginning it is better to use weights that are too light rather than too heavy. A good rule of thumb is to make the smallest possible increases from week to week, unless those small increases don't properly tax the muscles. One way you can tinker with this program to make each workout more tailored to your strength level on any given day is to move your target weight up, or even down, 5 or 10 pounds after your *first* target-weight set. By doing this, you can adjust the resistance so that it is appropriate to your strength level. This should make your second and third target-weight sets what they should be — tough but achievable.

Two other questions that should be answered here are how long to rest between sets and how much weight to use on warm-up and intermediate sets. The answer to the first question is that you should train as fast as you *comfortably* can. Obviously, you shouldn't do 10 reps with your target weight and immediately do 10 more. As a matter of fact, you shouldn't be *able* to do this since it would imply that you were using too light a target weight. A good guideline is to take your next set as soon as you feel able to lift the weight the designated number of repetitions. As soon as your breathing begins to return to normal, take the next set. You'll soon learn how long you need to rest. The key is to rest as little as possible and still use substantial weight.

The answer to the question of what weights to use on your warm-up and in intermediate sets can vary, but good ball-park figures are 65 to 70 percent of your target weight on your warm-up set and 80 to 85 percent on your intermediate set. If you've stretched properly, you'll already be fairly well warmed up, so 65 to 70 percent should be a safe warm-up weight. Finally, if you're really pushed for time and you feel well warmed after your first set, you *can* skip your intermediate set. We don't recommend this, however, as it lessens your overall workload and consumption of calories.

To give you a little more understanding of how to choose poundages, we made a chart of a full ten-week cycle for a man who's never trained with weights before. Joe Average is forty-five, weighs around 150 pounds and has done no regular exercise for the past ten years. Joe will use the basic program described in Chapter 17.

## Joe Average's Training Log

Age: 45        Body weight: 150

(Note: Log entries follow the Weights-Repetitions-Sets format.
125 × 10 = 125 pounds for 1 set of 10 repetitions.
125 × 10 × 3 = 125 pounds for 3 sets of 10 repetitions.)

---

### HYPERTROPHY

**Week One**

Monday — Heavy

*Flexibility:* Did all 11 stretches twice; held each for 10 count both times

*Squats:* Did 2 sets of free squats, 1 set with 45-pound bar

*Bench Press:* 45 × 10 × 3

*Rows:* 45 × 10 × 3

*Sit-ups:* 10 reps

Thursday — Light
- *Flexibility:* Repeated 11 stretches twice; held for count of 10, then count of 20
- *Squats:* No weight × 10 (warm-up)
  45 × 10 × 3
- *Bench Press:* 45 × 10 × 4
- *Rows:* 45 × 10 × 4
- *Sit-ups:* 12 reps, 10 reps

## Week Two

Monday — Heavy
- *Flexibility:* Repeated 11 stretches twice; held for count of 10, then count of 20
- *Squats:* No weight × 10 (warm-up)
  45 × 10 (intermediate)
  60 × 10 × 3 (target)
- *Bench Press:* 45 × 10; 55 × 10; 60 × 10 × 3
- *Rows:* 45 × 10; 55 × 10; 60 × 10 × 3
- *Sit-ups:* 15, 10, 8

Thursday — Light
- *Flexibility:* 11 stretches × 15 count; then 20 count
- *Squats:* No weight × 10; 45 × 10; 50 × 10 × 3
- *Bench Press:* 45 × 10; 50 × 10 × 4
- *Rows:* 45 × 10; 50 × 10 × 4
- *Sit-ups:* 15, 10, 10

## Week Three

Monday — Heavy
- *Flexibility:* 11 stretches × 20 count; then 25 count
- *Squats:* 55 × 10; 65 × 10; 75 × 10 × 3
- *Bench Press:* 50 × 10; 60 × 10; 70 × 10 × 3
- *Rows:* 55 × 10; 65 × 10; 70 × 10 × 3
- *Sit-ups:* 18, 12, 10
- *Leg Raises:* 10, 8

Thursday — Light
- *Flexibility:* 11 stretches × 20 count; then 25 count
- *Squats:* 45 × 10; 55 × 10; 65 × 10 × 3
- *Bench Press:* 45 × 10; 55 × 10; 60 × 10 × 3
- *Rows:* 50 × 10; 55 × 10; 60 × 10 × 3
- *Sit-ups:* 20, 15, 12
- *Leg Raises:* 10, 10

**Week Four**
    Monday — Heavy
        *Flexibility:* 11 stretches × 25 count; then 30 count
              *Squats:* 60 × 10; 75 × 10; 95 × 10 × 3
      *Bench Press:* 55 × 10; 70 × 10; 80 × 10 × 3
                *Rows:* 60 × 10; 70 × 10; 80 × 10 × 3
            *Sit-ups:* 22, 18, 15
        *Leg Raises:* 12, 10

    Thursday — Light
        *Flexibility:* 11 stretches × 30 count, twice
              *Squats:* 60 × 10; 70 × 10; 80 × 10 × 3
      *Bench Press:* 55 × 10; 65 × 10; 70 × 10 × 3
                *Rows:* 60 × 10; 65 × 10; 70 × 10 × 3
            *Sit-ups:* 25, 20, 20
        *Leg Raises:* 15, 15, 10

---

## BASIC STRENGTH

**Week Five**
    Monday — Heavy
        *Flexibility:* 11 stretches × 30 count, 11 × 30 count
              *Squats:* 65 × 10; 95 × 5; 115 × 5 × 3; 90 × 10
      *Bench Press:* 60 × 10; 80 × 5; 90 × 5 × 3; 65 × 10
                *Rows:* 65 × 10; 85 × 5; 95 × 5 × 3; 70 × 10
            *Sit-ups:* 25, 25, 25
        *Leg Raises:* 15, 18, 12
              *Twists:* 25, 25

    Thursday — Light
        *Flexibility:* 11 stretches × 30 count × 2 sets
              *Squats:* 65 × 10; 90 × 5; 100 × 5 × 3; 80 × 10
      *Bench Press:* 60 × 10; 70 × 5; 75 × 5 × 3; 55 × 10
                *Rows:* 65 × 10; 75 × 5; 80 × 5 × 3; 60 × 10
            *Sit-ups:* 25 × 3
        *Leg Raises:* 20, 15, 15
              *Twists:* 35, 25

**Week Six**
    Monday — Heavy
        *Flexibility:* 11 stretches × 30 count × 2 sets
              *Squats:* 75 × 10; 110 × 5; 125 × 5 × 3; 95 × 10
      *Bench Press:* 65 × 10; 85 × 5; 100 × 5 × 3; 70 × 10

> *Rows:* 75 × 10; 95 × 5; 105 × 5 × 3; 75 × 10
> *Sit-ups:* 25 × 3
> *Leg Raises:* 20 × 3
> *Twists:* 35, 30

Thursday — Light
> *Flexibility:* 11 stretches × 30 count × 2 sets
> *Squats:* 75 × 10; 95 × 5; 105 × 5 × 3; 80 × 10
> *Bench Press:* 65 × 10; 75 × 5; 85 × 5 × 3; 60 × 10
> *Rows:* 70 × 10; 80 × 5; 90 × 5 × 3; 65 × 10
> *Sit-ups:* 25 × 3
> *Leg Raises:* 25 × 2, 20
> *Twists:* 50, 35

## Week Seven

Monday — Heavy
> *Flexibility:* 11 stretches × 30 count × 2 sets
> *Squats:* 95 × 10; 125 × 5; 135 × 5 × 3; 95 × 10
> *Bench Press:* 70 × 10; 90 × 5; 105 × 5 × 3; 75 × 10
> *Rows:* 80 × 10; 100 × 5; 110 × 5 × 3; 80 × 10
> *Sit-ups:* 25 × 3
> *Leg Raises:* 25 × 3
> *Twists:* 50 × 2

Thursday — Light
> *Flexibility:* 11 stretches × 30 count × 2 sets
> *Squats:* 90 × 10; 105 × 5; 115 × 5 × 3; 80 × 10
> *Bench Press:* 70 × 10; 80 × 5; 90 × 5 × 3; 65 × 10
> *Rows:* 75 × 10; 85 × 5; 95 × 5 × 3; 70 × 10
> *Sit-ups:* 25 × 3
> *Leg Raises:* 25 × 3
> *Twists:* 50 × 2

## Week Eight

Monday — Heavy
> *Flexibility:* 11 stretches × 30 count × 2 sets
> *Squats:* 95 × 10; 130 × 5; 145 × 5 × 3; 100 × 10
> *Bench Press:* 75 × 10; 95 × 5; 110 × 5 × 3; 80 × 10
> *Rows:* 80 × 10; 105 × 5; 115 × 5 × 3; 85 × 10
> *Sit-ups:* 25 × 3
> *Leg Raises:* 25 × 3
> *Twists:* 50 × 2

Thursday — Light
 *Flexibility:* 11 stretches × 30 count × 2 sets
 *Squats:* 90 × 10; 115 × 5; 125 × 5 × 3; 90 × 10
 *Bench Press:* 70 × 10; 85 × 5; 95 × 5 × 3; 70 × 10
 *Rows:* 80 × 10; 90 × 5; 105 × 5 × 3; 70 × 10
 *Sit-ups:* 25 × 3
 *Leg Raises:* 25 × 3
 *Twists:* 50 × 2

---

## POWER

### Week Nine

Monday — Heavy
 *Flexibility:* 11 stretches × 30 count × 2 sets
 *Squats:* 100 × 10; 130 × 3; 145 × 1; 160 × 3 × 3; 115 × 10
 *Bench Press:* 80 × 10; 90 × 3; 105 × 1; 115 × 3 × 3; 80 × 10
 *Rows:* 90 × 10; 110 × 3; 120 × 3 × 3; 85 × 10
 *Sit-ups:* 25 × 3
 *Leg Raises:* 25 × 3
 *Twists:* 50 × 2

Thursday — Light
 *Flexibility:* 11 stretches × 30 count × 2 sets
 *Squats:* 95 × 10; 115 × 3; 135 × 3 × 3; 95 × 10
 *Bench Press:* 70 × 10; 90 × 3; 100 × 3 × 3; 70 × 10
 *Rows:* 75 × 10; 95 × 3; 105 × 3 × 3; 75 × 10
 *Sit-ups:* 25 × 3
 *Leg Raises:* 25 × 3
 *Twists:* 50 × 2

### Week Ten

Monday — Heavy
 *Flexibility:* 11 stretches × 30 count × 2 sets
 *Squats:* 100 × 10; 140 × 3; 155 × 1; 170 × 3 × 3; 120 × 8
 *Bench Press:* 85 × 10; 100 × 3; 110 × 1; 120 × 3 × 3; 85 × 10
 *Rows:* 90 × 10; 115 × 3; 125 × 3 × 3; 90 × 10
 *Sit-ups:* 25 × 3
 *Leg Raises:* 25 × 3
 *Twists:* 50 × 2

Thursday — Light
 *Flexibility:* 11 stretches × 30 count × 2 sets
 *Squats:* 100 × 10; 130 × 5; 145 × 3 × 3; 100 × 8
 *Bench Press:* 75 × 10; 95 × 3; 105 × 3 × 3; 75 × 10
 *Rows:* 80 × 10; 100 × 3; 110 × 3 × 3; 80 × 10
 *Sit-ups:* 25 × 3
 *Leg Raises:* 25 × 3
 *Twists:* 50 × 2

**Weeks Eleven and Twelve**       **REJUVENATION**

Please remember that the sort of fitness you can achieve through periodization has very little to do with strength for the sake of strength. Your aim is to increase your level of fitness in every way — flexibility, muscular endurance, cardiovascular condition, psychological health, *as well as strength*. Periodization can help you with all of these areas and at the same time not be so terminally boring that you find it hard to decide whether to go to the gym or clean out the septic tank. Overcoming the mental routineness of any sort of training program is tough, but going to the gym and doing the same exercises for the same number of repetitions week after week after week is deadening. And if you're bored, you'll find yourself stopping to talk to your fellow trainers — when you should be pushing ahead, trying to keep your pulse elevated — or skipping certain exercises that you particularly dislike or, what's worse, avoiding the trip to the gym altogether.

The important things to remember with periodization are:

**1.** Choose weights that are heavy enough to "stress" the muscles without being so heavy you miss any repetitions.

**2.** Never increase to a heavier weight unless you were able to do all 3 sets of 10 with the target weight for the day the previous week.

**3.** Make sure to keep your light days "light" by using around 85 percent of the poundage you used on your heavy day.

**4.** Be patient. Even if you feel really strong, resist the urge to "max out" unless it's the very last workout of the cycle. Then, if you like, do some singles to see what your limits are. Otherwise, train progressively so that your body has time to adapt muscularly and psychologically to the heavier poundages.

**5.** Be sure to Rejuvenate before you start your next cycle. This is critical.

**6.** When you start your second cycle, start Hypertrophy at a higher level than you did the cycle before. You don't have to move that first target weight up much from where you started the previous cycle, just enough that you continue to stress the muscles properly.

**7.** Always remember to do a "down set" of 10 repetitions during the Basic Strength and Power phases of training to maintain your hypertrophy.

**8.** And, finally, while you are scheduled to do only 3 sets with your target weight, don't forget that you are supposed to also do a warm-up set and an intermediate set before you hit the target. For safety's sake don't neglect these. Even if you're working with a light weight such as 55 pounds, do 45, 50, and then 3 sets at 55. Remember that the *total* workload is important.

# 14 / Safety

EVEN though, statistically, weight training is among the safest forms of sport or exercise, we still want to take a couple of pages to talk about safety and injury prevention. We've both trained for years, yet neither of us has ever suffered any serious injury while training. We're proud of that fact not because we feel we were blessed with injury-free bodies, but because we suspect our training methods are effective *and* safe. We've had an occasional ache and pain through the years, but by warming up properly, varying our training loads through periodization, and using good old common sense while we were in the gym, we've avoided major injuries and continued to enjoy and maintain our physical well-being. So can you.

First of all, no matter what your age, we urge you to have a thorough checkup by a physician before you begin working out. Make sure you explain that you plan to begin a new fitness program and that you'll be doing some weight training. If you've had any history of heart disease, high blood pressure, arrhythmia, emphysema, diabetes, or had any serious back, knee, or other joint problems, we recommend that you see not just a GP but a sports medicine or cardiac specialist for this initial assessment. Even if you do have one of the conditions mentioned above, in nine out of ten cases you'll still be able to train with weights. But you do need to be a bit more careful about starting out on your training and you should continue to check with your doctor periodically. Research shows that exercise has many curative powers, and while we can't give you a hard-and-fast guarantee without knowing your particular set of circumstances, we won't be surprised if after a few months on the weights you report to your doctor a lowering of your blood pressure and an increase in your energy level.

If high blood pressure and cardiac disease *are* among the problems you're now facing, we *strongly recommend* that you include an aerobic component such as rapid walking or cycling to your workouts. Talk to your doctor about this and take a look at some of the current books out on aerobics, as well as our suggestions later in this chapter. And while you're doing your weight work, move rapidly through your sets so that you get an aerobic effect from your weight training. This rapid exercising may mean you need to back off on the amount you lift a bit — but that's okay. Once you've "cured" yourself, you can concentrate on heavier poundages from time to time.

Another thing to remember is that if at any time you feel dizzy while you're training, stop exercising immediately until you've recovered. Likewise, don't ever hold your breath while exercising. This applies not just to those who have blood pressure problems but to *all* weight trainers. Breathe normally throughout the movements, or breathe as we have recommended in the descriptions of the exercises, so that your pressure doesn't rise abnormally while you're lifting. Holding your breath can also make you lightheaded, which can lead to dropped barbells.

## Backaches and Barbells

The most common excuse we hear for not training with weights is lower-back problems. Literally millions of Americans are plagued by chronic lower-back pain, much of which is of undetermined origin. While a good percentage of these back problems are the result of slipped discs, pinched nerves, and spinal malformations such as scoliosis and kyphosis, a high percentage of lower-back pain is the result of weakened and atrophied muscles that allow the spinal column to slip out of line. Another source of trouble surfaces when unconditioned muscles in the back are called upon to lift something suddenly, causing them to tear, to go into spasm, or to allow the vertebral column to get out of proper alignment. Anyone with a history of lower-back problems should proceed very cautiously in any exercise in which the back muscles are involved. As you gradually strengthen these muscles, you'll be able to handle heavier poundages, but at first, start out light and concentrate on using good form. *And remember,* if an exercise causes pain in your back when you try to do it, put the weight down immediately and try to find a substitute exercise.

You should also pay close attention to your flexibility work before each training session and make sure you do abdominal work if you have back problems. Much lower-back pain is caused either by inflexibility or by a weakened abdominal wall that allows a swaybacked posture to develop, causing unnecessary stress on the lower back. By strengthening the abdominal sheath, your internal organs will be better protected, you'll stand straighter, and your clothes will "hang" as they should. Stretching will help you relieve tightness in the back, as well as bring blood into the back muscles, which has been shown to limit further injuries. Also, keep your back warm at all times while training. In fact, if the place where you train is especially cool, you might also apply some sort of analgesic balm, such as Ben-Gay or Icy-Hot, before you begin your stretching.

The main thing to remember if you have back problems is to use your head when it comes to the weights. For instance, there's no reason you can't train the bench press pretty hard, even if your back is a bit on the blink, because the bench press is an exercise in which your lower-back muscles are relatively uninvolved. If something *is* painful, *don't do it.* If squats bother your back, try leg presses or extensions and leg curls, exercises in which your back is stationary. Even if your back does bother you, you should make some effort to come up with *some* exercise — try hyperextensions for a starter — that you can do regularly, *without pain,* to begin strengthening the area. And, don't forget to keep checking with your doctor.

## The Knee

Another weak link in our structure seems to be the knee. In years past many physicians forbade patients with knee injuries from doing any sort of exercise, particularly weight training, because they felt exercise would place undue stress on the injured joint. In the early stages of knee injuries this is certainly true, but these days, as soon as the initial trauma is under control, doctors and physical therapists recommend certain weight-training exercises as therapy for injured knees. They know that by strengthening the muscles around the knee and by increasing the diameter of the tendons and ligaments that hold the knee together, stronger knees less prone to injury will be produced.

This book is not the place to prescribe a series of exercises to rehabilitate your knees any more than it is a place to prescribe a course of therapy for lower-back pain. Each case is individual, and without seeing you and your injured area and assessing your situation, it's impossible to make a prescriptive judgment. What we do suggest, however, is that if you have knee problems, you should consult a doctor before you begin any sort of exercise program. Then, if he agrees to let you train, you should proceed slowly in those exercises that require flexion of the knee joint. Naturally, if you feel pain during the performance of an exercise, stop immediately. As we suggested in our discussion of back problems, try an alternate exercise if one we've listed continues to cause you pain.

And, finally, a word about squats. Squats have gotten a bad rap in a lot of circles because of their supposed ability to create knee problems. The fact is that the most up-to-date research findings indicate that the connection between squats and knee injuries is nonexistent as long as two principles are followed. First, don't go all the way to the "bottom" as you squat. Stop partway down so that the knee is not forced into an extreme position. Second, don't descend rapidly and try to bounce out of the bottom position. It's the sharp, sudden movements that can cause ligaments to tear. We'll talk more about this when we explain how to do squats, but for now just keep in mind that, properly done, *squats are safe.* We've squatted for many, many years, often with record weights, and our knees are all four fine.

Here are some additional guidelines for safe, injury-free workouts.        **Safety Tips**

**1.** If you can, train with a partner. Be especially certain to have someone close by when you do bench presses, squats, incline presses, or any of the exercises in which we suggest you use a "spotter."

**2.** Make sure you read each exercise description completely. Don't simply look at the illustrations and attempt to imitate what you see. We've written detailed descriptions for each exercise because *positioning* is crucial to your success and safety. When the instructions say, "Look straight ahead," make sure you look straight ahead. When they say, "Keep your back flat," make sure that you do so. If you're not sure that what you're doing is correct, have your training partner check it for you against the photos and in the text. If you train alone, use a mirror.

**3.** Pay attention to what you're doing. We don't mean to sound overly paternal, but a large percentage of gym accidents are the result not of muscle "tears" or faulty equipment, but someone not paying attention at the right time. Never talk while exercising. Talk all you want between sets, but when it's your turn to lift, bear down on what you're doing and think, "Is my body in the right position? Is my head up? Back flat? Am I breathing properly? Do I feel the 'pull' in the right muscles?" Likewise, give your training partner attentive silence when he or she is lifting.

**4.** Pay especially close attention when you load and unload the bars. Don't remove all the plates from one side at once if the bar is resting on a bench or squat rack. Take a few from one side, then a few from the other, and so on, until you've gotten the weight down to where you want it. This will save you on bridgework, because exercise sets are notorious for flipping over and hitting people when all the weights are pulled from one side at once.

**5.** You should also pay attention to what the people training near you are doing if you decide to train in a gym. Make sure as you walk across the room that you don't bump into anyone. Many gyms are overcrowded, and it's easy to inadvertently hit someone as they're exercising.

**6.** Be aware at all times of how your body *feels* as you lift weights. *Always* warm up with stretching before you begin your exercises, and if you *still* feel cold, ride an exercise bike for ten minutes or jog in place for a bit until you feel ready for the weights. Your body should feel both loose and warm before you begin. Never start with heavy poundages. Always follow the periodization schedule and start with a light weight for a warm-up set.

**7.** Make sure you tune in to any aches and pains you feel as you exercise. If you experience any sharp, sudden pains, especially if you hear a loud "pop" at the time of the pain, you may well have torn something. You should see a doctor immediately if the pain persists. Place ice on the area at once to reduce swelling. If you can't get to the doctor that day, keep icing the area for at least fifteen minutes, every hour. By all means, if there is any discoloration, swelling, or continued pain, *check with your doctor* before training again.

**8.** Keep in mind that rapidly gaining and/or losing weight is not something that either we or the AMA recommends. Though we've both gained and lost a great deal of weight over the past years, neither of us did it rapidly, and we were at all times conscious of the effect such changes had on our blood pressure, skin, and homeostasis. If you're seventy-five pounds overweight, you *could* lose fifty pounds over the next two months, but we certainly don't recommend that as a procedure. We especially disrecommend rapid weight gain. Lose or gain your weight slowly. A pound a week is plenty — more than two is too much.

Throughout the text are other caveats or warnings that deal specifically with particular exercises or aspects of our program. We don't want to sound alarmist about the safety aspects of weight training, for it is, indeed, a very safe activity. However, you are using tools that have the capacity to harm as well as to help and we want to help you avoid some of the snags that might produce problems. We realize that a lot of our safety tips seem so self-evident that you're beginning to wonder whether, instead of being big strong weightlifters, we're really a pair of old maids. Well, in a sense, we're both. The caution and protectiveness most people associate with a stereotypical old maid are precisely what has enabled both of us to become both big and strong, and then smaller and strong, safely. This has kept us robust and uninjured for a lot of long years. Never make fun of cautionary old maids. They generally outlive the rest of us.

# 15 / Preparing for Your First Workout

WHETHER you decide to train at home or at the gym, there are some common denominators that need to be considered. The first of these is training clothes. Keep them loose and simple, and, before you buy any clothes specifically for weight training, consider what you already have on hand. Those old gray sweat pants in your bottom drawer may not have quite the style of the latest Gilda leotards but they will keep you warm. They should be more than adequate for the job, especially if the job is to be done in the privacy of your home. We generally train in T-shirts and sweat pants, sometimes a sweatshirt, too. If the workout area is cool, make sure you keep either a sweatshirt or a jacket around to wear between your sets or until you're thoroughly warmed up. The warmer your muscles stay while you're training, the less chance there is of an injury.

The second thing to consider when choosing clothes is the sort of exercise routine you'll be following. If you plan on incorporating some running or cycling (either indoor or outdoor) into your routine, workout clothes that will let you move from the weights to your next activity or vice versa not only saves time but laundry as well. Most advanced trainers wear some sort of running shoes in the gym, and we recommend this practice to you, although any flat-soled, nonslick shoes will suffice. One word of caution. Try to find a shoe for your training that is neither so curved through the toe and heel area (as many jogging shoes now are) nor so spongy that when you plant your feet to lift you lack a solid base. Many of the ultracomfortable running shoes on the market are now so heavily padded that they are less than ideal for lifting purposes. You want stability as well as comfort in your shoes — especially as the weights begin to increase for you.

Finally, you may want to get a weightlifting belt. Wearing the belt helps to support the midsection when you lift, and it also serves to psychologically

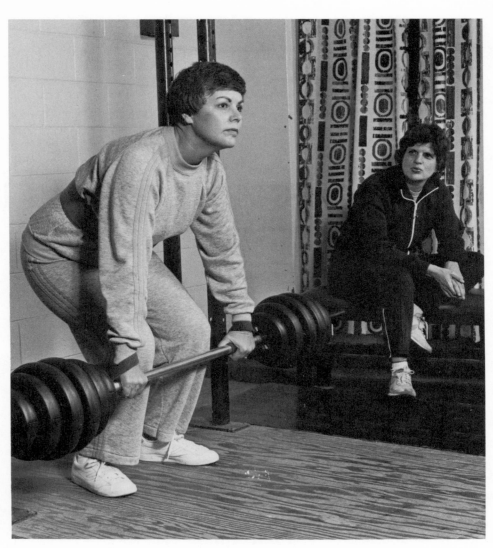

*If the place where you train isn't uncomfortably hot, a warm-up suit of the sort worn here by Kathryn Pilgrim of our women's study group is a good idea.*

ready you for your lifting. A belt isn't an absolute necessity, but they are relatively inexpensive ($20 or so), and they help impart a certain seriousness and purpose — girding your loins and all that. There is some disagreement in scientific circles as to their actual benefit, though almost all lifters swear by them, feeling that they help to support the back during lifts such as squats, deadlifts, and overhead presses of one sort or another. Belts do create a feeling of tightness in the midsection, which makes you feel more solid. They give you something to push against with your abdomen as you lift. We both wear belts when we train and admit to feeling a bit naked in the gym without them. We don't tighten them in all exercises, however, only in those such as squats or rowing motions, in which the back is centrally involved. We loosen them as soon as we've finished the exercise so that we can breathe normally as we recover, and we wear them loosely buckled when we do such exercises as bench presses, in which the back is only very minimally involved. In short, belts can't hurt you, unless you buckle them so tightly you cut off your wind, and they very well may help you by making you feel more secure and stable as you lift.

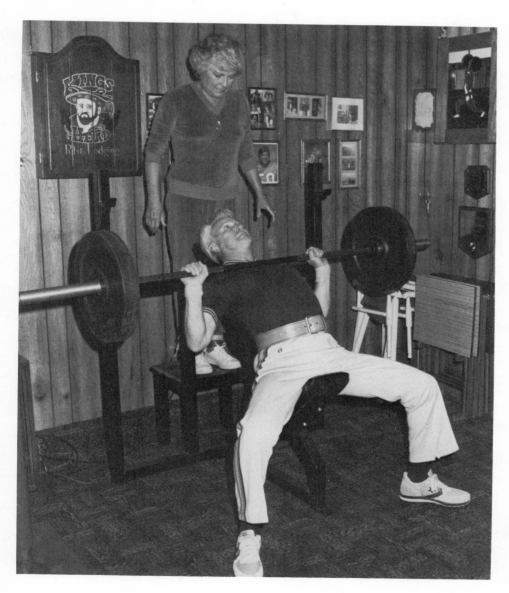

*Training partners are a help in many ways, such as the "spotting" Eleanor Curry gives to her husband, Bill, as he grinds out a tough set.*

The next thing you'll need for your workouts, if you can arrange it, is a training partner/spotter. If you train at home, the ideal training partner, of course, would be your husband, wife, or roommate, but if you lack one of those, try to find an interested friend. Training partners play a very important role in successful weight work. They help to spot you on the heavier and more difficult exercises, they help to motivate you to train harder and to not miss workouts, and they keep you from getting bored. If you get a friend or two together to train, you'll find the camaraderie, the support, and the competition very gratifying. Even if you can't get someone there for all your workout sessions, try to make sure to have someone with you as often as possible. In fact, heavy bench presses — where you use weights near your limit — should not be done alone. If you either need or prefer to train alone, however, you can take workouts that are both safe and effective if you simply exercise a little common sense as you exercise your body.

While many people seem to think that training partners should train exactly the same, set for set, such is not the case. We have been training partners, for instance, for the past twelve years, yet we've usually done very different workouts. And even during the times when we've done virtually the same workouts, we've used dramatically different poundages. Yet we're training partners, in the best sense of the term. What you mainly need is not a shadow who'll follow you set for set, but a good friend who'll help you plan your workouts, offer suggestions on technique, and who'll pause momentarily to spot you when you need assistance. It's important that you learn to be independent about your training — to learn to direct yourself and to take charge of your body — but don't be so independent that you rule out the positive aspects of training with someone. If you're training in a gym, you'll have little trouble getting someone to help you bench press and squat. But if you'll be working out at home, try to have someone else there besides yourself. Perhaps even one of your children would like to train — the weights can do wonders for them, too.

Another thing that will help you, regardless of where you train, is a diary or training log. Working with a great many people over the years, we've found the use of a training log to be one of the best motivators for continued progress. In a small notebook that will easily fit into a workout bag, we both logged every set of every workout that we did during our years of competition. This may sound like a chore, but it's a very useful training tool, and if you'll just keep your book open to the proper page during your workouts, you'll find that you can jot down your sets and reps and poundages while you're resting. A standard day-by-day calendar appointment book is excellent because it allows a full page per day of writing space. You should keep track of your body weight, any feelings of soreness or injuries, and, from time to time, make notations about the lifts themselves.

These extra notations can mean a lot to you later, when you sit back at the end of the cycle and assess your progress. If you pulled a hamstring on the tennis court, causing you to slow down on the squats for a week or so, *and* you noted this in your book, you'll remember why you decreased the poundages during that period. At times, we've also kept track of our food and vitamin intake to see if there were any differences in the way we felt and progressed.

The main reason for keeping a log, though, is to help you remember week to week how you're doing. Periodization, as we've said, requires planning for it to be successful. Since you'll be using a percentage of one day's exercise for your target weight on another, writing down the poundages will make the process much easier.

**Jan:** "Here's a sample page from one of my books of last year. Note that I wrote the poundage first, then the number of repetitions. Since we trained then on a "kilo set" of weights, the numbers may seem a bit odd, unless you're used to converting kilos to pounds. Also note that I mentioned my stretches and abdominal work. Don't neglect to keep track of these as well."

---

Tuesday, January 18 Body wt: 154.5
Stretched for five minutes before beginning. Trapezius and lat muscles sore from Sunday's workout.
*Bench Press:* 88 × 10 repetitions, 121 × 5, 137 × 2, 154 × 1, 171 × 3 (easy), 176 × 3, 176 × 3 (PR) *
*Incline Press with Dumbbells:* 43 × 5, 50 × 3, 55 × 3, 55 × 3, 55 × 3, 43 × 10
*Incline Fly with Dumbbells:* 25 × 5, 30 × 5, 30 × 5, 30 × 5, 30 × 5, 28 × 10
*Decline Press with Dumbbells:* 43 × 5, 50 × 3, 50 × 3, 50 × 3, 50 × 3, 43 × 10
*Decline Fly with Dumbbells:* 35 × 5 × 5, 30 × 10
*Abs: Crunches:* 3 sets of 25; Leg Raises: 3 sets of 20; Twists: 200

*PR means personal record

---

By keeping a log, you can always check to see where you are. Patterns begin to develop, and you can make better progress and perhaps avoid past mistakes. The historians are fond of saying that those who know no history are doomed to repeat it, and this is certainly true of athletics, especially lifting. A log is also an excellent motivator because, though you sometimes may feel you're not making much progress, a glance through your log book will help you appreciate your gradual improvement. In this regard, a log book is rather like a bankbook. As a matter of fact, training regularly is a *lot* like making regular deposits in your savings account or IRA. In both cases you are providing for the future. An ant would understand.

# 16 / Stretching and Warming Up

I N some respects, the most important minutes you'll spend working out will be those first 5 to 10 minutes when you stretch and warm up, before you ever touch a weight. Warming up — bringing blood into the areas to be exercised — is especially important among older trainers. As we discussed earlier, the increasing lack of flexibility we all encounter as we age is among our most serious problems. Unless we continue to work at flexibility, it will gradually diminish, along with our nimbleness, our strength, and our appearance. Stretching is of primary importance to every workout because the stretching movements we suggest and explain on the following pages will prepare you — warm you up — for your workouts.

The stretches we recommend allow you to direct blood flow into the specific areas to be stretched and subsequently exercised; they not only warm up the tendons and joints but the muscles as well. If at the end of the stretching period you still feel stiff and cold, however, ride a stationary bicycle or run gently in place until you begin to perspire lightly. Always remember that you want to be warm when you begin your workouts. If it's cool in the area where you train, make sure to leave your sweat pants and jacket on *at least* until you've done all your stretches and your body feels loose and supple. If you have trouble staying warm, rub some analgesic balm on your back and shoulders to make sure you remain warm while you train.

There's an awful — truly awful — lot of misinformation floating around about how to stretch properly. Anyone who graduated from high school anytime between the thirties and the sixties, and even into the seventies, was probably taught in gym class that to loosen up you should "bounce" into positions of increased tension (as in toe-touching) and then bounce right back out. The truth is that we now know that bobbing up and down is the *wrong* way to loosen the muscles. Physiologists refer to this bobbing as "ballistic" stretching, and, according to them, when a person bounces — stretching the muscles further than is comfortable — a "stretch reflex" is triggered, causing the muscles to contract. This is an unconscious protective reaction to keep the muscle tissues from tearing. As Bob Anderson says in his excellent book, *Stretching*, "Any time you stretch the muscle fibers too far (either by bouncing or overstretching), a nerve reflex responds by sending a signal to the muscles to contract; this keeps the muscles from being injured. Therefore, when you stretch too far, you tighten the very muscles you are trying to stretch. . . . These harmful methods cause pain, as well as physical damage due to the microscopic tearing of muscle fibers. This tearing leads to the formation of scar tissue in muscles, with a gradual loss of elasticity."

What Anderson and most physiologists now recommend is the technique called "static stretching." Static stretching involves the progressive and *slow* application of pressure to other muscles and tendons to make them lengthen beyond their normal resting length. In other words, you reach for greater and greater positions of flexibility until you feel a tight, slightly burning sensation in the muscle group being stretched. This position is then held in stasis for 8 to 10 seconds and then released. There should be no "pain," just a feeling of tightness in the area as you hold the position. Then, the position is resumed and, if possible, extended a bit. This method of stretching is far safer than the ballistic variety because the muscles are kept under control at all times.

We've included eleven stretches for you to do as a warm-up prior to your weight work. These eleven exercises work most of the major joints in the body, though if you feel the need for extra flexibility work, Anderson's *Stretching* contains dozens of other stretches.

We recommend that each stretching movement be repeated at least twice and that you attempt to reach a slightly lower or deeper position on the second try. Don't push yourself to the point of pain, however. You should feel a tightness and the beginnings of warmth as a result of blood coming into the area, but the muscles, even when in full stretch, should feel soft to touch; they should not be contracted. If they feel overly tight, back off a bit and begin your count again. In the beginning, you will probably only want to hold these for 10 to 15 seconds at a time. As you become more familiar with these positions, try to hold the second position longer — ideally at least 30 seconds. You'll notice, as the positions become more natural for you, that the feeling of tightness will diminish the longer you hold the position. This is exactly what you want to happen. This means that the muscle is relaxing and allowing itself to be stretched. It further means that blood has come into the area, blood carrying extra oxygen to the muscle cells so they will be able to work for longer periods of time once you begin to exercise. The additional warmth also helps to make the muscles less "brittle" and more supple so that they will be more resistant to muscle tears. Try to breathe rhythmically while you're in the stretches: *do not hold your breath*. Move slowly from position to position so that the feeling of relaxation can be maintained during the entire 10 minutes or so as you stretch. Finally, stretching *following* a heavy workout can be a wonderful way to cool down and let your body return to normal. Most of us rarely have the time; we're always running somewhere else after we've been to the gym, but if you can make yourself take the time, it's very beneficial. The slow movements bring both your heart and your mind back to normal, and we've even found that we seem to be less sore on the days following a heavy workout when we've taken a few extra minutes to restretch those muscles we've worked most heavily.

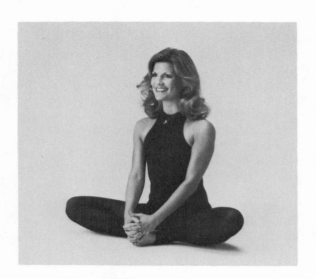 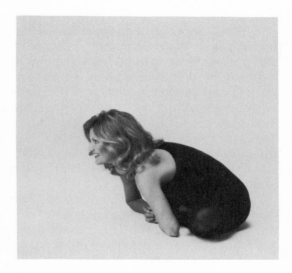

**Position 1**    *Stretches the groin, low back, and inner-thigh muscles*

Sit on the floor and put the soles of your feet together. Grasp your toes with your hands and pull your heels toward your body until you feel a stretching sensation in the groin area. Hold this for 10 seconds while you keep your elbows on the outside of your legs. Keep your knees wide and as close to the floor as is comfortable. Relax. Again resume the position and increase the intensity by pulling your feet closer to your body and by bending forward from the hips. *Try not to round your back.* Pick a point on the floor several feet ahead of where you're sitting and look at it as you move your upper body forward. Do not look down at your feet. Hold this position for 15 to 30 seconds and then move to the next position. Remember, breathe steadily throughout the stretches, and back off from your attempted position if you feel true pain — not simple tightness. And don't be surprised during the second part of this and all of the other 10 remaining stretches if the feeling of tightness subsides during the second stretch — this is desirable and indicates that you are performing these properly. Once it does subside, however, don't change the position until you've finished the full count. Then, if you feel you can do more, assume an even greater position of flexibility and repeat again. Do this and all the other stretches at least twice, more if you still feel tight in an area.

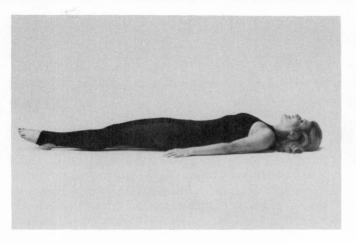
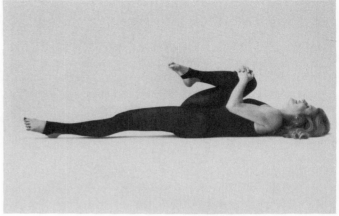

*Stretches the backs of the thighs and the hips*

**Position 2**

Lie on the floor with your legs extended and relax. Then draw your right leg toward your chest and grasp your shin with both hands. Pull the leg as close to the chest as possible and hold for 10 seconds. Replace the leg on the floor and bring the left thigh to the chest and repeat the stretch. Keep your head on the floor at all times. Lower your left leg back to the floor and repeat the stretches again, this time holding each leg at the chest position for 30 seconds.

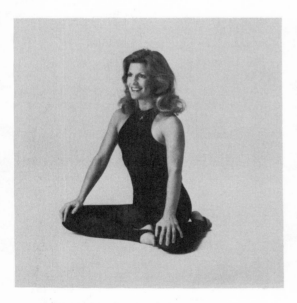
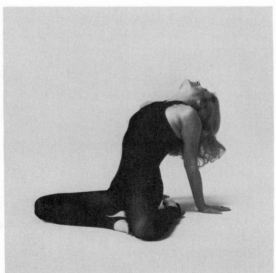

*Stretches the tops and insides of the thighs*

**Position 3**

Sit on the floor and bend your left leg back so that the heel of your left foot is as close to your left hip as possible. Place the sole of your right foot against the inside of your left thigh. From this position, lower yourself slowly backward until you feel a tight sensation in the quadriceps of your left leg. Remember to keep your left heel close to your hip as you move backward and place your hands behind you for additional support. Hold for 10 seconds and repeat for the right leg. Then, assume the left leg position once again and try moving a little further back. If you like, allow your head to relax and fall backward as shown in the photo, or continue looking straight ahead. Hold for 30 seconds and then repeat for the right leg.

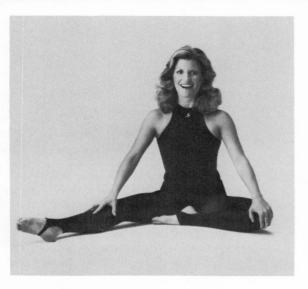
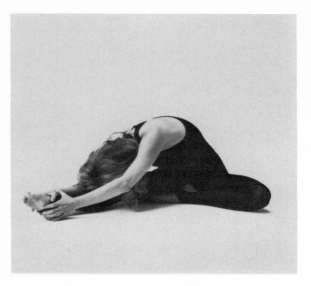

**Position 4**   *Stretches the hamstring and lower back*

Sit on the floor with your legs extended in front of you and place the sole of your left foot against the inside of your right thigh. Lean forward from the hips, keeping the back relatively flat, and grasp your right shin or foot. Hold this position for 10 seconds, relax, and stretch out the other leg in the same manner. You should feel a stretching sensation in the back of your thigh as you do these, and in your lower back. Don't attempt to stretch too far and force the hamstrings to contract, however. Repeat the stretch again for both legs, holding this time for 30 seconds.

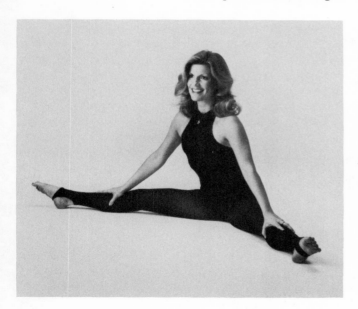
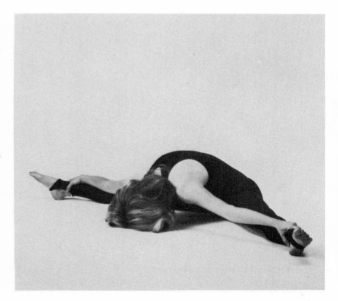

**Position 5**   *Stretches the lower back and the inner thighs*

Sit on the floor and spread your legs as far apart as is comfortable. Then, keeping the back straight, lean forward from the hips and hold for 10 seconds. Keep your toes pointed upward and try to keep your back flat. Return to the erect position, try to spread your legs slightly wider, and again bend forward as far as possible, grasping your legs for support. Hold for 30 seconds.

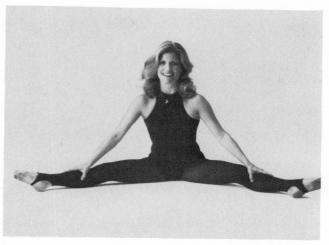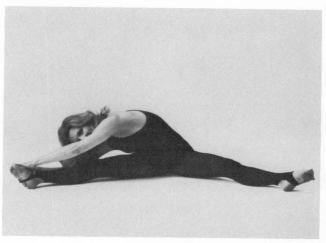

*Stretches the hamstrings, the shoulders, and the back*
Sit on the floor and spread your legs as far apart as possible, toes pointing upward. With your right hand, reach forward and grasp either your left shin or the outside of your left foot and hold for 10 seconds. Relax and repeat for your opposite side. Then, going back to your right arm, hold the stretch again for 30 seconds, remembering to bend from the hips, before repeating for your left arm.

**Position 6**

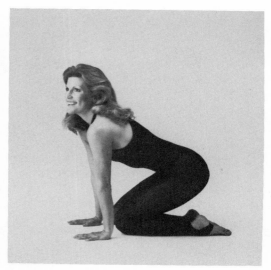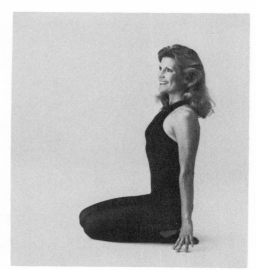

*Stretches your ankles and the tops of the thighs*
Kneel on the floor and then sit back on your haunches with your feet pointing directly behind you underneath your hips, your hands on the floor next to your knees. Then, remove your hands from the floor and lean backward until you feel a stretching sensation in your thighs. Hold for 10 seconds, relax, and then repeat, trying to stretch slightly further back on the second, 30-second stretch.

**Position 7**

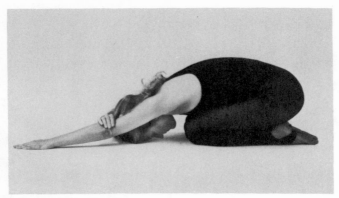

**Position 8**     *Stretches the shoulders and the sides of the back*

Kneel on the floor again, lean forward, and extend one arm as far as possible in front of you. Bend the other arm and place it either on the floor in front of your head or use it to hold on to the elbow of the extended arm. You'll look a bit like a Muslim at prayer. Lower your upper body until you feel the stretching sensation throughout the shoulders and sides of the back and hold for 10 seconds. Repeat for the opposite arm. Do a second stretch for each side, holding these for 30 seconds each.

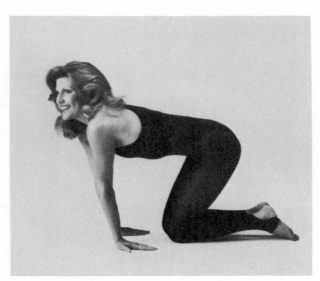

**Position 9**     *Stretches the forearms and wrists*

Kneel on the floor and place your hands so that your fingers point directly back toward your knees. Keep the arms straight as you slowly lean slightly backward until you feel the stretching sensation in the arms. Hold for 10 seconds, relax, and hold again for a 30-second stretch.

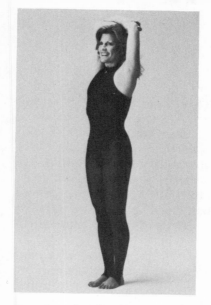

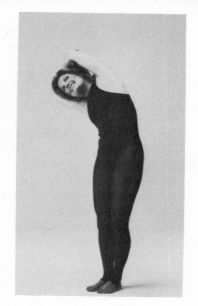

*Stretches the shoulders and the upper arms*

**Position 10**

Stand erect and fold your arms over the top of your head, holding your elbows with your opposite hands. Keep looking straight ahead as you lean slightly to the left and pull downward on your right elbow with your left hand. Hold for 10 seconds and repeat for the other side. Relax for just a second and then repeat, holding the second series of stretches for 30 seconds each.

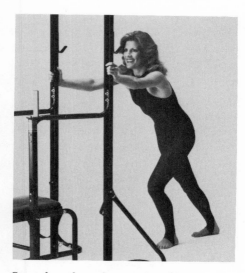

*Stretches the calves and ankles*

**Position 11**

Place both hands against a wall or other stationary object, with your feet about 24 inches from the wall. Move your right leg in close to the wall and place your head against your hands or the wall while keeping the back straight. Your back foot should remain flat on the floor with the toes pointed forward. Shift your weight so that you feel a stretching sensation in the calf of the back leg and hold for 10 seconds. Repeat for the opposite leg. For your 30-second stretches, move further back from the wall, lean slightly farther forward, and repeat on both legs. Be careful that you don't overstretch your calves — if the stretching sensation does not subside after several seconds, move the back leg closer to the wall. But above all, keep your feet flat on the floor, with the toes pointed directly ahead.

A new method of stretching now being used by a few athletes is called Proprioceptive Neuromuscular Facilitation, or PNF. PNF involves going through similar stretching motions with the help of a partner who, when you reach your maximum stretch positions, resists you as you use near-maximal pressure to come out of the low positions. We caution you to be careful with this method, but if you have a willing training partner and you'd like to try PNF, proceed with care and work up to a near-maximal push or pull in the maximum stretch position only after several sessions of experimentation. A simplified version of the training theory behind PNF is that it not only allows you to gradually increase your flexibility but that it also helps you strengthen your muscles and tendons, in these extreme positions of stretch, more effectively than static stretching.

Whichever method of stretching you decide to try, proceed with caution and patience. And remember — we recommend stretching not only for its antiaging qualities but also because it facilitates injury-free training. Whether the 10 to 15 minutes you'll spend going through these stretches will enable you to put your toes back in your mouth remains to be seen, but if you stretch regularly you'll definitely find your posture improving, your aches and pains diminishing, and grace and ease returning to your daily life.

# 17 / Training at Home with the Basics

Before you begin to train, you'll need to make a major decision: whether to train at home or at a health club. Training at home does have much to recommend it; for a relatively small, one-time investment, you can purchase the basic equipment you'll need to get a thorough weight workout. You'll thus not only save money by not having to pay annual gym membership fees, but you'll also save in transportation and time. Having a gym at home is one of the easiest ways to make weight training a permanent part of your lifestyle. You need never fight traffic to get to the gym, you won't have to wait in lines to use the equipment, and you'll be able to train in privacy.

**Jan:** "I can still remember how self-conscious I felt during my first gym workouts. Weights weren't at all chic then as they are now and I didn't want anyone to see me working out. I admit to having been embarrassed about it. But as I saw the improvements in my appearance and strength, I gradually came to terms with the weights and myself, but it might have been easier had I been able to train at home in the beginning."

If you do feel awkward about training, perhaps working out at home would really suit you. But even if you aren't at all self-conscious, there is still the matter of convenience. There are few excuses you can muster for not training when the weights are right there in the corner of your den. You'll be able to train before work, while the kids are taking their nap, or even during the evenings as you listen to the radio or watch television. The basic equipment we recommend won't take up much space. You can put weights and bench in your den, bedroom, garage, basement, or — in the summers — on a porch or patio, where they'll be outdoors but still protected from the weather. Just make sure your training area has enough space so you can train without hitting other pieces of furniture.

The rest of this chapter assumes you have decided to train at home and invest the minimum amount of money necessary to get a good workout. Your first step should be to check your local newspaper for sales on weight-training equipment. Sears, Kmart, JC Penney, and most sporting-goods stores now carry a full line of lifting equipment. So shop around as you would for any major purchase and don't be afraid to ask questions. How much weight will the bench safely hold? Will the store assemble it for you? What sorts of collars come with the barbell set? Are extra plates available for the weight set? And so on. You can, naturally, spend a lot of money on heavy-duty equipment, but you don't have to. If you are at all unsure of your commitment to training, we recommend that you begin with less expensive equipment and see how it all feels. Just as a Lamborghini is more exciting to drive than a Volkswagen, expensive benches and barbells are more pleasant to use than less expensive equipment designed for home use. *However,* just as the VW will take you where you want to go, so will less expensive weight-training equipment. So don't feel as if you can't begin a weight program because you don't have hundreds of dollars to spend on gym memberships or equipment. You can get everything you need for good, basic workouts for less than $100.

## The Benches

A flat, nonadjustable bench can generally be found for less than $40, and for several dollars more you should be able to locate one that will adjust so you can do incline work. If possible, buy a model with adjustable racks that will allow you to put the bar at shoulder height for squatting and overhead pressing movements. You can, of course, get by with a basic, flat bench, but if you can afford the more expensive combination bench-incline-squat rack, go ahead and buy it from the first. Remember, even the least expensive weight-training equipment will last you a very long time — with care, probably a lifetime — so invest in equipment that will satisfy more than one purpose. You won't regret the extra expense.

## The Weights

How much weight you'll need to begin is sometimes hard to say because you need almost no resistance for some exercises and quite a lot for others. The weights themselves come in a variety of shapes and materials. If you'll be setting up a gym in a large room where your equipment will not be shifted around every time company comes to visit, and if you think you're going to make a serious commitment to training, you may want to invest from the very beginning in a set of Olympic-style weights such as those used in lifting competitions. These sets, with their heavily constructed bars and big iron plates, will last a lot longer than you will and will also have a good resale value if you decide at some later time not to train at home. Olympic sets are generally calibrated in kilos (due to the requirements of the international lifting federations) and the basic 308-pound set (including bar) will retail for somewhere between $325 and $450 depending on the make and type of bar you choose to buy.

Most people, however, would not want to begin with such an expensive set, and we recommend that you consider buying a standard exercise set as your first barbell. Exercise sets, as they are called, have barbell plates in two basic materials — cast iron and a vinyl-covered composition substance. A cast-iron set will generally cost almost twice what the vinyl ones do since the plates are thinner, but you can get more weight on the bar at one time. They are also indestructible. However, if you plan to train in an apartment building or are thinking about working out while your kids take their afternoon nap, you should consider the fact that cast iron is more noisy and if you ever drop a weight, you, all your neighbors, and your floor will definitely know about it.

In the early days of vinyl-covered plates there was a problem with their breaking, but you'd need to really try to break one now. The heaviest set of vinyl-covered plates weighs 165 pounds, although if you buy extra plates in the heavier range you can load this set to slightly over 200 pounds. Another thing to consider is that composition weights won't rust as cast iron sometimes does, making them cleaner for home use, and they won't cut your carpet if you drop one while training in the living room. Their primary advantage, however, is their price. When vinyl-covered plates were first developed some 20 years ago, they were more expensive than iron weights, but the dramatic increase in the price of iron ore has reversed that situation. The standard 50-kilo set (110 pounds) handled by the major department-store chains sells for less than $50 and can sometimes be found on sale for as little as $30.

## The Big Three

Now that you have your weights, your lifting gear, and your log book, let's put that first free hour to good use. We've already explained periodization (Chapter 13) and how it applies to training for fitness, and what we want to do now is give you a *very basic program* for your *very basic equipment*. We've reduced the number of exercises to the minimum, but make no mistake — this program will get the job done. It will stimulate all your large muscle groups, and, used with a combination of dedication and discretion, it will make you stronger, leaner, more enduring, and more flexible.

The exercises we've chosen to call the Big Three are the squat, the bench press, and the bent-forward rowing motion. The squat has often been called, with good reason, the single most result-producing exercise in all weight training. It forms the core of the training programs of most athletes as it places such great stress on the leaping muscles of the body — the thighs, hips, and lower back.

As for the bench press, it is no doubt the most popular of all weight-training exercises, and a moment's thought will reveal why. It's fun, for one thing, and you can use fairly heavy weights. You get to stretch out on your back and just pump out those reps. You work the large muscles in your chest and shoulders with the bench press, and you can really feel the work — the pump.

The final exercise, the bent-forward rowing motion, works the muscles that almost exactly oppose the muscles you work with the bench press. The rows work all the muscles in your back as you pull the bar to your chest in almost the same groove you use to push the bar away *from* your chest in the bench press.

If you're *really* pressed for time, use the program we've outlined below. It calls for only two workouts a week, but two a week done properly can still generate the sorts of positive changes you want in your appearance. We sometimes even suspect that it might be best if all relative newcomers to lifting would start with a very simple, short program and then, as interest, commitment, and condition improve, go on to more advanced training. All too often, beginners try to squeeze too many exercises into their programs and wind up sore, discouraged, and anxious to find excuses to skip workouts.

Before you begin this program, reread the periodization section and be instructed by it. Make sure to look over Chapter 16, Stretching, again before you start the routine, and include at least ten minutes of stretching movements before you begin training. Also, familiarize yourself with the muscle chart that appears on page 305. Don't rush into the exercises — ease into them. Take a few weeks to reach the point at which you're doing the full workout. Ultimately, you'll *save* time this way, not waste it. And before you begin each workout, don't forget to warm your body up with stretching movements. Look back at the discussion of the sedentary women's study and see how these women, who hadn't exercised in years, gradually accommodated themselves to their new stretching and weight routine.

When you use this twice-weekly schedule, be sure to have at least two rest days between sessions. In other words, train Sundays and Thursdays, Mondays and Fridays, Tuesdays and Saturdays, or in some similar pattern — not Tuesday and Thursday, for instance. Your body needs time to recover from the stresses you're placing on it, but not *too* much time or your muscles begin to shrink or atrophy. And, as much as possible, be regular in your schedule. Try to train not only on the same days but at more or less the same time each training day. Assuming a Monday and Thursday pattern, your bare-bones basic workout would be:

**Monday**
  **Squat — Heavy**
      1 warm-up set                                10 repetitions
      1 intermediate set                           10 repetitions
      3 heavy sets at target weight                10 repetitions each
  **Bench Press — Heavy**
      1 warm-up set                                10 repetitions
      1 intermediate set                           10 repetitions
      3 heavy sets at target weight                10 repetitions each
  **Bent-Forward Rowing Motion — Heavy**
      1 warm-up set                                10 repetitions
      1 intermediate set                           10 repetitions
      3 heavy sets at target weight                10 repetitions each

**Thursday**
  **Squat — Light**
      1 warm-up set                                10 repetitions
      1 intermediate set                           10 repetitions
      3 sets at target weight                      10 repetitions each
        (85% of Monday's weight)
  **Bench Press — Light**
      1 warm-up set                                10 repetitions
      1 intermediate set                           10 repetitions
      3 sets at target weight                      10 repetitions each
        (85% of Monday's weight)
  **Bent-Forward Rowing Motion — Light**
      1 warm-up set                                10 repetitions
      1 intermediate set                           10 repetitions
      3 sets at target weight                      10 repetitions each
        (85% of Monday's weight)

There it is in all its primitive splendor. You should stick with this workout for 4 weeks, trying to use slightly heavier weights every Monday. Then, having completed Hypertrophy, increase your target weights on both days and decrease your reps to 5 per set, except for one final light set. As we explained in detail in the section on periodization, this sudden change prevents physical and mental boredom and it allows you to move forward more rapidly toward your goal of total physical wonderfulness. Then, after 4 weeks on sets of 5 reps, drop to sets of 3 repetitions (again, increasing the weights) for 2 weeks before taking a week or two off and then starting all over again with sets of 10. Written out in workout shorthand, the second and third parts of your training cycle would look like this:

## Second Phase: BASIC STRENGTH

**Monday**
**Squat — Heavy**

| | |
|---|---|
| 1 warm-up set | 8 to 10 repetitions |
| 1 intermediate set | 5 repetitions |
| 3 heavy sets at target weight | 5 repetitions each |
| 1 light set | 10 repetitions |
| (70% or so of weight just completed) | |

**Bench Press — Heavy**

| | |
|---|---|
| 1 warm-up set | 8 to 10 repetitions |
| 1 intermediate set | 5 repetitions |
| 3 sets at target weight | 5 repetitions each |
| 1 light set | 10 repetitions |
| (70% or so of weight just completed) | |

**Bent-Forward Rowing Motion**
Same pattern as for squat and bench press

**Thursday**

Use the same pattern indicated for Monday, only use 85% of the weight used on Monday for your 3 sets of 5 at the target weight (as you did in your first month) and be sure to add a final light set of 10 repetitions with each exercise.


## Third Phase: POWER

**Monday**
**Squat — Heavy**

| | |
|---|---|
| 1 warm-up set | 8 to 10 repetitions |
| 1 intermediate set | 3 repetitions |
| 3 heavy sets at target weight | 3 repetitions each |
| 1 light set | 10 repetitions |
| (70% or so of weight just completed) | |

**Bench Press — Heavy**
Same as squat routine
**Bent-Forward Rowing Motion — Heavy**
Same as squat routine

**Thursday**

Use the same pattern indicated for Monday, only use 85% to 90% of the weight used on Monday for your 3 sets of 3 and be sure to add a final light set of 10 repetitions.


## Fourth Phase: REJUVENATION
**Two weeks**

# The Big Three Defined

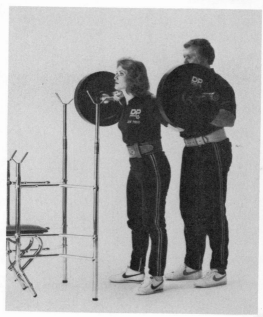

**Muscles worked:** Quadriceps, hamstrings, gluteus maximus, spinal erectors. The squat is an excellent exercise for strengthening and toning the thighs and buttocks. It is especially recommended for would-be athletes of any age who are interested in increasing their power and leg strength.

**Directions:** Place the bar across your back just below the point at which the neck joins the torso. Make sure that the bar is not resting on your seventh cervical vertebra (the one that protrudes when you bend your head forward), as holding it too high on the neck will not only be painful for you, it will also decrease your ability to maintain a flat-backed upright position when descending with the weight. Place your feet shoulder-width apart, toes pointed slightly outward, and focus your eyes on a fixed point on the opposite side of the room. Keeping your eyes on this spot, take a deep breath and lower your body slowly until the tops of your thighs are roughly parallel to the floor. When you have reached this position, reverse gears, and push yourself back upward as quickly as possible, keeping your back flat, your eyes fixed on the spot on the opposite wall, and the weight under control at all times. At the top, breathe out, take another deep breath, and repeat.

**Tips:** Though they look easy, squats are hard for many people to do because of a lack of the necessary flexibility or even balance. Make sure to stretch out well before you begin the squat portion of your workout, and do at least one set of deep knee bends with no weight at all as an extra warm-up. If you find it hard to keep your heels on the floor, place a one-inch board or a pair of barbell plates under your heels. Try to use as little extra height as you can, however, as the higher your heels are elevated, the more the stress of the exercise is thrown onto the quadriceps muscles *alone* and away from the hip, thigh bicep, and low back muscles. Experiment with your foot stance during the early stages of your training. Sometimes, slightly widening the stance or turning your toes further out will solve your balance problems.

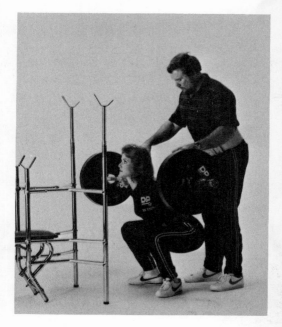

If you don't have a bench with a squat rack attached, your main problem will be getting the bar to your shoulders to do the lifts. Your training partner is important here, as he or she can either lift the weight to your shoulders for you or help you put it in place yourself. Training partners should also be alert for uneven positioning that will make the bar seem heavier on one side than the other. When in the proper position, the bar should rest just below the top of the deltoid muscles on the *back,* not on the shoulders.

As for the lift itself, take a full chest of air at the top and hold it throughout the descent. When you pass the midpoint of the upward part of the push, exhale. Then, take another full breath before you do your second repetition. Don't be surprised, as you use heavier weights, if you find yourself taking 2 and even 3 breaths between your reps. Squats will make you puff — and puff hard—which is one of the reasons so many coaches and physiologists recommend them to athletes. If you do your sets quickly enough, you'll find yourself feeling as if you just finished a series of 50-yard dashes, so be sure to allow your body time to recover before going on to the next set or the next exercise.

## The Bench Press

**Muscles worked:** Pectorals, deltoids, triceps. The muscles of the forearm are slightly involved in stabilizing the weight.

**Directions:** Lie on the bench in a supine (face upward) position and grip the bar, as it rests in the rack, approximately at shoulder width, palms facing forward. With the aid of your spotter, remove the bar from the rack and hold it at arms' length directly over your sternum (center of your chest where the ribs join). From this position (*not* with the bar at arms' length over your face) lower the bar to the chest to a point at the lower end of the sternum (women should lower the bar to the point on their chest immediately beneath their breasts) and then push it upward until it is again at arms' length over the chest. As with the squats, take a full breath of air in the starting position, hold it through the descent, and exhale after you've passed midway on the upward push. Make sure that your feet stay planted firmly on the floor and that your buttocks and shoulders do not lift off the bench.

**Tips:** The bench press moves in a slight arc from the point on your chest where you touch the sternum to the lock-out position. In the early going, with light weights, you will probably not notice much arc at all, as you can easily push the weights directly up over your chest. However, as the weights get heavier, you'll need to concentrate more on the technique of the lift. Try to visualize a path of movement from the chest up that brings the bar back toward the face. It will help if you bring the elbows close to the body at the bottom of the lift and then "flare" them out as the bar glides back up the grooved arc. Try to hit the same place on your sternum with each repetition and make sure that you touch the chest each time in order to get the full range of movement from the lift.

Two other things to keep in mind are your position on the bench and your grip on the bar. Most lifters try to arch their backs slightly when

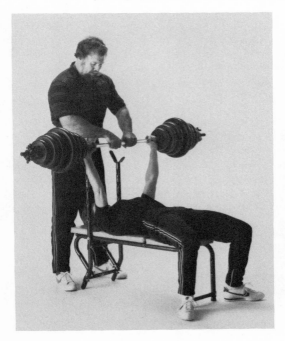 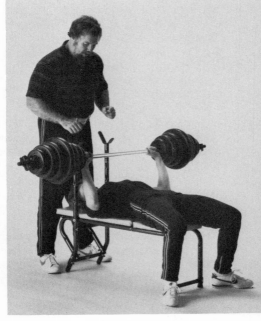

they are lying on the bench. The arching of the back makes the chest "taller," which means you have a shorter distance to push the bar. Presto, heavier weights. However, you should also do your bench presses with your back flat some of the time as this will give you a bit more muscular work, even though you can't lift quite as much weight, since you have to push the bar further. Also, be careful to position yourself far enough down the bench so that when you push the bar to lock-out you won't hit the uprights, or catchers, on the bench. Sometimes, on really heavy lifts, you may feel a slight cramping sensation in your lower back as you push the bar upward. This is not abnormal, and is the result of your arched back position. Make sure to warm your back up properly, as well as your shoulders, before you bench and you should avoid the problem. However, if you do cramp, pull your knees into your chest to stretch out the back muscles and allow the cramp to relax before you do your next set.

For your own safety, always have someone hand off the weights to you so you can set up well away from the racks. If you must bench alone, *never* attempt to lift weights near your limit and *always* leave the collars off the bar so you can tip it to one side and let the plates slide off in case you happen to get stuck at the bottom. The alternative involves being pinned under a heavy bar, which will quickly result in severe oxygen deprivation, a sure way to spoil your day. As for your grip, start training with a shoulder-width grip; a few people do use extremely wide hand-spacings to increase the work on the pectorals — the wider the grip the more the "pecs" are worked, the closer the grip the more the shoulders and triceps are worked. You should vary your grip from time to time to prevent mental and physical staleness. But be careful to warm up well if you significantly alter your grip from one workout to the next.

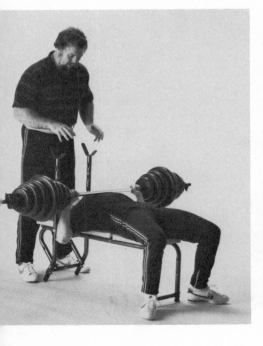 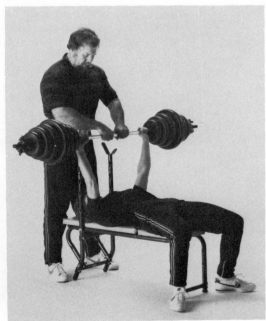

## The Bent-Forward Rowing Motion

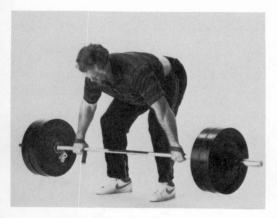

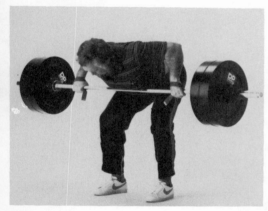

**Muscles worked:** Latissimus dorsi, biceps, trapezius, spinal erectors. Rowing motions strengthen the upper back and shoulder-girdle region and are an important exercise for people with posture problems or those who play sports, such as golf and softball, in which upper back strength is important.

**Directions:** Place the barbell on the floor in front of you and bend down to it, placing your hands 6 to 8 inches wider than your shoulders and taking an overhand grip. Then, slightly bend your knees and, keeping your back flat and in a fixed angle in relationship to the floor, pull the bar to your chest to the same point at which you touched your bench presses. Lower the bar to arms' length and repeat.

**Tips:** Rowing motions are rather like upside-down bench presses and, like bench presses, they require some concentration on technique. Make sure to keep your knees bent slightly and your back flat to decrease the stress on the lower back. When you lower the bar from the chest, lower it in a controlled manner so that you don't jerk your body out of position. Pull your elbows high when you reach the chest, as this helps in the contraction of your back muscles. With light weights you should be able to maintain your leg and back position easily, but as the poundage increases you may find yourself using your knees as springs — bending them slightly as you pull the weight to the chest and allowing them to act as shock absorbers as you lower the weight back to arms' length. There is nothing wrong with this; just make sure not to overdo it. Use the legs only when the "lats" and the other muscles alone can't quite pull the bar for the last few reps.

An additional training aid often used with rowing motions is the hand strap (see photos on this page). Straps simply allow you to concentrate on the exercise itself and not on whether your grip might give way if you pull really hard. Straps can be purchased from a number of mail-order houses or can easily be made from a yard or so of 1-inch cotton webbing, such as that used in military belts. Cut the webbing into two lengths and stitch a loop in one end just large enough for your hand to pass through fairly easily. The "tail" is then wound around the bar and held by the hands while doing the lift. If you have your straps on properly, you should feel a pull not in the palms or fingers when the bar is lifted but at the wrist. Straps should only be used in those exercises requiring quick pulling movements, such as rowing motions. On other lifts it's better to work without straps, as you strengthen your grip and forearms by holding the weights naturally.

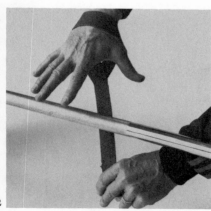

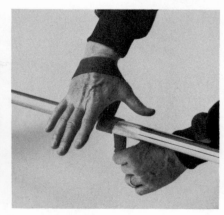

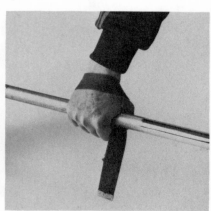

# Adding On, Basically

There are, of course, a number of other exercises you can also do with your two basic pieces of equipment, and after you've completed your first training cycle, you may wish to add a few exercises.

Below is a list — arranged according to the areas of the body worked — of some of the many exercises that can be done with your basic equipment.

## Lower-Body Exercises

### The Deadlift

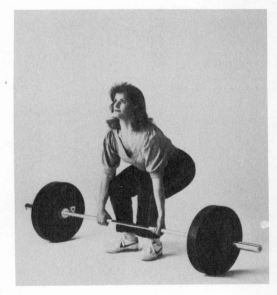

**Muscles worked:** Lumbars, gluteus maximus, hamstrings, trapezius, latissimus dorsi, quadriceps, forearms

**Directions:** Place the barbell on the floor in front of you about an inch from your lower legs. Your feet should be about shoulder-width apart. Bend your knees, keep your back flat, and grasp the bar in an overhand, shoulder-width grip or in a reverse grip with one hand over and one hand under (see photos on this page). The reverse grip is used with heavy weights to keep the bar from slipping from your hands. Whichever grip you choose, make sure it is even by checking to see that your hands are equidistant from the center of the bar. Then, look upward at a point on the opposite wall, push with your legs, keeping your back flat and your hips down, until you are standing erect with your shoulders back and the barbell resting across the front of your thighs. To do your repetitions, bend your knees, lower the bar in the same flat-backed position, and repeat. If you're using an exercise set, with plates that are smaller in diameter, we recommend that you not touch the floor on every repetition. Do your repetitions by going only about halfway down your lower leg before you begin the upward pull for the next repetition.

**Tips:** Over 50 percent of all weight-training exercises use the deadlift to get the bar into the proper starting position. For this reason, learn to do it properly. The flat-backed, heads-up position used here is critical. Also, don't "yank" the weights off the floor. Use your legs to generate the starting force and remember to keep the bar moving in a straight line upward, close to your body. The further in front of your body the bar gets the "heavier" the weight will seem, because of unfavorable leverage. Never look down when deadlifting. Keep your eyes straight ahead — even slightly upward — and your back will stay flat, your hips will stay down, you'll lift more weight, and your body will respond to the exercise.

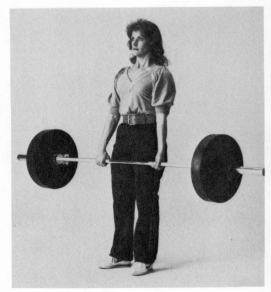

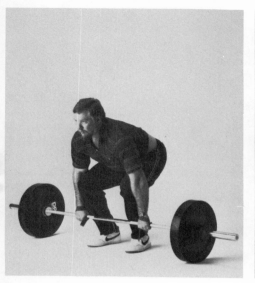 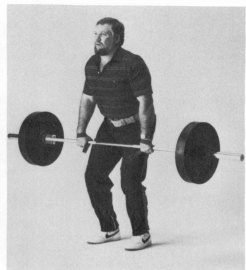 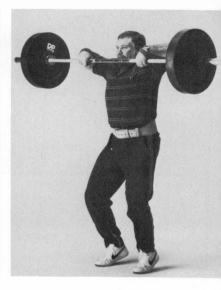

**The High Pull**  **Muscles worked:** Calves, hamstrings, quadriceps, gluteus maximus, lumbars, latissimus dorsi, trapezius, biceps, forearms, etc. The high pull is one of the finest exercises a person can do, *especially an athlete,* as it involves almost every muscle in the body, working together.

**Directions:** Assume the starting position for the deadlift, using an overhand grip of shoulder width. (Because high pulls are explosive, quick movements, you may wish to use your hand straps.) Flatten your back, raise your head, and, taking a full breath of air, pull the barbell from the floor as if you were doing a deadlift — only more quickly — until the bar is just past your knees. Then, without stopping the bar, shift your hips forward quickly and continue to pull even higher, extending the body by rising onto your toes with your elbows flaring out to the sides as high as they can be pulled. At the top position, which you will maintain only momentarily, your elbows will be high, the bar will be in front of your chest with your palms facing downward; your body should be fully extended and straight, and you will be standing on tiptoe, your eyes looking slightly upward. From this top position, lower the bar to your thighs, dipping slightly at the knee to catch the weight as it comes down, and then straighten your back and legs to assume a finished deadlift position. To do your second repetition, lower the bar just below the knees (not all the way to the floor) and begin the upward pull again.

**Tips:** Though a bit difficult to learn, this exercise is well worth the trouble. We strongly recommend that you incorporate it into your routine at some point. High pulls work almost all of the muscles of the body, they make your heart and lungs pump, and they're fun. The bar almost floats at the top when they're done correctly. Think about jumping as you do these, though you shouldn't actually come off the floor. But try to get that sort of momentum and speed going as you go through your repetitions.

**The Power Clean.** We recommend the high pull and *not* the more commonly done "power clean" because we feel the high pull is a somewhat less dangerous yet equally result-producing exercise. But for those of you who want to know, any time a weight is "cleaned" it is pulled from the floor to the shoulder in one movement. Power cleans are done exactly like high pulls except that at the top of the movement, the elbows are shifted forward, the hands turn over, and the bar is allowed to stop and rest across the top of the clavicles before it's lowered to the thighs for the next repetition. Stopping the bar, however, creates several problems. For one thing, when the wrist is bent backward into the position necessary to hold the weight at the shoulders, some people experience discomfort, and sometimes injuries and tendinitis develop. Another problem arises as the weights get heavier: it becomes harder and harder to pull the weight high enough to "catch" it at the shoulder. So, people start arching backward, thrusting their hips forward under the bar, and sometimes splitting their legs to the sides during the performance of the lift, all of which causes the back to lose its upright position, thus opening the door to injuries. With the high pull, however, the bar is pulled as high as possible on each rep and then allowed to go back down. Nonetheless, you still get good work from those movements as long as the bar is being pulled as high as possible and the body is being extended fully. Olympic lifters perform this exercise in a slightly different way, but the differences and the reasons for them are beyond the scope of this book.

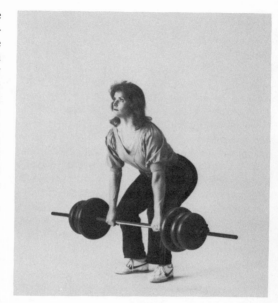

The big trick in doing either the high pull or the power clean is to learn to do the "pull" properly. Start the pull with the arms straight and don't bend them until the bar is well past the knees. At all times, keep the bar as close to your body as possible — no more than an inch away from your legs and torso — and remember that this is a lift for speed and explosion. Once the bar has passed the knees, shift the hips forward rapidly as you begin the upward pull. This shifting should provide the impetus for getting the bar to your chest and getting your shoulders back. As in all other lifts, keep your head up when you're doing these, even when you're returning the bar to the thighs to begin the second repetition. And, finally, always reset your back — flatten it — before you begin the next rep.

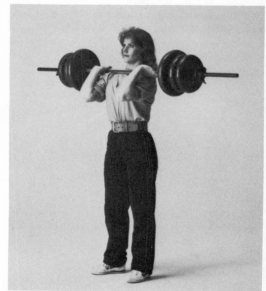

# The Lunge

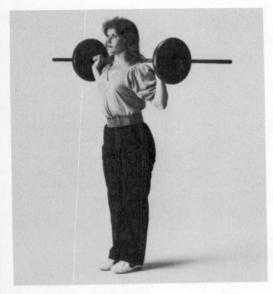

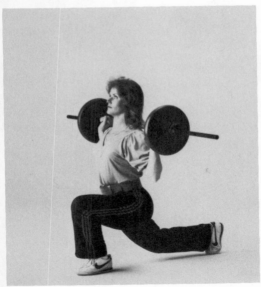

**Muscles worked:** Gluteus maximus, hamstrings, quadriceps, calves

**Directions:** Place a light bar across your shoulders and stand with your feet together. Raise your right foot and step out forward, allowing your left heel to raise upward, left toes pointed directly ahead. As you step forward, lower yourself into a deep split with your right knee bent and your left (or back) leg kept fairly straight. You should feel a stretching sensation in your hips and the back and inside of your front thigh and a stretch on the inside of your back thigh. Then, push with your right leg and raise upward as rapidly as you can — using only one thrust to return your body to the starting position. Reverse your legs and repeat. Throughout the lift try to stay as upright as possible and keep your back leg from touching the floor.

**Tips:** Let us warn you, these will make you very sore the first couple of times you do them. In fact, do no more than 10 repetitions per leg on the first day with *no* added weight. Add weight *only* when you can do several sets of 10 reps easily with no weight. The reason they produce such soreness is because they work all the hip and thigh muscles so completely, which is why we highly recommend them as an addition to your routine. To help yourself stay upright, put a broomstick across your shoulders until you have gained enough strength so that you can use the barbell. Lunges require good flexibility, but like other flexibility movements they can be worked into gradually.

Don't be discouraged if you can't go very low in these at first. Just make sure to work a little lower each time you do them and to keep your back leg almost straight — not touching the floor. Keeping your back upright will also help you get lower. One final word. Your back foot should always point straight ahead. Your heel will come up, of course, but the toes should be pointed in the same direction as you're facing. Don't turn the back foot out to the side, as this significantly lessens the effect of the exercise. You may find it hard to balance, but stick with the toes-ahead position, even if you hold on to something the first day or two while you get used to the movement.

**Muscles worked:** Hamstrings, lumbars, gluteus maximus

**Directions:** Using a *light* barbell, deadlift the bar as usual, using an overhead grip. From this top position, lower the bar by locking the knees and bending forward at the waist. Do the lift slowly and bend forward as far as possible while keeping the knees locked. Return to the upright position and repeat for the desired number of repetitions.

**Tips:** This is the only exercise in which we'll ever tell you to lift a weight with your legs straight. The locking of the knees puts almost all of the strain on the hamstrings on the back of the thigh and the lumbar muscles in the low back, so be sure to use light weights in this exercise and to do the reps slowly and with good control. As your flexibility increases, you may want to do these while standing on the end of your bench or on a large block of some sort so that you can stretch down even further than the plates will permit you to do while standing on the floor. A large dictionary or phone book should give you enough extra height, at least for awhile. If you have had back trouble, we recommend that you avoid this exercise.

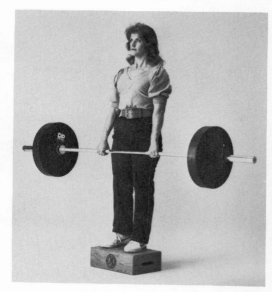

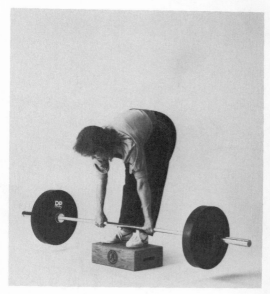

# The Good Morning

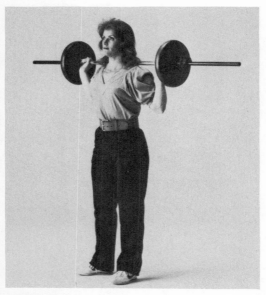

**Muscles worked:** Lumbar muscles of the lower back

**Directions:** Place a light barbell across your shoulders and stand as if you were ready to do a squat — shoulders back, chest out, eyes looking straight ahead, feet about shoulder-width apart. Very slightly bend the knees — more than is shown in the photos — and then bend forward at the waist until your upper body is parallel to the floor. Keep the bar tight across your shoulders and don't allow it to roll onto your neck as you do these. Once you've reached parallel (*not* lower) reverse the movement and resume the erect position before starting again.

**Tips:** Like stiff-legged deadlifts, good mornings are exercises requiring care, and they should be avoided if you tend to have back trouble. They should be done with weights light enough so that your back can stay fairly flat throughout the entire range of movement. By keeping your head and eyes pointed straight ahead, even at the bottom part of the lift, a flat back is much easier to maintain. This exercise was designed to build the muscles of the lower back — the lumbars — though how they came to be named "good mornings" is unclear, unless it was a carry-over from the early days of free-hand calisthenics done upon rising, before an open window, breathing ever so deeply at each bending of the waist. A perverse sense of humor may also have had something to do with it.

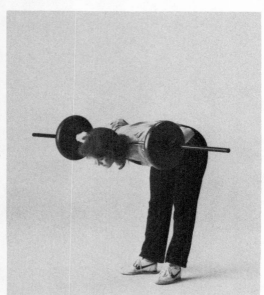

**Muscles worked:** Gastrocnemius and soleus muscles of the lower leg

**Directions:** Place the barbell across your shoulders and place the ball of your foot on a thick board or something similar (four inches high or more is best). The heel portion of your foot should hang off the edge so you can get a full stretch — or extension — of the muscles in the calf. Slowly raise onto your toes, feeling the contraction in your calves, then lower yourself all the way down so your heels go below the board and you can feel a stretching sensation. Repeat for the desired number of repetitions.

**Tips:** Bodybuilders will tell you to hold the contraction at the top for a second to make sure to get the best work from the movement. Since calf raises require moving the weight only a short distance, don't be afraid to use fairly heavy weights. An inexpensive board can serve as a toe block for calf work by taking a 36-inch-long piece of 2 x 4 board, cutting two 8-inch sections from it, and then nailing the remaining 20 inches to the centers of the two 8-inch pieces. This should allow you to reach a full stretch and is more stable than simply using a 4-x-4-inch board alone.

**Variations:** Calves can be worked in a number of ways. You can do them one leg at a time (with no added weight), holding on to your bench or something stable with the hand opposite the leg you're working. They can also be worked in a seated position by placing your toe block at the end of the bench. Sit with your toes on the board and place a loaded barbell across your knees, then push upward and stretch downward just as if you were standing. A towel will pad your thighs a bit if the bare bar is uncomfortable. You can also vary your calf work by turning your toes inward and then outward on the alternating sets, shifting the emphasis back and forth from the inside to the outside of the calves. Also, use high reps in all calf work for best results.

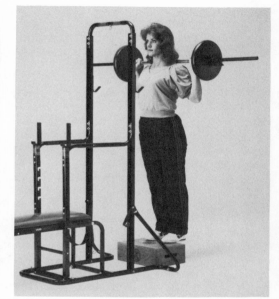

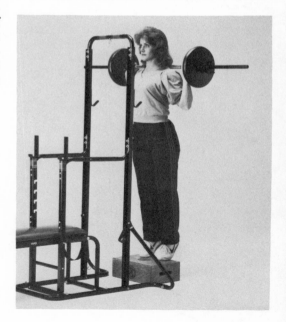

# Jumping Squat

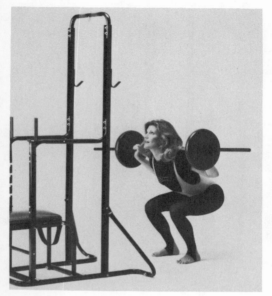

**Muscles worked:** Quadriceps, calves, hamstrings, glutes, lumbars, heart and soul

**Directions:** These are done in exactly the same manner as your regular squats except that at the bottom of the lift when you begin your ascent, you must try to rise upward as quickly as possible, as if you were going after a rebound in basketball. At the top you should come slightly off the ground (or at least up onto your toes) before resetting and starting over again. Make sure to use very light weights, or no weights at all, for this exercise so you can keep from losing your balance when you've finished your jump.

**Tips:** These are great exercise for athletes and others who desire explosiveness and power. However, jumping squats should be done without "bouncing" out of the bottom position. Also, you must use a good flat back throughout the entire lift in order to minimize the chances of a possible injury. You would be well advised to stop after each jump and assume the starting position again before you perform your next repetition.

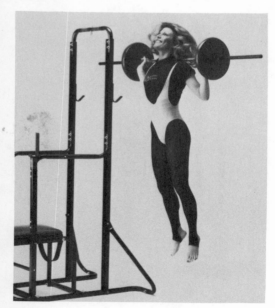

## Upper-Body Exercises

**Muscles worked:** Trapezius, deltoids, biceps

**Directions:** With the bar on the floor in front of you, take a slightly closer than shoulder-width grip — hands spaced about 8 inches apart. Then deadlift the bar, stop, and pull it to the top of your shoulders in a slow, controlled motion. At the top, your elbows should be pulled as high as possible, letting you feel a contraction of the muscles in the shoulders and upper back. Remember to keep your back flat as you lower the bar to arms' length and repeat the movement.

**Tips:** Unlike high pulls, which are done with a wider grip and more explosively, upright rows are to be *controlled* throughout the entire movement — though you should pull the bar up quickly. Don't just jerk it up. Remember to keep your eyes fixed on a point on the opposite wall and maintain a straight back in all parts of the exercise. Don't stop the weight at the top overly long. Pull it up till you feel the contraction (the bar should be at neck level) and then lower it.

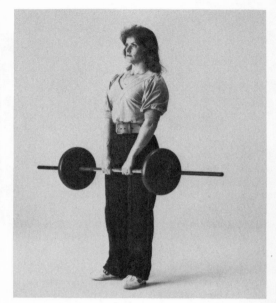

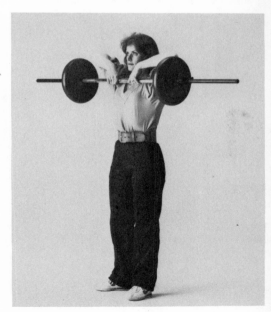

## Standing, or Military, Press

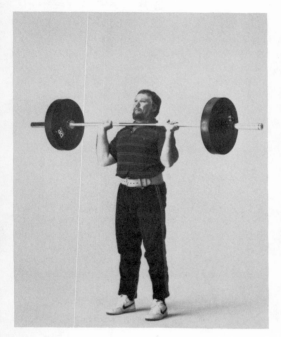

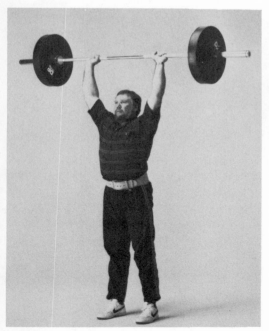

**Muscles worked:** Deltoids and triceps

**Directions:** Place your feet shoulder-width apart and, with an overhand shoulder-width grip, deadlift the bar until it rests against the front of your thighs. Next, bend your knees slightly and pull the bar quickly from your thighs to your shoulders, turning your palms upward at the shoulder so that the bar rests in the palms, across the clavicle area. Anytime you pull the bar from the floor to your shoulders, in one movement, it is said that you have "cleaned" the weight. This simply means that you have lifted the weight "cleanly" — without touching the body — to the final position. In many rural areas, particularly in the South and Southwest, you still hear people speak of someone lifting something "clean over his head." Used this way, "clean" has come to mean "all the way," whereas in the old days it was used to distinguish between a "clean" lift and one called a "continental" lift, in which the bar touched the body one or more times on the way up.

Anyway, now that the bar is at your shoulders, push it straight up, keeping it close to your face until it is locked at arms' length overhead. Lower the bar to your chest and repeat the movement for the desired number of repetitions. Once you've completed the set, lower the bar to your thighs, bend your legs, keep your back flat, and return the bar to the floor.

**Tips:** Stability is important in this lift, so make sure you have on good sturdy shoes. Clinching or contracting the muscles of the thighs and hips also helps. You should also wear your lifting belt. You can bend back a bit as the bar goes up, but don't bend so far back that you are no longer basically "upright." You can cause undue back strain by bending back too far. You'll also not get as much benefit from the presses. Finally, make sure the ceiling is high enough to do these. A young friend of ours in Canada once put a sizeable hole in his family's living room ceiling when he decided to show his girlfriend how much he could lift over his head.

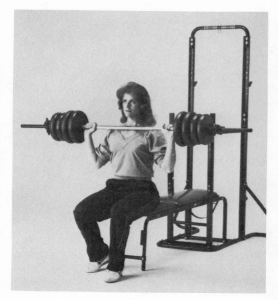

**Muscles worked:** Deltoids and triceps

**Directions:** Seated presses are done the same way standing presses are except you are seated on your bench. To get the bar to your shoulders, you have two options. You can "clean" the weight as you did for the standing press and then sit down to do the actual presses, or you can straddle the bench, facing the bench-press racks, and take the bar off those. In either case make sure that you straighten your back before you begin your presses.

**Tips:** Many lifters prefer to do seated presses because they feel the seated position allows them to "isolate" the muscles in the arms and shoulders, making them do the lift more strictly. There *is* less chance to cheat by dipping your knees or by bending backward to help you get the weight up when you're seated, and thus many bodybuilders favor the seated position. One thing that's commonly done to insure a straight-backed position is for a lifter's training partner to sit back to back with him, thereby providing a brace. The person lifting the weight can often lift quite a bit more weight braced in this manner and you might want to try it if the lift seems awkward to you. Don't be surprised if you have to use less weight in the seated press than you can lift in the standing press. Even though you plant your feet as firmly as possible you won't have quite as much leverage for the lift, seated, as you had standing — though you'll isolate the deltoid muscles more completely and, perhaps, get better results.

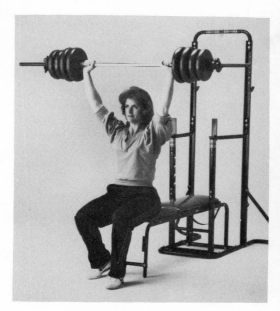

# The Shoulder Shrug

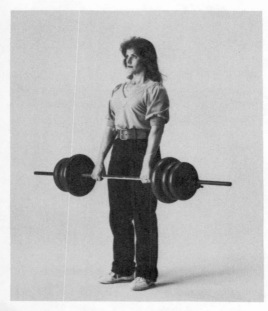

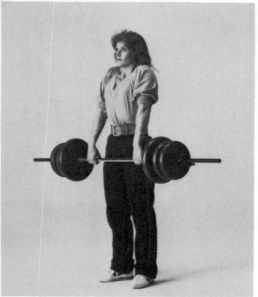

**Muscles worked:** Trapezius primarily, though the other muscles of the shoulder girdle have some involvement

**Directions:** Deadlift a relatively heavy barbell using an overhand grip, with your hands and feet about shoulder-width apart. Keeping your arms straight, pull your shoulders upward as high as you can, contracting the muscles in the back of your neck and shoulders. Try to touch your ears with your shoulders before you relax and repeat the movement for the required number of repetitions.

**Tips:** Shoulder shrugs are an exercise used by a lot of powerlifters and Olympic weightlifters who want additional pulling strength. They directly work the large, triangular trapezius muscles located at the very top of your back. The "traps" are important in all pulling movements such as deadlifts or cleans of one sort or another, or even hauling out the garbage. It is best to use fairly heavy weights when doing shrugs, as the relative shortness of the movement and the power of the muscle group both allows and requires large poundages. Wear your hand straps when doing these so you can concentrate on the contraction at the top and not on your grip.

Doing shrugs is very important to your general fitness. The trapezius muscles are the wheelhorses of the shoulder-girdle group that holds the shoulders in an upright, nonrounded position. As we age, we all have a tendency to slump more, but working the trapezius muscles with shrugs and other "pulling" movements will dramatically offset that tendency. If you do incorporate them into your program, you may also want to try a slight variation from time to time. Once you have pulled the shoulders as high as possible, roll them backward and downward (sort of like the cancan girls used to do for Maurice Chevalier) before starting the upward contraction again. This rolling motion helps to develop the back of the "traps" as well as the top, and will work your shoulder girdle over a slightly greater range of motion.

**Muscles worked:** Deltoids, triceps, trapezius

**Directions:** Start with the bar resting across the front of your shoulders as if you were ready to do a standing press. Then press the bar overhead and lower it to the back, bringing it down to the base of the neck. You will need to bring your head forward half an inch or so as the bar comes down, but as much as possible maintain your flat-backed position whether seated or standing. From the base of the neck, push the bar upward to arms' length and lower it again for each repetition. The bar should be directly overhead when your elbows are locked. After you've finished your reps, lower the last one to your chest and replace the bar on the floor or bench.

**Tips:** You should use a wider hand spacing for these than you would for regular presses. Try not to go *too* wide, however, as you decrease the range of motion.

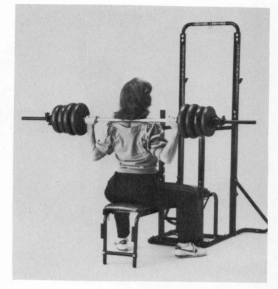

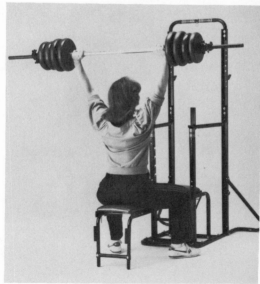

# The Close-Grip Bench Press

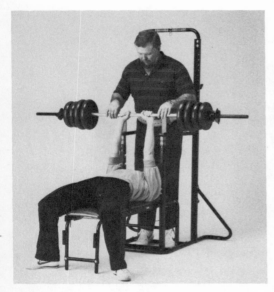

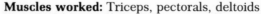

**Muscles worked:** Triceps, pectorals, deltoids

**Directions:** Lie on the bench with your feet flat on the floor and take an overhand grip, your hands 6 to 8 inches apart on the bar. Have your spotter lift the bar off the rack to you, then lower it to your chest to the same place you touch when you do your regular bench presses. Push the bar upward to arms' length and repeat for the desired number of repetitions.

**Tips:** Close-grip bench presses are an assistance exercise to develop the front part of the deltoids as well as the triceps muscles in the back of your arm. The closer you grip your hands, the more the workload is thrown onto the triceps muscles and away from the pectorals and, with an extremely close grip, even away from the deltoids. If you add "close grips" to your routine, do them after your benches and before any other triceps exercises. Because the triceps is a relatively small muscle, it tires rather quickly and often dramatically when isolated in this way. So, be sure to have your spotter stand by when you do these, as the muscles often "pump" so quickly that you can fail *unexpectedly* with a weight, which is, of course, dangerous without a spotter. As with regular benches, keep your hips, feet, and shoulders stationary during the lifts.

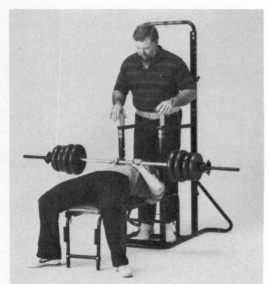

**Muscles worked:** Triceps

**Directions:** Using an overhand grip, with the hands approximately six inches apart, place the barbell overhead in the locked-out position of a standing press. Then, keeping your arms close to your head, lower the barbell slowly behind your head, *keeping the elbows pointed upward and the upper arms in a fixed position.* When the bar touches the back of your neck, return the bar to the locked-out position. At the completion of the repetitions, return the bar to the floor as you would for a standing press, or to the bench.

**Tips:** The most important thing to remember in the performance of this lift is to keep the upper arms stationary. Keep your elbows pointed at the ceiling and your arms close to your head in order to place the full stress on the triceps in the back of the upper arm. Don't try to use a lot of weight at first; learn to do this lift properly, from the beginning, before you add poundage.

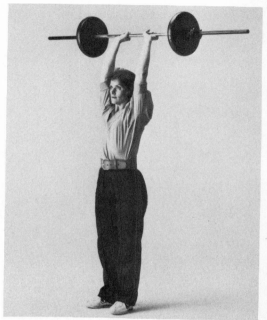

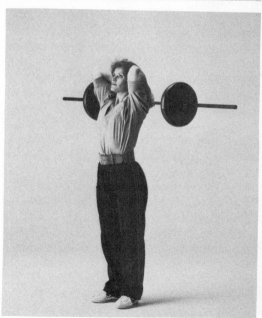

# The Front Raise

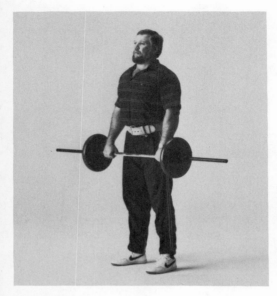

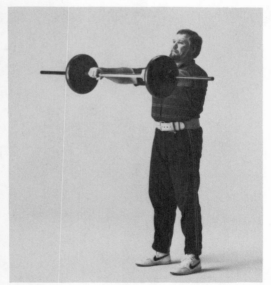

**Muscles worked:** Deltoids

**Directions:** Take the bar in an overhand shoulder-width grip and deadlift it so that it rests across the tops of your thighs. Then, with your elbows bent *ever so slightly,* raise the bar from thigh to shoulder height so that your arms are extended directly in front of you. Slowly return the bar to the thighs and repeat for the desired number of repetitions.

**Tips:** You should feel this exercise in the front of your shoulders, where the deltoid muscles are prominent. Move the bar quickly to the top, without jerking, then control it on the way down. Maintain a good rhythm through the repetitions and keep your back straight and head up at all times. This is an isolation exercise, meaning that you are working primarily one muscle (rather than a group of muscles), so don't be surprised if you tire quickly. Women, in fact, may want to start by holding a 5- or 10-pound barbell plate in their hands rather than using the exercise bar, which normally weighs around 20 pounds. To use the plate, hold it in front of you with your palms facing one another. Grasp the sides of the plate, which should be perpendicular to the floor. As with the bar, don't raise the plate past shoulder height; you lose the stress on the deltoid when you do, and what we're trying for here is a concentration on that particular muscle.

**Muscles worked:** Serratus, latissimus dorsi, triceps

**Directions:** Grasping a barbell in both hands, position yourself on a bench with your feet on the floor. Put the barbell at arms' length over your chest and lower it behind your head, with your arms almost completely straight. Take a full breath of air before you begin to lower the bar and hold your breath until the bar is behind your head. Then, shift gears, moving the bar upward in the same arc as you exhale. At the top, take another full breath and repeat the movement for the desired number of repetitions.

**Tips:** You should expect to feel a pulling sensation in your chest as you do this exercise. Pullovers are designed to stretch and lift the rib cage and improve your posture, as well as to exercise the jagged little serratus muscles that lie along the sides of your chest and help you with your breathing. You don't need to use very heavy weights, but you do need to remember to keep your arms fairly straight. A slight bend is necessary — but make it very slight so that you get maximum stretch. Pullovers can also be done with a barbell plate.

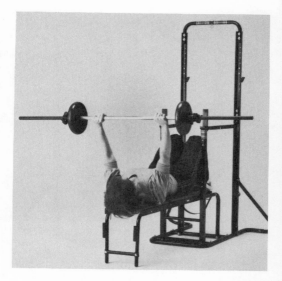

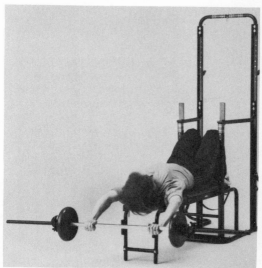

# The Bent-Arm Pullover

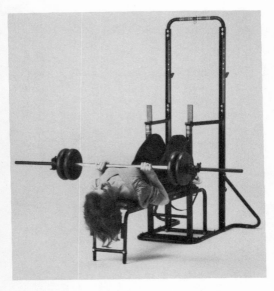

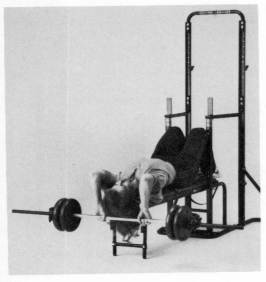

**Muscles worked:** Latissimus dorsi, pectorals, triceps, and deltoids

**Directions:** Lie on the bench with your feet at the end where the uprights are and extend your head over the opposite end. If this proves uncomfortable, bend your knees and place your feet where your head would normally rest when you do bench presses. Have your spotter hand the bar to your chest. Take an overhand grip with your hands about 8 inches apart. Your palms should be facing away from your eyes and your arms should be close to the sides of your body. Push the bar slightly off the chest and back over your face in an arc to a point just slightly below the back of your head. Return the bar to the chest in the same semicircular pattern, being sure that the bar goes about 2 inches above your face as you return to the starting position. Repeat for the desired number of repetitions.

**Tips:** As you can see, the close proximity of the bar to your face makes this a somewhat dangerous lift. Make sure your spotter is close at hand when you do these and use a weight you can handle with confidence. And never force the bar further behind your head than is comfortable. At the bottom, the elbows should still be bent. The object is not to touch the floor but to move the bar through a semicircular range of motion.

**Muscles worked:** Triceps

**Directions:** Lie on the bench with your feet at the end where your head would normally be, with your feet either resting on the floor or with your knees bent, feet on the bench. Have your spotter hand the bar to your chest. Take a slightly less than shoulder-width grip with your palms facing toward your face. Push the bar to arms' length, lock your shoulders, and slowly lower the bar down *behind the head* by bending the elbows until the bar is an inch or two below the very top of your head. With the upper arms fixed, reverse the movement and repeat for the desired number of repetitions. Remember, concentrate on keeping the elbows close together, the upper arm stationary.

**Tips:** Keep your upper arms in a fixed angle with your torso as much as possible. Your elbows should be over your mouth, approximately. Always lower the bar behind the head — not to your nose or forehead — as the quick fatiguing of the triceps muscles makes such variations dangerous. As with other triceps extension exercises, keep the weights fairly light and the form good and you'll soon see the results of your efforts. It will keep the arms firm and reduce the flabbiness along the back of the upper arm.

**Variations:** This can also be done in exactly the same manner but with a pronated (overhand) grip rather than the supinated one just described above. This slightly changes the effect of the exercise, and more weight can be used. However, some people find that the exercise as shown in the photos places less strain on their elbow joints; we prefer it.

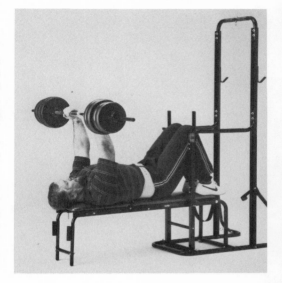

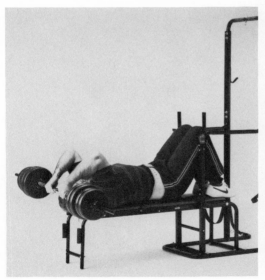

# The Curl

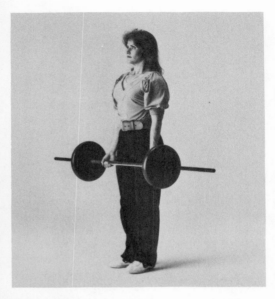

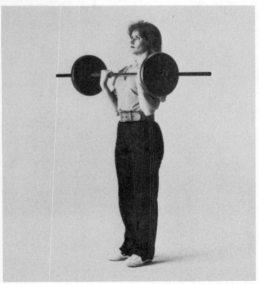

**Muscles worked:** Biceps, brachialis, and related flexors

**Directions:** Grasp the bar in a supinated (underhand) grip, roughly shoulder width, and place it across the front of your thighs while standing erect. Keep your elbows against your body and move the weight upward through a semicircular range of motion until it rests against your chest and your elbows are fully bent. Lower the weight slowly to the bottom position — keeping your elbows against your sides — and repeat for the number of repetitions needed.

**Tips:** Barbell curls should be done while standing and with a weight light enough to be moved through the range of motion using *only* your arm muscles — not the thrust of your hips or legs. Curls should be done in a controlled manner with the eyes fixed on a point on the opposite wall and the back and legs stationary. Don't jerk the weight upward. Let the lift come from the biceps, where you want to see the effects of the training. If you have trouble remaining stationary, brace your back against a wall or post. Also, be sure to start the curl with your wrists. You should never let your hand or knuckles get lower than your wrist. Notice how the wrists are "cocked," or flexed, in the photo.

**Variations:** Reverse curls are done in the same manner, using an overhand or pronated grip. Take a shoulder-width grip and move the bar through the full range of motion. Again, let the generating force come from the biceps, not the back and legs. Reverse curls place more emphasis on the brachialis muscle near the elbow and are a good addition for those who want exercise in both the upper and lower arm. They are also a very good exercise for golfers and people who play racquet sports.

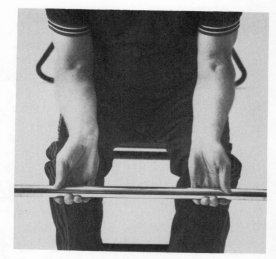

**Muscles worked:** All of the flexor muscles of your forearms and your fingers

**Directions:** Sit upright at the end of your bench with your forearms resting on your thighs, the bar in an underhand grip, your hands extending past your knees. Bend the wrist backward, allowing the bar to descend for several inches, and then "curl" the weight upward, bending the wrist as fully as possible at the top while keeping the forearm securely on the thighs. You should feel a sharp contraction at the top of the lift before you return to the bottom position and start again.

**Tips:** Keep the forearms firmly on your thighs. Don't hurry these, just pump out the reps. As with calf work, wrist curls and other forearm work should be done with two or three times the repetitions used on other exercises because the forearm muscles have a higher percentage of slow-twitch fibers and seem to respond better to higher repetitions.

**Variations:** These can also be done with an overhand grip, thus placing the emphasis on the extensor muscles of the forearm. If you'd like to strengthen your grip as well, there's another variation that's excellent. Using the underhand grip described initially, allow the bar to descend to the bottom position as usual. However, instead of curling the weight immediately, allow the hand to open, letting the bar roll down into your *curled* fingers before rolling it back up into your palm and doing the rest of the curl as usual. Be sure to use moderate weights with this variation until you get used to opening the hand at the bottom.

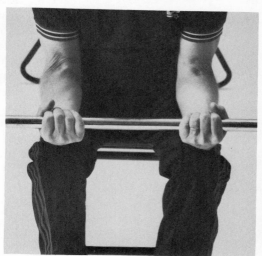

# Abdominal Work

No workout — even a basic one — would be complete without a little "ab" work. Take the time to do it because the 10 minutes or so you'll spend each day on your abdominal exercises will be among the most important minutes in your entire workout. A trim, firm waistline can make a greater difference in your appearance than any other change you and the weights can manifest. But you must exercise restraint at the table for your ab work to have its best effect. No matter how much you train the abdominal muscles, you won't see a lot of difference if you continue bad nutritional habits. Both men and women store a large portion of their fat reserve on the abdominal wall and though you can strengthen the underlying muscles, you can't "tighten" fat.

Besides improved appearance, there is another reason to train the abdomen — especially as you age. Our internal organs are situated inside a cavity primarily composed of muscle, and if these muscles are not kept strong and resilient, the internal organs will not be held in proper position and imbalances will occur. In some cases the organs even function less efficiently as the abdominal wall continues to weaken with advanced age and as gravity continues to make the stomach protrude.

A secondary result of a weakened abdominal wall is the condition known as lordosis — being swaybacked. If the spinal erector muscles are not counterbalanced by strong abdominal muscles, the greater lumbar strength can cause the pelvis to tilt, causing back pain and an even more protruding stomach.

Many different muscles make up the abdominal sheath, though for simplicity's sake most trainers say they're working the "upper abdomen," the "lower abdomen," or the "obliques" (sides). These muscle groups can be trained in two ways — with or without added weight. Adding weight to these movements by holding a barbell plate in your hands or by using a pair of leg weights (not part of your basic equipment, but a good investment nonetheless) will make the muscles respond more quickly, just as adding weight to a deep knee bend will make the muscles in your legs and hips strengthen more quickly than if you did the squats without added weight. As a beginner, however, don't worry about adding any weight to your ab exercises until you can do at least 25 repetitions, for at least 3 sets. Then, you can either add weight or you can increase the number of sets or increase the number of repetitions per set. Adding weights, of course, takes the least amount of time. However, high-repetition waist work has much to recommend it, since it will not only tone and strengthen the abdominal muscles but will whittle away extra calories at the same time, creating even more of a change in the way that new pair of jeans fastens.

Below we've listed several basic abdominal exercises. As with all other exercises, start out slowly, doing only a few repetitions until your body adjusts. Your abdominal muscles have just as much capacity for soreness as any other muscle group and they need a chance to adapt to the new workload just as your legs and arms do. We recommend that you start with one or two of three different abdominal exercises — the bent-leg sit-up, the leg raise, and the standing twist. You should do 2 sets of 10 repetitions for the first week. Some of you will be unable to do a full set of 10, so do as many as possible, then rest a few minutes and go again. Even though you'll decrease reps on your *lifting* exercises during the cycle, you should *increase* the reps on your waist work, therefore burning more calories. If you have the time, try to get to the point at which you can do least 3 sets of 25 repetitions in the sit-up, 3 sets of 25 in the leg raise, and 3 sets of 100 in the standing twist *per workout*. When you've reached this level of abdominal fitness you can add an additional exercise and up your *total* number of repetitions so that you're doing around 600 repetitions per day. We know this sounds like a lot, and it is, but the abdomen can stand a lot of high-rep work. Play the radio or the stereo to help keep your mind busy. If you're short of time, however, or bore easily, add weight and not reps.

# The Bent-Leg Sit-up

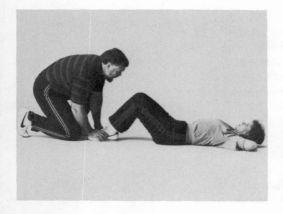

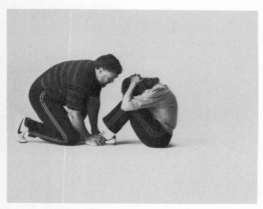

**Muscles worked:** Upper abdomen and hip flexors

**Directions:** Lie on the floor and secure your feet under the edge of a couch or under a loaded barbell, or have your training partner hold them flat on the floor. Lie so that your knees are bent at least to a 90-degree angle, your legs are together, and your fingers are laced with your palms against the back of your head. Tuck your chin against your chest and slowly raise your body upward by "curling" the torso until your elbows touch — or closely approach — your knees. Don't jerk your body off the floor and don't swing your arms to help unless you must in order to sit up. Try to keep your fingers locked behind your head and concentrate on using your stomach muscles to do the lift. Return your body to the floor in the same curling motion. Repeat for the desired number of reps.

**Tips:** If you can't do a full set of 10 with your hands behind your head, cross your arms and place them on your chest, holding a shoulder in each hand. This makes the movement easier, but as soon as you can do 10, move your hands back behind your head. Make sure to do sit-ups on a carpet or pad to protect your backside and make sure that your feet are held down firmly. Always do sit-ups with the knees bent, *never with your legs extended straight in front of you.* We were both taught in gym class to do them that way, but physiologists now feel that straight-leg sit-ups place undue strain on the lower back and can cause injuries. Keep your knees bent, please.

**Variations:** To add weight, place a barbell plate behind your head and grasp it firmly with both hands. Or, hold a plate against your chest in the crossed-arms position. Another excellent variation is to twist at the top of the sit-up, alternating right elbow to left knee, left elbow to right knee. You can either do one sit-up per twist, or you can come up and twist to both the left and the right before lowering yourself to the floor.

**Muscles worked:** Lower abdomen

**Directions:** Lie on your bench and grasp either the bench itself or the uprights behind you. Position your hips so that they are at the very end of the bench, your slightly *bent* legs extending away from you. Slowly raise your legs above your body until you feel the movement become easier. Don't go past perpendicular before slowly lowering the legs back to horizontal. Repeat for the desired number of reps.

**Tips:** Do these *slowly* — both upward and downward. You should feel a definite pulling sensation throughout the movement, especially as your legs return to the starting position. If you feel any discomfort in the lower back, place your hands, palms down, underneath your hips or use a small pillow to change the angle. There is no need to pull the legs past perpendicular, as you then have no stress on the abdomen. You really don't even need to go *that* high.

**Variations:** Most physiologists now recommend that you do leg raises with your knees slightly bent to reduce the possibility of lower-back strain. We concur. However, once you fix the angle of your legs don't change it. Keep them in the same slightly bent position throughout the entire movement. Don't pull the knees to the chest. The best variation for leg raises is to do them on an incline. Place the end of your bench on some bricks or a cement block and grasp the uprights behind your head as you do the same slow up and down movements. The incline position adds additional stress to the lower abdomen. To make these an even more intense exercise, add a pair of light leg weights.

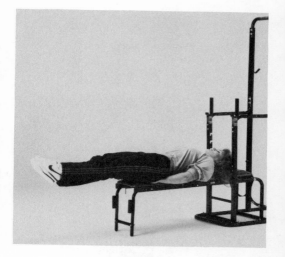

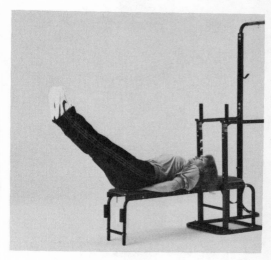

# The Standing Twist

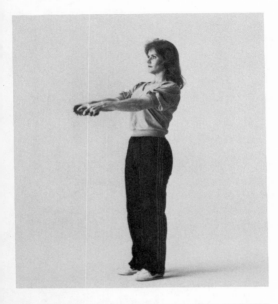

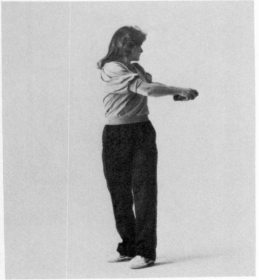

**Muscles worked:** Sides of the abdomen

**Directions:** Hold a 5-pound barbell plate in your hands, with your slightly bent arms almost fully extended in front of you, about 3 inches above waist level. Grasping the plate firmly, twist your upper body from side to side without moving your feet or hips. As you turn, try to look as far behind you as possible and attempt to turn slightly further with each repetition while maintaining your same foot position. A complete twist to both sides counts as one repetition.

We learned this exercise from Bruce Randall, the former Mr. Universe who, because of job pressures, had to find ways to train while on the road. Though simple, the exercise *is* effective, especially when done in high repetitions. Bruce advises you to keep the plate just slightly above the waist and to try and look over your opposite shoulder as you twist to the back. We saw him taking a workout recently and he did 2000 of these, *without stopping,* as his final exercise for the day.

**Tips:** The more traditional way to do standing twists (or seated twists, for that matter) is to use a light broomstick or wooden rod about 5 feet long placed across the shoulders. You can also use light barbells for your twists, though most bodybuilders argue that adding weight to the twist movement causes the oblique muscles to thicken, making the waist appear wider.

**Variations:** The Bent-Forward Twist is done by holding a broomstick across the shoulders. With the legs almost straight, bend at the waist until your upper body is parallel to the floor. Then, twist your torso from side to side as far as possible, keeping the legs in the same position throughout.

**Muscles worked:** Lower abdomen

**Directions:** Knee-ins can be done in three different ways: seated on the very end of a flat bench, lying on a flat bench, or lying on an incline bench. To do them seated on the end of the bench, sit on the end of your bench (where else!) and grasp the bench behind your hips. Lean your upper body slightly back and extend your legs straight in front of you as shown in the illustration. Then, bend your knees and pull your legs as close to your chest as possible. Lower the legs — toes pointed — and repeat for the desired number of reps. Lying knee-ins (both on the flat bench and on the incline) are done in the same way. Extend your feet away from your torso, toes pointed, and pull them as close to your chest as you can, as shown in the accompanying photos. On the incline bench (put your bench up on your calf block), grasp the uprights firmly and position your legs in the same general way as in the lying knee-in.

**Tips:** These are considered a low-intensity abdominal exercise — meaning you need to do a lot of them for them to do you much good, since at least 50 percent of the "pull" in these come from the hip flexors, not the abdominals. However, if you do them at the end of the workout — after you've done your three main abdominal exercises — they can be beneficial in providing that last, and crucial, pump.

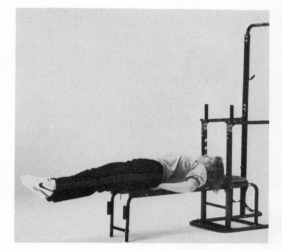

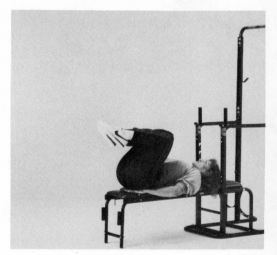

# The Crunch

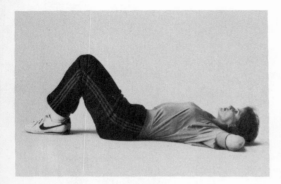

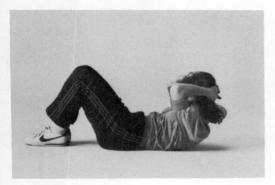

**Muscles worked:** Upper abdomen

**Directions:** Lie on the floor with your knees bent and feet secured as if you were going to do a bent-leg sit-up. Tuck your chin against your chest, place your hands behind your head and roll or curl your head and shoulders — only your head and shoulders — off the floor. At the top of the crunch, before you "uncurl" and repeat the movement, you should feel a tightening sensation directly below your rib cage.

**Tips:** Many physiologists feel that crunches and their several kinfolk are the most effective exercises available for strengthening the upper abdomen. Crunches are intense — they require good concentration — and should be done with a pause at the top of each repetition so that the stomach muscles can be fully contracted. Remember to roll just the head and shoulders off the floor and to tuck the chin against the chest on every rep. This exercise is especially recommended for pregnant women.

**Variations:** A highly effective variation of the crunch movement can be done by lying on the floor with your lower legs resting on the top of your bench. Place your hips as close to the side of the bench as possible and perform your crunches in the same way you would have done them with your feet on the floor. Three-time Mr. Olympia Frank Zane is especially fond of this variation and even recommends that the isolation be accentuated by raising the hips at the same time as you raise the shoulders. Crunches can also be done with added weight; hold the plates either behind the head or in front, on the chest. You can also make them even more difficult by alternately crossing your bent legs. This throws even more work onto the abdominal muscles.

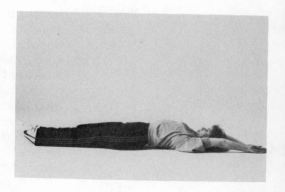

**Muscles worked:** Both the upper and lower abdomen

**Directions:** Lie flat on your back on the floor with your hands extended backward over your head and your toes pointed. Then, and quickly, simultaneously raise your slightly bent legs to perpendicular and pull your upper body completely off the floor — attempting to touch your toes, momentarily, with your fingertips. Return to the starting position and repeat for the desired number of repetitions.

**Tips:** This is an *advanced* abdominal exercise. Don't try these till you've developed good basic abdominal strength and even then be prepared to be sore for the first couple of times you try them. Their degree of difficulty comes from the fact that you're using both your upper and lower abdominals at the same time, something few other abdominal exercises can offer. Don't be surprised if it seems hard to learn this movement. They're hard for everyone, and even now, when we've done them for years, we still find ourselves out of rhythm on these when our abdominals are already fatigued. If you do add these, do them as your first abdominal exercise to give yourself a fair chance at them. Also, if you find them at all uncomfortable, just skip them. But, don't skip *all* your ab work. Do it, even if you need to keep it *basic*.

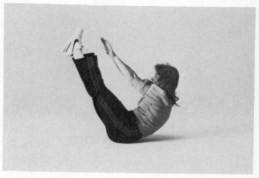

If you have time, you may wish to add a few exercises to your workouts to concentrate on particular areas of your body. Women often feel they need more leg and hip work; men often want to add size to their shoulders and arms, which is why we've included all these exercises — *all of which can be done with your two basic pieces of equipment.* If you do want to expand your workout, do a little experimentation and then select one extra exercise, maybe even two, to go with each one of the Basic Three. We suggest that you increase the number of exercises you do slowly, just as you worked into the program in the beginning slowly, so that both your body and your mind have time to get used to the extra demands of the increased work load.

Here's a program you might try that is predicated on the Big Three, but expanded to include additional exercises that work the various major muscle groups in slightly different ways. Although the order of the Big Three is the same, the "assistance" exercises for each of the three movements are done immediately following so that the already warmed-up muscles will get the full benefit of the extra work. The number of repetitions and periodization approach would be used in the same way as for the basic program: 5 sets of 10 for four weeks, 5 sets of 5 for four weeks, 5 sets of 3 for two weeks and then two weeks off the weights before beginning all over again.

**Expanded Workout**

Squats
Lunges (See page 156 for a complete description.)
Bench Presses
Seated Presses (See page 163 for a complete description.)
Bent-Forward Rowing Motions
Curls (See page 172 for a complete description.)
Bent-Leg Sit-ups
Leg Raises

As you become familiar with both the exercises themselves and the way your body responds to the weight work, you can experiment with different exercises on different cycles to see which combination will produce the results you want.

# 18 / Training at Home with the Works

THIS chapter presupposes that you have either trained before or that you have done the basic workout outlined in the previous chapter for at least one full twelve-week periodization cycle and, having done that, have decided to invest in a fully equipped home gym that will allow you to do a wider variety of exercises than you can do with just your bar and bench. It also presupposes that you've decided to set aside a room or part of a room that will be a permanent workout area. Finally, this chapter presupposes that you are neither rich nor poor and that you have a space in mind that is smaller than a basketball court and larger than a broom closet.

## Free Weights or Machines

The key to resistance training is to provide stress for the muscles as they go through a range of motion. The stress or resistance can be provided by another body part, a barbell, a rock, an ankle weight, or by one of the many machines on the market such as the Nautilus and Universal machines. Machines, of course, aren't new, and there is an old and dishonorable tradition of quackery in the exercise-device field. Many people, in fact, have built machines with more of an eye to building their bank account than building the bodies of the folks who buy or use the machines, yet machines exist that are safe and, when used properly, result-producing.

At present, a huge controversy is raging in coaching and physical fitness circles as to the relative benefits of exercise on machines and exercise work using "free weights," and while many of the machines in question are too expensive for most people to consider for home use, we'd like to briefly explain the controversy because *some* machines, while not costing an arm and a leg, can help you develop those two body parts and lots more besides.

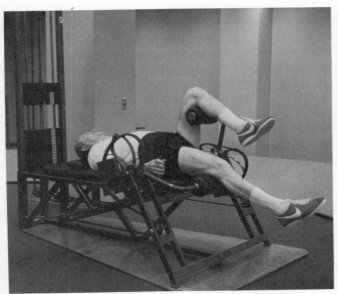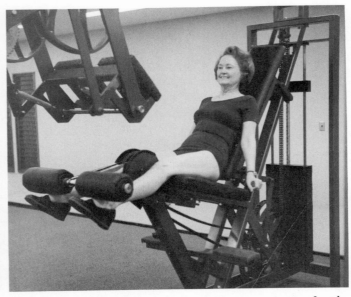

LEFT: *The Nautilus Duo Hip and Back Machine provides full range exercise for the gluteal muscles of the hips.* RIGHT: *Pat Peterson of Atlanta, Georgia, does the Nautilus Leg Extension Machine for her frontal thighs.*

To the credit of machines, many people who probably never would have trained with barbells have become devoted fitness buffs since the invention of the Nautilus machines and the extraordinary promotional campaign that their originator, Arthur Jones, has mounted over the last fifteen years. What the Nautilus machines and other similar systems offer is a relatively safe, clean, sophisticated-looking method of resistance training. Part of America's fascination with Nautilus stems from the futuristic look of the machines. Whereas barbells have long been associated with dirty jocks and narcissistic he-men, the Nautilus machines look sleek, businesslike, and modern. For this reason, perhaps, many women who would never think about training with barbells will jump right into a Nautilus program. Self-image, of course, does have a lot to do with our willingness to start and continue an exercise program, and all the evidence seems to indicate that the Nautilus or machine "image" has a lot to offer in this regard.

One thing some physiologists feel Nautilus and other machines don't offer, however, is freedom of motion in all the standard weight-training movements; an example sports scientists often cite to demonstrate the physiological differences in working out on a machine as opposed to working with a barbell is the case of the bench press. Many of you will have had the experience of doing bench presses on a multistation Universal machine, and if you recall the experience, you'll no doubt remember that when you had the handlebars in the bottom position for the press the handle did not rest on the chest. Depending on your body size, and the height of the bench you were using, the bars might have been anywhere from 2 inches below to 3 inches above the top of your rib cage. Because of this, if they didn't reach your chest, you moved the weight through a lesser range of motion on the machine than you would have with a regular barbell.

Another important difference lies in the pattern of motion that the bar travels. This pattern is always the same on the machine, while on a bench with free weights the upward and downward pattern will vary *according to your own body's structure, your grip, and your own desire to vary the pattern*. Some bodybuilders, for instance, do part of their benches to the upper chest or even to their neck to get a full "stretch" in the pectoral area — a difficult, sometimes impossible, thing to do on some machines. Another factor that physiologists feel makes machine bench presses, for instance, less effective than the barbell bench press is that a number of stabilizing muscles used to balance the barbell as it is lowered to the chest and lifted for the repetitions are only minimally involved when benching on a machine because there is no "balance" to worry about.

Despite their drawbacks, some machines do have advantages that you may want to consider for your home gym. For one thing, they are relatively safe because there's no way the bar can fall on you or pin you. And if you have children and would like to involve them in training, a machine can be a good, safe way to get kids started. For another thing, machines make it easier to change the weights, which is helpful if you're training alone or with someone who has a different strength level than your own. Also, there are some exercises that simply cannot be done using only barbells and dumbbells. From the earliest days, some exercises have always been done using pulley systems and weight stacks. Lat pulldowns, for instance, simply cannot be duplicated by a barbell nor can some of the exercises for the inner and outer thigh that are done by using a low cable attached to the ankle. Our suggestion is that you go to a sporting-goods department and take a look at one of the lower-priced machines made for home use. Ask to try it out and see if it feels the way you think it should.

The machine you'll see in the exercise photos accompanying this section consists of a weight stack and an assortment of handles and attachments that will allow you to do quite a few different exercises. It comes fixed with several different pulleys so that cables can be used to allow such exercises as lat pulldowns, seated cable rows, leg lifts using the ankle strap, and tricep extensions. At the time of printing, this machine sold for less than $300. Heavier-duty machines cost more, of course, and if you can afford a better machine, we urge you to buy it, as it should last longer and you'll not "outgrow" it or wear it out. In the exercise section that accompanies this chapter we've tried to give some examples of how exercises can be done with this device. Remember, when you begin to invest in exercise equipment, think carefully about what you really need. Then, buy the very best equipment that you can afford. If you have a good bankroll, we strongly recommend buying a heavy-duty lat machine with seated pulley attachment, a heavy-duty cable set-up for leg work and cross-chest cable work, a chinning bar, a heavy-duty leg-curl/leg-extension machine and a heavy-duty leg-press machine. By "heavy duty" we mean heavily constructed equipment such as you'd find in a regular, commercial gym. Taken together, the machines will work far better than any inexpensive multipurpose home gym, but they do cost more. In short, if you've got the funds — and the space — it's obvious that you'd get more results and pleasure from the individual machines.

## Benches and Squat Racks

Regardless of whether you decide to invest in any sort of machine for part of your resistance training, there are other items without which no fully equipped home gym would be complete. The first is a combination flat and incline bench that may or may not also include a set of squat racks attached to the rear. The model we've pictured in the accompanying exercise photos is a relatively inexpensive, designed-for-home-use model that includes an attachment for doing leg curls and leg extensions. If you've already purchased a bench that adjusts into an incline, what you need to shop for now is a pair of sturdy squat racks. Simple as this sounds, regular sporting goods and department stores generally don't sell freestanding squat racks — they're almost always attached to a bench of some sort. But get the freestanding racks if you can — they're much better. If there's no one in your area with a pair for sale, and no one who manufactures gym equipment, call your local health spa and they'll generally let you know what's available. But make sure, whether you're buying squat stands alone or a combination bench-incline bench-squat rack, that your squat racks can be adjusted so that you can take the bar off at a height about an inch or so below your shoulders. If other members of your family are also going to train, make sure the racks can be adjusted to their heights. As for the incline bench, the more positions or angles possible, the better. Almost all incline benches adjust to three or four different angles, though we've seen some that don't adjust at all. The different angles possible on an adjustable bench allow the muscles to be worked in slightly different ways; the effect of the exercise changes when you change the angle of the incline, and it helps prevent boredom of either the mind or the body.

## Barbells

If you made it through the first twelve weeks with your basic exercise set and bench, you probably noticed that while perfectly functional, the smaller, less expensively made exercise sets do have a few disadvantages, especially when compared to a larger set of weights. For one thing, you can't get much over 200 pounds on the bar because of the thickness of the vinyl-covered plates. For another, the shorter height of the plates puts the bar in a lower and less than ideal starting position for the deadlift and other pulling movements. And if you're a man, you may have felt that the gripping surface of the bar was too narrow when you squatted or benched; you may have found your hands butted up against the sides of the plates, making it uncomfortable for you, especially in the squat. And you may have discovered that the collars holding the plates on the bar sometimes don't tighten as effectively as they should and so the plates slip at inopportune times. These are the common complaints one hears about the smaller, less expensive weight sets, and there's a ring of truth to each.

So, if you can spring for good, heavy-duty equipment that'll last you the rest of your life, go ahead and buy yourself an Olympic set, such as the one shown in the previous chapter. They do have advantages. The plate height is better for exercises that begin with the bar on the floor, you can load more weight on the bar, and the greater length of the bar (7 feet) allows you to experiment with a wide variety of hand spacings; but the most important difference between the two types of sets is in the way Olympic-style bars revolve as you lift the weights. Whereas exercise sets consist of a steel bar with a metal tube, or sleeve, that fits over the bar for your hands to grip, an Olympic set is constructed so that the gripping surface *is* the bar itself. Etched into the bar is a heavy crosshatch pattern called "knurling," which assists you in gripping the bar tightly. The ends of an Olympic bar — where the plates are placed — are made of a heavy steel cylinder placed over the actual end of the bar so that as you raise the bar the ends don't revolve as the bar in your hand does. This allows you to defeat centrifugal force and makes a tremendous difference in the ease with which a weight can be lifted. This allows the bar to rise directly upward. As we mentioned in the last chapter, there's little to depreciate with a barbell set, so even if at some later date you decide to close down your sweat shop, you'll almost surely be able to sell your set or sets without too much trouble and little or no money loss.

## Dumbbells

You won't believe how many, many exercises you can do with dumbbells. They add more variety to your workout than you would ever have thought possible, and they'll definitely allow you to work your muscles more thoroughly. There are some vinyl-covered composition type dumbbells on the market today that are fine to use, but they don't go much beyond 10 pounds in weight and even women will need more than 10 pounds in many exercises before very long. We suggest that you have metal dumbbells made for you by a welder, or that you purchase them from a gym equipment company in increments of 5 pounds. To make them up, buy the cast-iron barbell plates and then take them to a local welding shop to be made into fixed dumbbells.

If the primary trainer in your gym will be a woman, have a *pair* made for each 5-pound increment up to 40 pounds. For men, we recommend starting with 5-pound increments up to 50 pounds, then 10 pounds up to 80. We realize that sounds like a lot of weights but take our word that they'll get used. As you'll see from the exercise section that accompanies this chapter, you'll be using fairly light weights for some exercises like dumbbell flys, yet for dumbbell rowing motions, you need to use much heavier poundages. And if you do get a wide variety, you'll be better off in the long run. There are adjustable dumbbell sets available that allow you to add plates and change the weight just as you do with barbell sets, and there's nothing wrong with these except that if you include many dumbbell exercises you'll find yourself spending a great deal of time changing plates back and forth — something we've found to be a real nuisance when one of your training objectives is speed. If you do opt for the less expensive route and buy adjustable sets, get at least two pairs so you can set up at least two exercises before you start your training.

**Curl Bar**      This is a specialized piece of equipment used to isolate the biceps and/or triceps muscles more effectively when doing certain exercises, such as the curl and triceps press shown later in this chapter. It was first developed for curling, thus its name. It's not a necessity for your gym, but because of its cambers (it looks sort of like an elongated "W"), it allows you to hold the bar for curls and triceps work in a more comfortable position, and the wrists are not under the same strain as they would be with a straight bar. Curl bars come in several styles and are available for use with either Olympic-style plates or exercise plates. They are fairly inexpensive and most sporting-goods stores sell them.

**Lat Pulldown Machine**      The large latissimus dorsi muscles in the back can be worked fairly effectively using barbell and dumbbell rowing exercises, but you should also have a lat pulldown machine. Lat machines consist of a weight stack and a pulley affixed to the wall so that the bar, which in this case is attached to the cable at the top of the weight stack, can be pulled down to your chest or behind the head while you're seated or kneeling. This allows for almost complete isolation of the lat muscles, the muscles that hold your shoulders back squarely and help your posture so much. In choosing a lat machine for your home, try to find one that includes an additional pulley option at the bottom of the weight stack for seated pulley work. The one we've pictured with the exercises on pages 210 and 211 is set up in this way, giving you greater variety in your training.

**Slant Board**      Doing abdominal work on an incline allows for greater tension on the abdominal muscles and hence faster results. The slant board pictured later in this chapter is adjustable in height and is long enough so that leg raises, which require the entire body to be supported on the board, can be done. There are shorter slant boards available, which, for the most part, are also nonadjustable, but a board of the type we've chosen will be of greater benefit to your training.

Riding an exercise bicycle is an almost painless way to get good cardio-vascular work and it's a perfect adjunct to your weight work. Most physiologists and sports-medicine specialists feel that cycling is safer than jogging (especially for older individuals) because it does not strain the feet, ankles, and back as jogging does with its relentless pounding. Buy the most expensive bike you can afford.

## Exercise Bicycle

Through the years, rubber cable, or "strand" devices of many different sorts have been used to provide resistance. In fact, the aggressively marketed Soloflex machine actually has no weights at all — it is a series of cables that create resistance when the lifter pushes or pulls on the handle. In the old days, cable sets were very popular and hundreds of articles were published about cable training, and "strand pulling" contests were even held in the United States as they still are in Great Britain. But here in the United States, rubber cables or springs fell out of favor with the public, who wanted "real" weights. Over the past five years, cable training has begun to make a comeback, largely among the new breed of fitness-conscious businessmen who can't take their barbells with them on a business trip but *can* slip a pair of cables into their suitcase. There's even a new product on the market called the "Jump Stretch" (see photos this page and next), which carries the principles of cable training even further. The Jump Stretch apparatus pictured consists of a padded board and a series of heavy rubber bands

## Cables/"Jump Stretch"

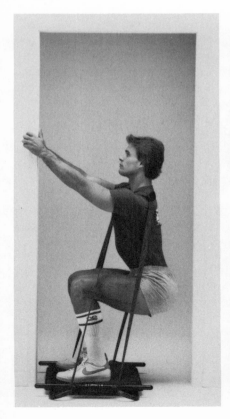
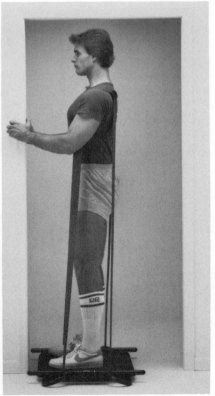

*Jump Stretch Squats. Here's an example of an exercise you can do using the newest form of cable training. By using the heavier bands that come with the set, or by increasing the number of bands used, you can get a good workout for your thighs as you do this version of the squat. Make sure to hold on to something solid as you go up and down.*

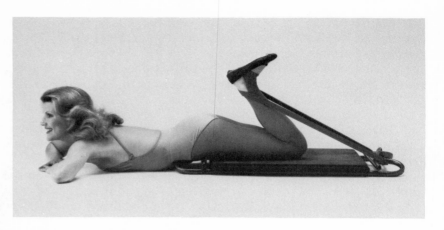

*Leg Curls can also be done with this device, as shown in the photo. Make sure to shorten the bands to get the proper resistance.*

in varying widths and lengths that are used to provide resistance. The bands can be attached to the board in a variety of ways that allow a person to perform squats, pulls, bench-pressing movements, curls, and so forth. We're not about to argue that the Jump Stretch is as effective as, or will ever take the place of, the barbell for producing maximum gains, but the early evidence on the new version of this "old" system of training does indicate that it is effective — especially for leg development. Many world-class athletes use such cables in their leg training. We recently conducted a study on it at the university and eight weeks of twice-weekly training produced a gain in the vertical jump of over two inches in two classes of undergraduates. Not bad at all.

Our main reason for mentioning the system, however, is to suggest it to the person who has to travel periodically yet doesn't like to miss workouts. The system is portable enough to be taken with you in a car if you go away for a few days, say, and while you might not be able to do all the stuff you can do at home with your fully equipped home gym, you won't feel as if you've done NOTHING either. Doing an altered workout is always better than skipping out — unless you're injured or ill.

As for the more traditional cable sets, be they spring or rubber, they too have a place in the traveling man's training. When buying cables, look for a set that's adjustable, making it possible to vary the resistance.

**Miscellaneous**     There are a few other items, familiar to most gyms, that you might wish to include as well. Ankle weights come in several sizes and are good for adding resistance when doing abdominal work and certain leg and hip exercises. We recommend getting two sets: a small set that weighs about two pounds apiece and a larger set in which each weight weighs about five pounds. Hardly anyone would ever need more than this seven-pound total per leg. And try, if you can, to buy ankle weights that have Velcro fasteners. They're easier to put on and they stay more securely in place.

Another addition you might want to consider would be an exercise pad for your warm-up stretches and abdominal work. An extra inch or so of foam rubber can make a significant difference in your comfort, even if your gym area is already carpeted. And it doesn't hurt to have a good jump rope lying around for cardiovascular work or for helping you to warm up before you start to train.

There are several mail-order houses we recommend that deal in a wide variety of exercise equipment and that have long, established reputations for building good, well-designed equipment. *Iron Man* magazine, owned and edited by Peary Rader, always carries 8 to 10 pages of advertising for their own equipment company, called Body Culture, as well as many ads from other companies, and Joe Weider of *Muscle & Fitness* and *Flex* always carries a full line of his own equipment. Another well-run firm is the Jubinville Equipment Company in Holyoke, Massachusetts, and don't forget the granddaddy of them all, the York Barbell Company. Addresses for all these companies can be found on page 320.

As you train, pick up from time to time one of the various lifting publications such as *Iron Man* or *Strength Training for Beauty* or *Muscle & Fitness* and take a look not only at the articles but also at the number of people advertising. There are more products to get you fit than you'd ever have imagined. But be careful. In ordering from mail-order houses, try to use the same discretion you'd use in buying in a store. Is this the best price? What will it cost to have this shipped? And, above all, how long will it take to get delivery? If you order gym equipment through the mail it's a good idea to phone and ask about freight costs and delivery. We've known people who've waited as long as six months for equipment ordered by mail, so make sure you check ahead of time.

## Training with Your New Equipment

Well, you've got it all in place. The new bars and benches have arrived, the lat machine's glowering at you from the corner, and the welder called this morning to let you know that the dumbbells were ready to be picked up. The gym's ready, but are you? Have you thought yet about *how* you're going to train on all this new equipment? Will you continue to do the basic two or three day a week routine we outlined in the last section or are you ready to do more? It's a good idea, before you have that first workout on your new cycle, to take a minute and give some thought to your training objectives. What physiological changes do you want to occur in the next three months? Do you want bigger arms? Smaller hips? Better posture? More endurance? Flatter stomach? Greater strength? All these things? A number of you would no doubt like to have them all. And there's absolutely no reason why you can't have any (or all) of these results with a little bit of work, some discretion with your eating, and the proper choice of exercises. Especially now that you have a fully equipped gym.

To help you, the exercise section that follows is divided into lower-body exercises, upper-body exercises, and abdominal exercises. And, as in Chapter 17, Training at Home with the Basics, we identify the major muscles used during each exercise so you have greater understanding of an exercise's effect. Most of you are probably unfamiliar with at least some of the formal names of the muscles we've talked about so far, such as the "latissimus dorsi" muscles, or the "gastrocnemius," but we hope you've begun to develop an understanding of how the physiology and biomechanics of your muscles determines which exercises you should be doing. Remember, some exercises work some muscle groups, while other exercises stress completely different areas. You can be a successful weight trainer without being a physiologist, but a basic understanding of which muscles are affected by which exercises *is* important. So, make sure to note, as you look at this next group of exercises, which muscles are being stressed, and refer to the muscle chart on page 305.

We've also tried to give you some further tips on how to order equipment, which exercises we've especially liked, and how effective individual exercises are at producing results. So, in looking through the book, check to see which muscles are used by an exercise and read the "Tips" on each one to further your understanding of how it will — or won't — work for you. One final word. The exercises in the basic section (Chapter 17) are not listed there because they are beginner's exercises. They're there because they can be done using only a barbell and bench. Furthermore, these "basic" exercises are among the most result-producing in this entire book, as many of them are multiple-muscle exercises. So don't overlook them in your desire for diversity. Ask any bodybuilder or weightlifter and he'll tell you that the foundation exercises used by all trainees are squats, bench presses, and some form of lat work. Make sure to keep these in your program as well.

Part Four contains detailed information about how to organize your training after you've gone through *at least one basic cycle* and one "expanded" basic routine as we explained in the last chapter. Then, if you wish to try a more difficult or personally tailored routine, do so only when you feel you've developed good endurance and recovery powers.

## Upper-Body Exercises

**Muscles worked:** Biceps of the upper arm, brachialis of the forearm

**Directions:** A curl bar looks like an elongated "W" when it is resting on the floor with no weights on it. Keeping this in mind, grasp the bar with a palms-up grip as shown in the photograph and assume the normal starting position for the curls. Keep the elbows tightly against the torso as you do your repetitions slowly, allowing the arms to completely straighten at the bottom of each repetition.

**Tips:** Curl bars vary greatly in the spacing of the various bends, depending upon the manufacturer. Exercise-type curl bars, such as used here, have fairly sharp angles bent into them, which may mean it would be more comfortable for you to use a wider handgrip than the one we've demonstrated here. Don't be afraid to experiment with the grip. Just find one that allows you to keep your elbows against your torso and to get a full contraction in the bicep. The advantage of using a curl bar, as noted earlier, is that it reduces strain in the wrist and elbows that often accompanies straight curling movements.

**Variations:** Reverse Curl-Bar Curls: Again, these are done in exactly the same manner as regular barbell curls with the exception of the grip. Take an overhand grip on the bar, using the closest hand spacing possible on the bends — probably the same spacings you used for the regular curls. Again, keep the elbows close to the body.

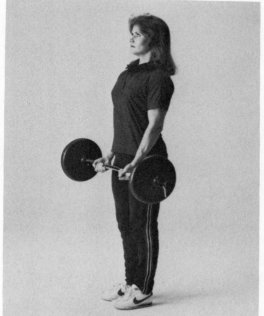

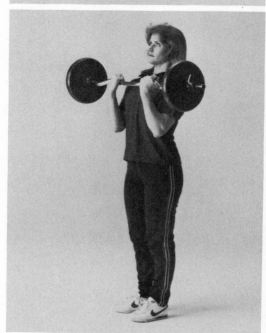

# Triceps Press

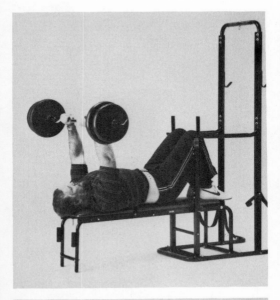

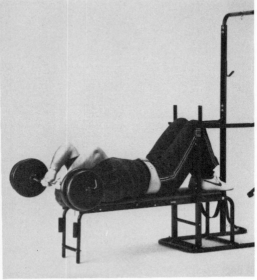

**Muscles worked:** Triceps of the upper arm

**Directions:** Lie on your bench with your head facing away from the rack, feet flat on the floor. Have your spotter hand you a loaded curl bar (make sure the collars are on tightly) and grasp it at the close hand spacing with your palms facing away from your face. Push the bar to arms' length over your chest and, locking the shoulders so that the upper arm will not move, lower the barbell to the back of the head by bending the elbows (see photos). Don't lower it to your face — just about halfway down the top of your head until you feel a stretching sensation in the back of your upper arms. Reverse and repeat for the proper number of repetitions.

**Tips:** If you're using relatively light weights with these, another approach to the start of the exercise would be to load the curl bar and to set it in the regular bench rack. Then, sit facing the rack and grasp the bar, holding it tightly against your chest. Lie down with the bar against your chest, push it to arms' length, and begin your repetitions. Only do this if you're handling weights well within your range. Any time you're doing an exercise in which the bar travels past your face you should be careful, but you should exercise even greater caution when doing triceps work, as the isolation causes the muscles to fatigue quickly. To replace the bar in the rack, lower it to your chest after the last repetition, sit back up — a bit harder than going down — and replace the bar.

**Variations:** Reverse-Grip Triceps Press: Perform the curl bar triceps press exactly as before, only use a reversed grip. Remember to keep the elbows locked. Another variation that works for both regular and reverse-grip presses is to perform the exercises while standing. It's best to do these in front of a mirror so that you can watch the angle of the arms, but Standing Triceps Presses are done by extending the bar directly overhead, locking the upper arms, and then performing the repetitions as usual, allowing the curl bar to descend to approximately the top of the neck.

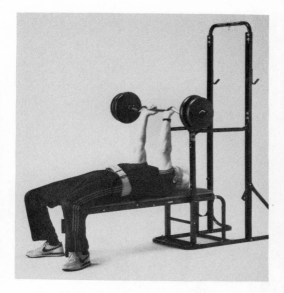

**Muscles worked:** Triceps, pectorals, and deltoids

**Directions:** Place the loaded curl bar in the rack on your bench and take a close grip on the bends of the curl bar. Have your spotter help you to position the bar directly over your chest, as shown in the photos, and then lower the bar to the chest as you would a regular bench press. Inhale at the top of the lift and exhale as you begin to press the bar back to arms' length. Try as much as possible to duplicate the same bench-press pattern that you normally use — only let the elbows flare out more to the sides.

**Tips:** "Close grips" done on a curl bar are an excellent way to pump the triceps without straining the wrists, as sometimes happens when people do close grips on a straight bar. Do close grips following your regular bench presses and/or incline presses rather than before them. Always remember to work your major muscle exercises first, then do your isolation exercises.

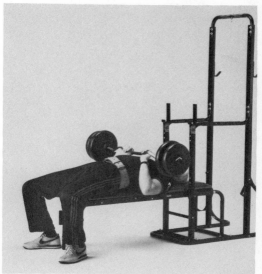

# Dumbbell Clean

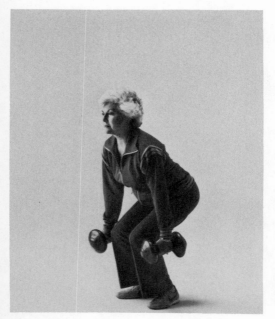

**Muscles worked:** Deltoids, trapezius, biceps

**Directions:** Grasp a pair of heavy dumbbells in each hand, palms facing in. Stand erect and, with your feet securely planted on the floor, dip your legs slightly, allowing the dumbbells to move backward for several inches before, keeping the back flat, you kick your hips forward and swing the dumbbells to the shoulders. Here, rather than moving the weight slowly as we've instructed you to do with curls and deltoid raises, the goal is to move the dumbbells rapidly upward, using the muscles of the hips and lower back to generate the upward thrust. Once at the top, carefully lower the dumbbells to your sides and repeat for the appropriate reps.

**Tips:** These are good exercises for getting the pulse rate elevated, as they involve most of the muscle groups in the body. Do them quickly, take little time between your sets, and you'll soon find you're making noises very much like those of a marathon runner coming down that last 100 yards. One limiting factor with these is your grip strength, so when you get into your "fives" and "threes," we recommend you tie your hands or use hand straps. If you can't fasten them on yourself, get your training partner to lend a hand.

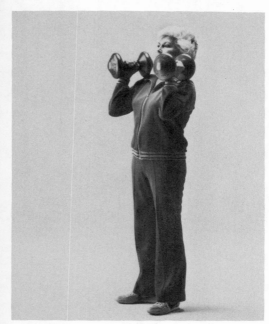

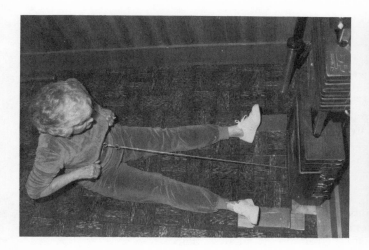
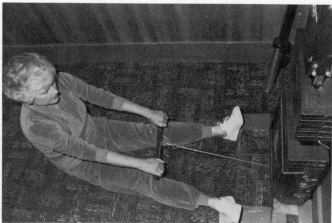

**Muscles worked:** Latissimus dorsi muscles of the upper back and other shoulder-girdle muscles

**Directions:** Attach the low pulley to your machine so that you can sit on the floor with your legs almost straight, your hands grasping the straight handlebars in an overhand grip. Fully extend the arms at the beginning of each repetition and then, keeping your back as straight as possible, pull the bar to your sternum. Return the bar slowly to the straight arm position and repeat for the desired number of repetitions.

**Tips:** You can increase the intensity of this exercise by placing several blocks of wood in front of the weight stack that will allow you to sit further back and stretch out the lower back, or lumbar, muscles on each repetition, as well as working the lats. As you back up 12 to 18 inches from the stack (but with your feet still braced) you allow your upper body to be pulled forward at the waist at the start of each rep and then, as you begin the backward pull, the lumbar muscles of the lower back will be worked as you return to the straight-backed position needed for the completion of the lift. This not only strengthens the lumbars but it increases your flexibility.

**Variations:** Some low wall pulleys are equipped with a set of double handles that allow you to pull your arms even further back, creating a greater contraction in the lat muscles.

## Cable Curl

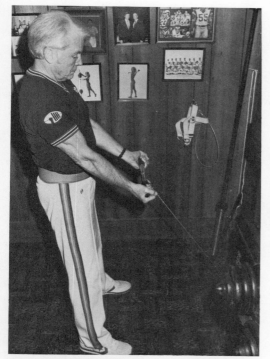

**Muscles worked:** Biceps muscles of the upper arm

**Directions:** Attach the low pulley to a short straight bar and stand erect, facing the cable machine, your arms straight at your sides, grasping the handlebar with an underhand grip. Keeping the back straight and the elbows against the side of the torso, raise the handle to the chest in a semicircular pattern until the bar is at the top of the pectorals and the elbows are fully bent. Slowly lower and repeat for the desired repetitions.

**Tips:** Cable curls are an excellent exercise to do on a home gym machine because the range of motion made possible by using the low cable is very close to that of a barbell or dumbbell. They can be done using both hands together, as shown in the photographs, or they can be done using a single handle that allows you to work one biceps at a time.

**Variations:** Reverse Cable Curls can be done by using an overhand grip on the short bar or on the single handle.

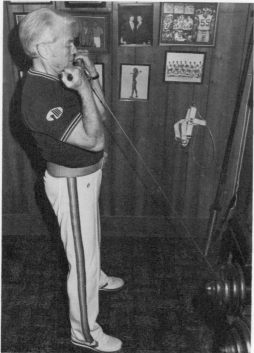

**Muscles worked:** Pectorals, deltoids, and triceps

**Directions:** Place the barbell in the rack on your incline bench, sit on the bench, and lie back so that you can take a grip approximately 6 to 8 inches wider than your shoulders. Remove the bar from the rack and hold it at arms' length for a second to make sure of the angle of descent. Then, slowly lower the bar to the top of the upper chest (the bar should touch the chest 3 to 4 inches higher than it would when bench pressing), and with your feet, hips, and head stationary, push the weight back to arms' length as you exhale. *Don't* try to bounce the weights as people often do with bench presses.

**Tips:** On this exercise, ask for a little assistance from your spotter. Since the bar has to be placed in the rack *behind* your head, it's impossible to see where the bar is supposed to land. Phrenologists say that creases in the head are supposed to reveal a lot about your personality, and working without a spotter on these is one way to develop creases that mainly reveal your lack of judgment. So, if you're using heavy weights, *don't work alone.* Incline presses stretch the muscles of the shoulders and chest, so to maximize the workload, keep the elbows well back, almost flared to the sides, throughout the reps, as we've shown here.

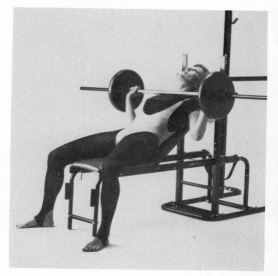

**Variations:** Dumbbell Incline Presses are done in exactly the same basic manner as barbell incline presses. A pair of moderately heavy dumbbells is "cleaned" to the shoulders before you sit down on the bench to begin your repetitions. The advantage in using dumbbells over barbells is that they allow each arm to work independently. Since many of us are stronger in one arm than the other you can't "carry" your weak arm along as often happens when using a barbell. Dumbbells also allow you to assume an even lower bottom position, causing a greater stretch in the pectoral-deltoid region. Just remember to use dumbbells as if they were a barbell. Lower them to the same area of the chest each time and raise them simultaneously. And, just as with the barbell, if you're using heavy weights, have your spotter stand by in case one arm fatigues before the other. You'll notice, by the way, that you'll lift less total weight when you use dumbbells. It has to do with balance difficulties, and shouldn't concern you.

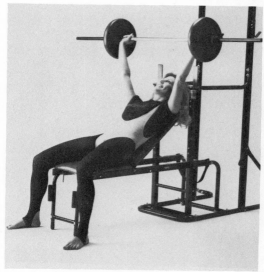

Both barbell and dumbbell incline work can be further varied by changing the angle of the bench. The more upright you are, the more the shoulder muscles are worked. The closer you get to the bench-press position, the more the pectoral muscles of the chest are involved. Most trainers do bench presses first and follow them with incline work done at a 45-degree angle to "fill in" the upper pectoral muscle and deltoid areas not reached by the benches. We suggest you try them in this order as well or do bench presses and incline presses on alternating workouts.

# Dumbbell Bench Press

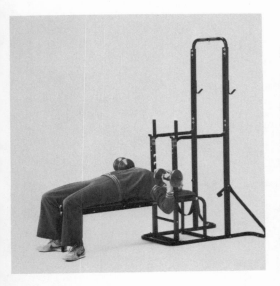

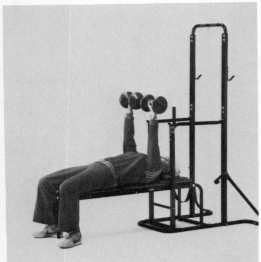

**Muscles worked:** Pectorals, triceps, and deltoids

**Directions:** Seated on the end of a bench, "clean" a pair of dumbbells to your shoulders and lie back on the bench in the exact same position you assume when benching. Push the dumbbells to arms' length over your chest and then, taking a full breath of air, begin to do your repetitions exactly as you would if you were doing a bench press with the bar. Keep your hands positioned so that the palms face away from you — the dumbbells forming a horizontal line across your chest. As with the barbell, try to bring the weights down to approximately the same position on your chest each time — roughly the area of the sternum.

**Tips:** Again, the advantage dumbbells have is that they allow a fuller range of motion because the elbows are lower at the bottom than they would be if you were using a barbell. Don't stop the dumbbells "on" the chest. Try to bring them down to the sides of your chest to get as much stretch as possible. And, if you're using heavy weights, have your training partner stand by to give you a spot. (With extremely heavy dumbbells, it's a good idea to let your training partner hand the dumbbells to you after you've taken your position on the bench.) Actually, dumbbell bench presses are usually thought to be safer because you can't be pinned by them as you can with a bar.

**Variations:** Some bodybuilders, as they lie on the bench with their arms straight, turn the dumbbells so that their palms are facing each other. Then, when they lower the dumbbells to the chest, the elbows are able to go lower than usual and a modified "fly" movement is created that further works to isolate the pectorals. Unless you decide to become a serious bodybuilder, however, don't worry about this refinement. Regular dumbbell bench presses are effective enough, and there's a greater risk of injury with this latter handgrip.

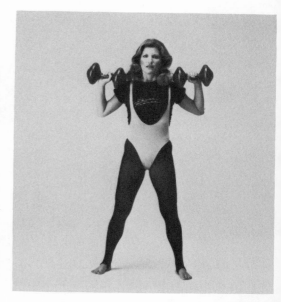

**Muscles worked:** Front and outer deltoids, triceps

**Directions:** Clean a pair of dumbbells to your shoulders and, with your back straight, turn the palms to face forward. Keeping the knees locked, push the dumbbells overhead to arms' length. Lower and repeat for the desired number of repetitions. As with barbell overhead presses, try not to lean back as you push the weights upward. Keep the torso straight and let somebody else have lower-back problems — not you. Wear your lifting belt to provide an extra brace.

**Variations:** Seated Dumbbell Presses are exactly what the name implies. Clean the dumbbells to your shoulders, sit on the end of your bench, and do your repetitions.

It's harder to "cheat" while doing seated presses, so they're a good variation to try. We prefer them. In fact, if you want to keep your back extra straight, sit in a solid chair with a straight back. And, as with dumbbell bench presses, you can also do these with the palms facing each other, which will vary the mechanics of the lift slightly. Finally, if your life doesn't already have enough variety, you can try doing these one arm at a time, while either seated or standing, in what we call Alternating Shoulder Presses, palms facing forward or palms facing in.

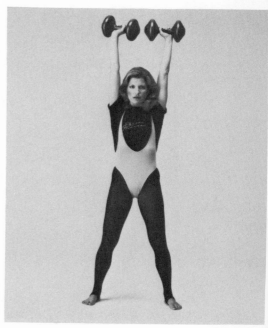

## Side Lateral Raise

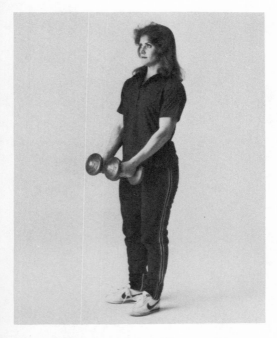

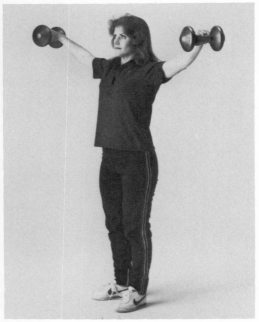

**Muscles worked:** Outer head of the deltoids

**Directions:** Stand erect, grasping a pair of light dumbbells in your hands, your palms facing your body. With your arms virtually straight, raise the arms to shoulder height until they are standing directly out to your sides, forming a parallel line with the floor. Slowly return the dumbbells to the bottom position, keeping the arms straight, and repeat.

**Tips:** Always keep your hands facing downward in these exercises in order to keep the deltoid in the optimum position. If you want width to your shoulders, work your delts and work them hard. Use light enough weights so that you can control the movement throughout the entire range of motion; simply swinging the dumbbells up and down isn't going to give you the look you want. Muscle the weights and they'll muscle you.

**Variations:** There are several variations you might want to try. You can do them seated, one arm at a time, but our special favorite is done standing with the elbows more fully bent, as shown in the photographs. At the top of these, rather than simply stopping the weight and lowering it to the bottom, flare the elbows upward and slightly outward, which should cause a cramping sensation throughout the muscles of your upper back. This little extra movement allows you to work the trapezius muscles as well as the deltoids and is an effective result-producer. Another good variation is to lie on your bench (or floor) and work the outer deltoids by raising one dumbbell at a time. Lie on your side and rest the dumbbell against your thigh. Keeping the palm of your hand always facing your legs, raise the dumbbell to shoulder level and repeat for the appropriate number of repetitions.

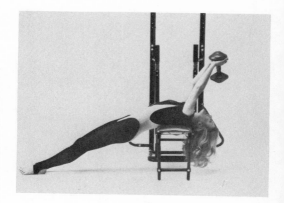

**Muscles worked:** Pectorals, intercostals, and serratus

**Directions:** Again, these are similar to barbell pullovers, except that with these you hold a single dumbbell in your two hands and your body is perpendicular to the bench. Remember to position yourself so that only your upper torso rests on the bench — your feet should point straight away from you in one direction, your head should be off the other side. Also remember to take a deep breath at the top position and to hold that breath until you've begun to return the dumbbell to the starting position.

**Tips:** The easiest way to hold the dumbbell for this movement is to wrap only your thumbs around the bar — one thumb resting on top of the other thumb — the flat parts of your hands against the face of the dumbbell plates. Remember the nifty butterflies you used to make when the movie was over, before the teacher got the movie projector turned off? That's roughly the hand position you're looking for.

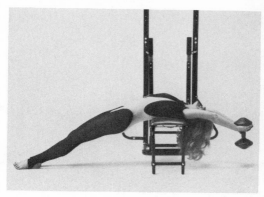

# Rear Deltoid Raise

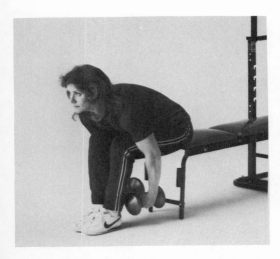

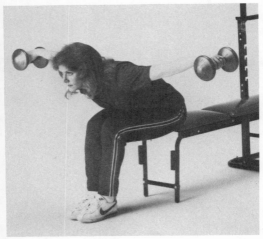

**Muscles worked:** Rear deltoids

**Directions:** Sit on the end of your bench with a pair of light dumbbells resting on the floor by your feet. Sit so that your feet are at least a foot away from the end of the bench, so that there will be room for the dumbbell to pass between you and the bench. Bend over so that your upper body is almost touching your thighs and grasp the dumbbells in an overhand grip, with your feet firmly planted on the floor. Keeping your torso as close as possible to your thighs, raise the pair of dumbbells in exactly the same motion that we described earlier for the barbell flies. Cock your wrists, slightly bend your elbows, and then move the weight as far back as possible until your wrists form a horizontal line with your shoulders. Inhale as you begin to raise the dumbbells and exhale as you lower them slowly back to the bottom. Don't go back to the floor between repetitions. Just bring the dumbbells down behind the knees and begin again. This keeps a constant pressure on the deltoid muscles, which you'll find will fatigue quickly when worked in this manner.

**Tips:** Once again, take these slow and easy for best results. Don't swing the dumbbells; concentrate on the way the back of your shoulder feels as you do your sets.

**Variations:** Bent-Over Rear Deltoid Raises are basically the same movement, done while bending forward at the waist with the legs slightly flexed. The main trick in doing these is to keep the upper body parallel with the floor. There is a tendency to raise the trunk as you raise the dumbbells, and for this reason many bodybuilders rest their heads on a bench or table so that they can maintain the flat-backed position. If you have a bench or table that's an appropriate height, try it; if not, we suggest you sit and do them as described above, sitting on the end of a bench. Although most folks choose to do these simultaneously, deltoid raises can be done one arm at a time. A further variation is the Lying Rear Deltoid Raise done by lying face down on a bench and allowing the weights to be at the "bottom position" when they are directly underneath the bench. If you have an incline rack large enough, you can also do Incline Rear Deltoid Raises by lying face down on an incline bench and going through the exact same range of motion. As with the curls discussed earlier, there are lots of variations, which generally result only in minute physiological differences. For this reason we usually mention the most common variations first.

**Muscles worked:** Biceps of the upper arm and the forearm flexors

**Directions:** Grasping two dumbbells, with your palms facing your body and your arms straight (underhand grip), stand erect with the dumbbells resting against your thighs. Slowly cock your wrists and move the dumbbells from the thighs to the chest through a semicircular range of motion. Move the dumbbells slowly, keeping the back and legs straight, and lower them to the thighs for the next repetition in the same controlled manner. Make sure to let the arms completely straighten at the bottom and to let all the "pull" come from the biceps — don't move your hips or thrust your legs forward to get the weight started.

**Tips:** In Bill Pearl's excellent book, *Keys to the Inner Universe*, he lists over 100 "curl variations" using only barbells, dumbbells, and curl bars. The biceps have always been an extremely important muscle in our culture, and so bodybuilders have, through the years, come up with lots of different ways to make them contract and grow. The variations we've listed, plus the next exercise described below, are, however, the most effective and, not surprisingly, the most commonly done variations. Try different variations on different cycles — or do one on your Tuesday workout and a different one on your Friday workout. Or, do as the bodybuilders do, and work two of them together doing first one exercise for one set, then another exercise for a set, then back to the first again, and so on, in what the bodybuilders call a "superset," so that you fully pump the muscle from several different angles.

**Variations:** Alternating Dumbbell Curls are done in exactly the same manner as described above except that one arm is worked at a time. Hammer Grip Curls are done while holding the dumbbells down to the sides of the body with the palms facing one another. Hammer curls place slightly different stresses on the biceps and brachialis muscles of the forearms and are often done following a set of barbell or curl-bar curls to hit the arms from a slightly different angle. Reverse Curls are done using an overhand grip (dumbbells forming a horizontal line with the floor).

With *all* of these variations, you have the further option of doing them seated or standing — alternately or both hands at the same time.

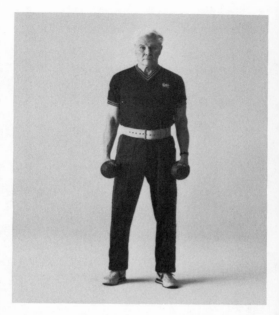

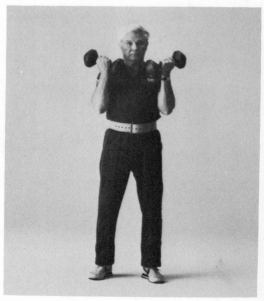

# Concentration Curl

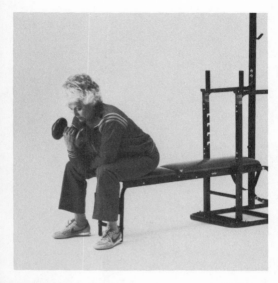

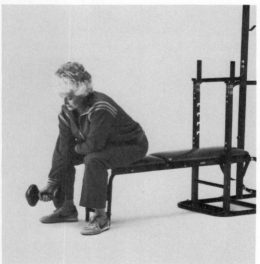

**Muscles worked:** Biceps of the upper arm

**Directions:** Holding only one dumbbell with an underhand grip, sit on a bench and bend your upper body forward until your upper arm is resting upon your inner thigh. Then, keeping the upper arm stationary, "curl" the weight from the extended arm position to the top, concentrating the entire time on isolating the biceps muscle. Turn your head to the side as the dumbbell comes to the top of the movement, to avoid hitting your face, and hold the dumbbell stationary for a second. Then lower the weight *very* slowly and repeat for the desired repetitions before you work your other arm.

**Tips:** If you plan to do two biceps exercises, do this one last. It's very intense and fatigues the muscles quickly. Again, keep the upper arm as stationary as possible as you do these. Don't be surprised if you need lighter weights for these.

**Variations:** Incline Concentration Curls can be done by standing behind your incline bench and resting your upper arm on the top of the pad. Again, keep the upper arm stationary as you slowly lower and raise the arm to contract the biceps muscle.

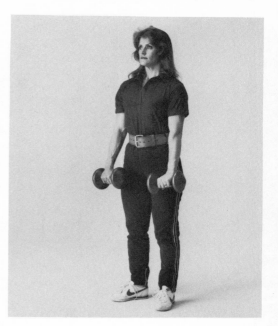

**Muscles worked:** Front deltoids

**Directions:** Grasping a pair of dumbbells in an overhand grip, stand erect and slowly raise the dumbbells to shoulder height while keeping the arms almost completely straight. Don't raise them as high as your face — just to shoulder height before you lower them back to the bottom. Repeat for the desired number or repetitions.

**Tips:** These can be done either seated or standing, but we personally prefer the standing version. Don't try to use a lot of weight with these — especially at first. It is far more important that you learn to do them without *swinging* the dumbbells. Let the pull come from the shoulder and concentrate throughout the entire movement on the pulling sensation there.

**Variations:** Alternating Front Raises are exactly as named. Raise one dumbbell while the other rests on your thighs. As the first one descends, raise the second, and so on. Don't forget that you count repetitions per arm, so 10 means 10 per arm, not 10 as the total of both arms.

Single Dumbbell Front Raises are done in exactly the same manner as the plate raises described in the previous chapter (page 168). To do these with the dumbbell, grasp it with both hands near the top of the short handlebar so that the sides of your fists rest against the plates. Then, with your arms *almost* straight, slowly raise it to shoulder height. Make sure to carry the weight equally between the two hands. If you feel one shoulder doing all the work, grasp the bar in a slightly different manner the next time so that you feel the stress on the other shoulder as well.

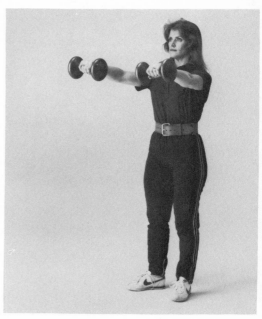

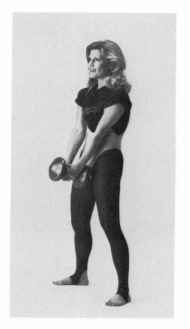

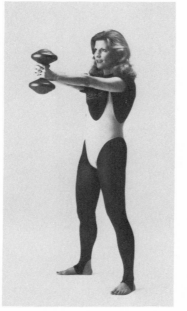

# Dumbbell Fly

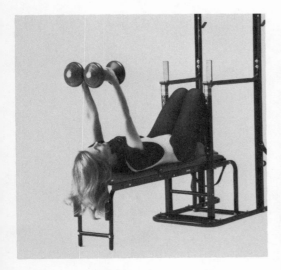

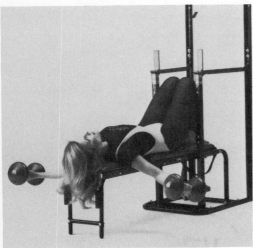

**Muscles worked:** Pectorals and front deltoids

**Directions:** Using a *light* pair of dumbbells, lie on your bench with your arms straight overhead, your feet, hips, and head stationary. Then, with your palms facing each other, cock your wrists outward as if you were going to do a wrist curl and move the dumbbells away from each other in a large semicircular pattern, so that at the bottom position your arms are extended out to the sides of your body, with your elbows slightly bent and your wrists still cocked. Reverse the circular motion to return to the top and repeat for the desired number of repetitions.

**Tips:** Flies should be done with slow, controlled movements so that in the bottom position you feel a burning sensation in the pectoral-deltoid region on each repetition that lets you know you are "stretching" far enough. This is not an exercise that calls for heavy poundages. Just use good form and work low on each rep. Since these are an isolation exercise for the pectorals, do these following your benches or incline presses so that the pectoral muscles will already be prefatigued. Then, the light, controlled movements of the dumbbell flies will help to really flush the pectoral muscles with blood, causing growth. This is one exercise that we especially recommend to women trainers. You can't do anything to change the size of your breasts, but you can change the pectorals underneath the breasts, and these are one of the better exercises for firming and enlarging them.

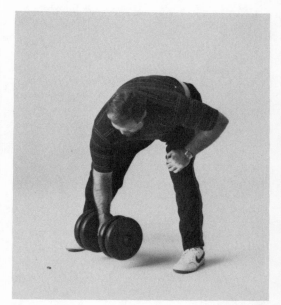

**Muscles worked:** Latissimus dorsi muscles, biceps, brachialis

**Directions:** Place a moderately heavy dumbbell on the floor at the end of your bench and grasp it with an overhand grip, your palm facing your body. Brace your upper body by placing your other arm on your knee so that at the start your knees are bent, your back is straight, one arm is grasping the dumbbell on the floor, and the other is braced against your thigh. If your back has a tendency to give you problems, this is a far better exercise than regular rows with a barbell. Then, keeping your back flat, pull the dumbbell from the floor to your chest, raising your elbow well past chest level until there's a contraction in the back of your upper body. Slowly lower the dumbbell until your arm is straight (just shy of the floor) and repeat.

**Tips:** This is one of our favorite exercises and we've both done thousands of them through the years. Even as many as we've done, though, we still have to watch ourselves because it's easy to "cheat" on these. Instead of pulling the weight with just your upper-back muscles, you give a little push by dipping and bending your legs. You can lift more weight that way, but it doesn't do you as much good. Try to watch your legs and let your back — not your thighs — get the benefit. Another thing you may want to remember as you increase your weights is to use a hand strap to help your grip. Just use one as you would when using a barbell. Wrap the strap firmly around the dumbbell handle before you begin your set. And finally, although you start with the dumbbell squarely in front of you, your palms facing your shins, your hand should turn at the top of the movement so that it ends up facing the side of your body. This allows you to pull the dumbbell and your elbow even higher, causing a greater contraction.

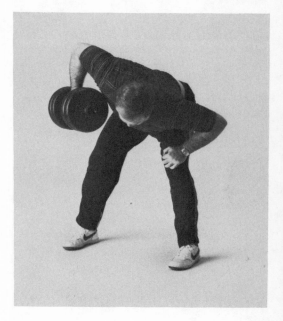

# Lat Pulldown

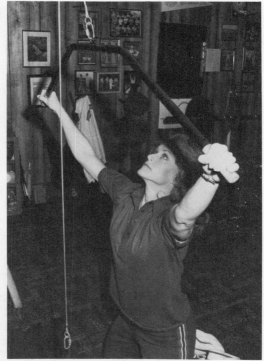

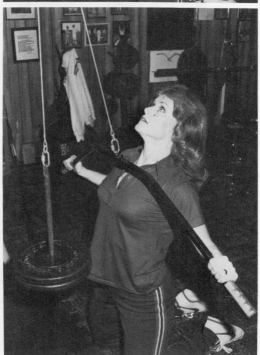

**Muscles worked:** Latissimus dorsi

**Directions:** Kneel on the floor in front of the lat pulldown machine so that the bar, when pulled to the chest, will be coming down from the top pulley at a slight angle. (You can intensify this angle by leaning slightly backward.) Take a wide, overhand grip on the bar and pull it to the top of the chest. It should touch the chest roughly 2 to 3 inches higher than your bench presses do. Keep the back arched slightly throughout the repetitions.

**Tips:** Some lat machines have seats affixed to them that will help to hold you in place. If there is no seat, however, you may need to ask someone to help brace you, as it is difficult to hold yourself down properly when using fairly respectable weights. To do this, get your training partner to press down lightly on the tops of your shoulders, close to your neck, where it will not interfere with the movement.

**Variations:** Besides the kneeling position, you might want to try these while seated on the floor. Sometimes, by sitting on the floor, you can brace yourself with your feet and not need a spotter to assist you. As with kneeling pulldowns, however, do not rock back and forth with each repetition. Allow your muscles to do the work — not your body weight.

Close-Grip Pulldowns: These are done in basically the same manner although the palms are turned upward and the hands are placed on the bar about 6 inches apart. Once again, pull the bar to the chest while keeping your back as stationary as possible.

Behind the Neck Pulldowns: Kneel in front of the lat machine with a wide overhand grip on the bar. Keeping the back straight, allow your head to drop forward so that the bar can be pulled to the top of the shoulders, *behind* the head. As with all other latwork, do these slowly, and control the bar as it moves upward. Don't be injured by being jerked upward.

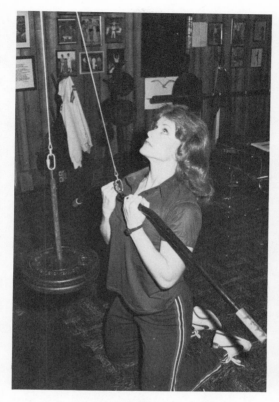
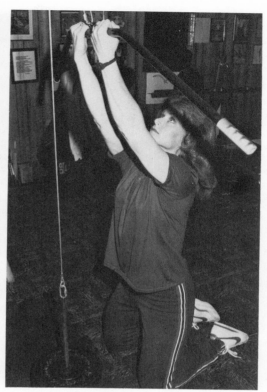
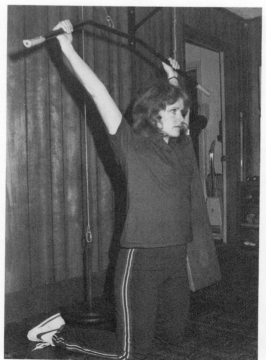
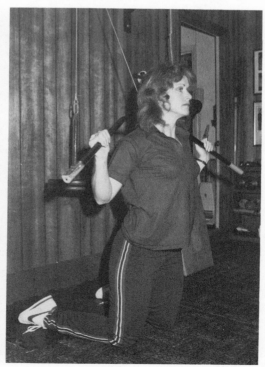

## The Power Snatch

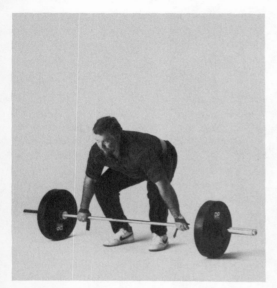

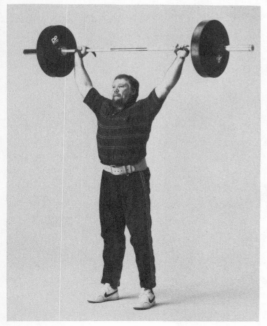

**Muscles worked:** Quadriceps, gluteus maximus, lumbars, deltoids

**Directions:** Place a loaded barbell on the floor in front of you and assume the deadlift position using an overhand grip about 36 inches apart. (You may wish to use your hand straps). Then, from the deadlift position, pull the bar swiftly from the floor (as you did in the high-pull movement described on page 154) until it is caught overhead with the arms fully extended. To lower the bar, unlock the elbows and allow it to travel downward, catching it on the thighs to break the downward descent. Reset (straighten) your back and start the next repetition by dipping the bar below the knees to midshin level and pulling it back overhead.

**Tips:** These are actually a *total* body exercise, and although their greatest effect is on the large muscles of the hips, thighs, and lower back — the muscles that pull the weight — they also straighten the shoulders and improve posture. Like high pulls, they should be done with speed and explosion. Remember, as the bar travels up past the thighs, the hips should kick forward, just as we explained in the high pull, to add momentum to the upward lift. At the top, the arms and shoulders should rapidly extend to their lock-out position so that the weight is not *lifted* or pushed at the top; it simply is caught, as the upward momentum will have carried it sufficiently high. As you increase the weight on these, you may find it necessary to dip under the bar as it travels overhead so that the arms catch the bar when locked.

One of the two competitive Olympic lifts is the snatch, and when done in competition style, the lifter generally catches the bar by squatting all the way down to the bottom of a deep squat before standing erect with the bar overhead. We don't advise you to use the squat-style snatch, however. The benefits of the power snatch are almost equal to those of the squat snatch but you don't run nearly the risk of injury that you do when you assume that ultradeep squat position. Just concentrate on pulling the bar from the floor to overhead in one continuous motion without pressing the bar at the top. You'll not only get a good overall workout — you'll be gasping for air by your tenth repetition — but you'll get some cardiovascular work into your workouts as well.

**Muscles worked:** Quadriceps, gluteus maximus, thigh biceps

**Directions:** Stand erect with a pair of moderately heavy dumbbells in each hand. As with barbell lunges, step out with one foot, keeping the toes of both feet pointed directly ahead. Lower your body by bending the forward leg as far as possible. Keeping the back leg as straight as possible throughout the movement, push the body back up quickly, returning the front foot to the starting point. Repeat with the other leg and continue alternating until the desired number of repetitions has been done *per* leg.

**Tips:** The main thing to remember when doing lunges is to keep the upper body straight. Lunges require a certain degree of balance, and it may take you a couple of exercise sessions until they feel comfortable for you. However, learn to do them properly from the first or you won't feel the benefits you should. These are an especially good exercise for women — especially women who want to shape up their buttocks and thighs. You don't need heavy weights with these, just stay with good form and stretch down as low as possible.

**Variations:** Dumbbell lunges can also be done by working one leg at a time. Do all 10 repetitions on your right leg, then all 10 on your left, before you repeat. This is a more intense method, often used by bodybuilders in search of the ultimate pump. Side Lunges are another method of lunging that more directly work the adductor / abductor muscles of the thighs, as well as the glutes and quadriceps. To do these, hold a pair of dumbbells at waist height to allow free leg movement. Then, step out as far as possible to the side, keeping your other leg as straight as possible, until the thigh of the first leg is virtually parallel to the floor. Push up firmly and repeat for the desired repetitions. These can also be done in the alternate manner described for regular lunges.

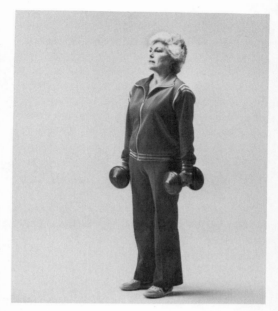

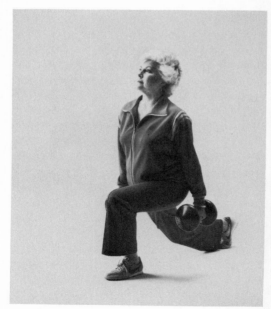

# Leg Curl

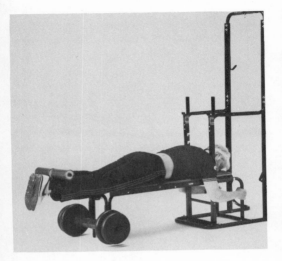

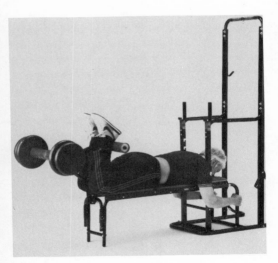

**Muscles worked:** Thigh biceps (hamstrings)

**Directions:** To do this exercise you will need a leg-curl machine of some sort. Traditional leg-curl machines are designed so that you lie face down on a flat bench and place your heels under a padded bar that is connected by a cable either to a weight stack or to a lever arm 'that allows you to lift plates that are loaded onto an attaching bar. In either case, the exercise principles are the same. Move the padded bar back toward your buttocks by contracting the thigh biceps (hamstrings) in the back of the thighs. This contraction will cause you to bend your knees, bringing the padded bar back until it almost but not quite touches your hips. *Slowly* lower the padded bar back to the start and repeat for the next repetition. Keep your hips on the bench at all times.

**Tips:** These are one of the best leg exercises available, and women, in particular, should try to include them in their routines. Don't be surprised if you can't lift much weight to begin with — most of us are very weak in the hamstring area until we begin to train the muscles. Also, try to concentrate on the muscles themselves when you do these; think about moving the weights slowly and deliberately so that all the muscle fibers get brought into play.

**Variations:** Some home gyms are set up with leg-curl attachments that require that the muscles be worked while standing upright. These are also effective; the only difference is that you must work one leg at a time. Follow the instructions in the training manual that comes with your home gym for these but remember to work them slowly for best effect.

**Muscles worked:** Quadriceps

**Directions:** Seat yourself on the leg-extension machine so that the fronts of your feet are placed against the padded bar. Keeping your upper body straight, slowly raise the lower legs until your feet are pointed directly ahead of you — the knees fully straightened. Hold for just a second at the top of the contraction and then slowly lower the weight back to the starting position.

**Tips:** To help brace your upper body, hold on to the bench near the back of your hips. Many bodybuilders will "superset" leg curls and leg extensions following their regular squat workouts. Since most machines are set up for doing both exercises, it is easy to do one, then turn over and immediately do the other, going back and forth in this manner until all the required sets are done. Remember one thing, however, when doing supersets: your quadriceps are generally much stronger than your hamstrings, so make sure you load properly for each exercise. Don't forget that you want to work each muscle to its fullest capabilities.

**Variations:** The only one that makes any sense is to work one leg at a time, but this is generally done only by very advanced trainers.

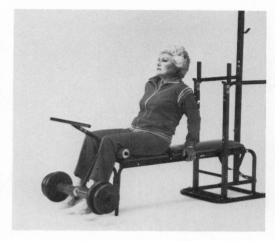

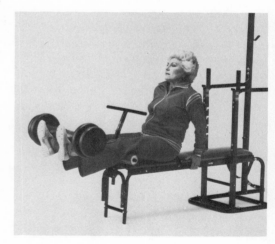

# Front Squat

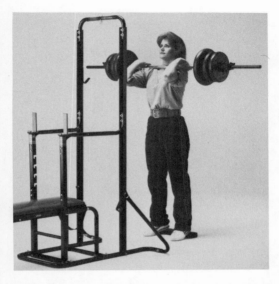

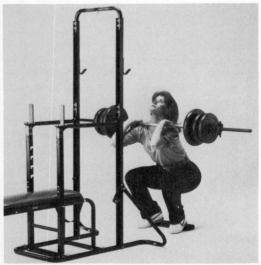

**Muscles worked:** Quadriceps, gluteus maximus

**Directions:** Place a loaded barbell in the squat racks and grasp the bar in an overhand grip that is *just slightly wider* than shoulder width. Then, step up very close to the bar and, by pushing your elbows forward, "rack" the bar on your chest, holding it across the tops of your shoulders. Back away from the racks and place your heels on a 2 x 4 or pair of barbell plates to do your squats. Keep the back rigid throughout the movement, and keep your elbows high as you go down into the squat position, before returning to the top.

**Tips:** Though these are an excellent — and we do mean excellent — result-producer, many people find them uncomfortable. They require good shoulder and wrist flexibility, for one thing, and for another, the pressure of the bar on the front of the chest is often painful. But, there are ways around both problems. To lessen the pain from the bar resting on your chest, place a folded towel across the tops of your shoulders before you rack the bar. If you feel pain in your wrists from the hands-back position, try a slightly wider spacing, or hold the bar on your chest by crossing your arms, keeping your elbows at about midneck level, and allow the bar to rest on the tops of the deltoids of the shoulders by simply balancing it with your hands.

**Variations:** Front Squats can be done without the 2 x 4 under the heels, of course. Elevating the heels simply throws more of the work load on the quads, which is the main reason people would do front squats rather than regular squats. Also, you can achieve slightly different effects by varying the foot spacing. Putting your feet close together allows you to concentrate more on the outer thighs, while a very wide, elevated foot stance will work the inner thigh more.

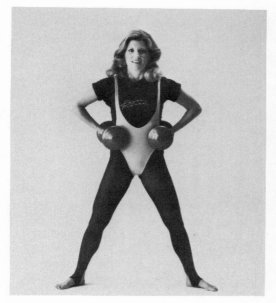

**Muscles worked:** Gluteus Maximus, quadriceps, abductors

**Directions:** These can be done using either barbells or dumbbells. If using a barbell, choose a light weight and hold the bar across your back. Hold the dumbbells either at the waistline or rest them on your shoulders. In either case, place your feet 30 to 36 inches apart (this will depend on your degree of flexibility) and point your toes outward as indicated in the photos. Then, lower yourself as far down as possible, keeping the back straight, the head up, and repeat.

**Tips:** As you may have guessed, this is another good exercise for women because it works the glutes so hard, but it should not be done in *place* of the full squat, but rather as an accompaniment. The depth you'll be able to reach will be determined by the degree of hip flexibility you've achieved. Don't go so low that your heels come up off the floor. Always keep your feet flat and simply try to work lower and lower with each successive repetition. Do not, however, go so deep that these are painful. Like your warm-up stretching exercises, work into these gradually — and stop if you feel any sharp pains.

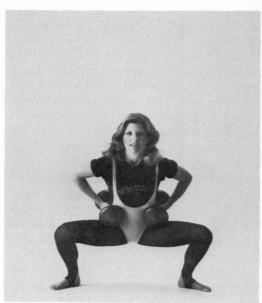

## Dumbbell Squat

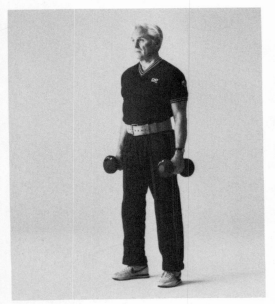

**Muscles worked:** Quadriceps, gluteus maximus, and lower back

**Directions:** Grasp a fairly heavy pair of dumbbells in your hands and stand erect, palms facing in. If you wish, elevate your heels by standing on a 2 x 4 inch block of wood, or keep your feet flat on the floor. Your feet should be about shoulders' width apart, your toes pointing slightly outward. Lower the body, the dumbbells held with the arms straight down, until the top of your thighs are roughly parallel to the floor. Keeping the back straight and the eyes fixed ahead, recover by pushing back upward until the legs are locked.

**Tips:** To really use enough weight to work your legs, you may want to use your hand straps so your grip won't be a limiting factor. As with the front squats, you can vary your foot spacing on these to suit your own training needs and comfort.

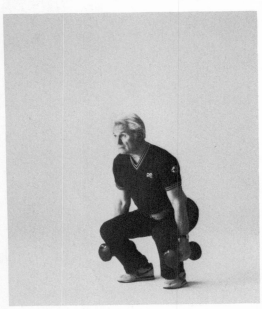

**Muscles worked:** Adductors

**Directions:** Attach the ankle strap to the low cable on your home gym and stand sideways to the weight stack. Brace yourself with the hand closest to the machine and slowly raise the attached leg as high to the side as possible. Keep your back straight and your other foot firmly planted while doing these. Then, slowly lower the weight back to the starting position and repeat. Reverse your position after you've completed one leg and repeat.

**Tips:** Cable work is especially effective at shaping and toning the adductors and abductors of the thighs. If you don't have a cable attachment, the same movement can be performed using ankle weights, although the cables do a superior job because they provide constant resistance throughout the movements.

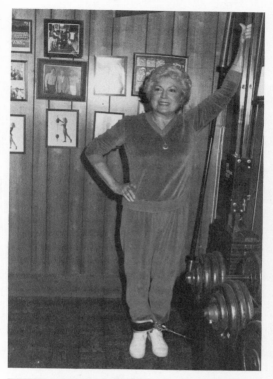

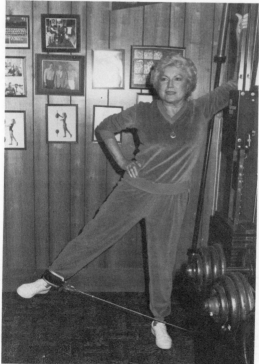

## Seated Cable Leg Pull

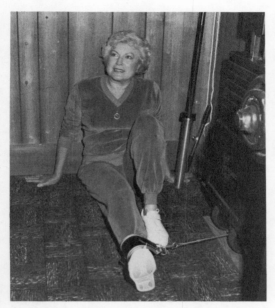

**Muscles worked:** Adductors

**Directions:** Sit on the floor to the side of your cable machine, your legs straight in front of you, ankle strap attached to the leg furthest from the machine. Brace yourself by placing your hands on the floor behind you, and, keeping the leg straight, swing the attached leg as far out as possible, raising it an inch or so from the floor. Keep the toes pointed, and return the leg slowly to the starting point. Repeat for the desired repetitions, then change sides and attach the other leg.

**Variations:** Inside Leg Pulls: Position yourself further away from the weight stack and attach the ankle strap to the leg closest to the machine. Spread your legs and pull the weighted leg toward your free leg by raising it slightly off the floor and swinging it inward. Keep the toes pointed and brace yourself by placing your hands on the floor behind you.

**Tips:** As you may have guessed, the Inside Leg Pull is designed to work the abductor muscles of the inner thighs. The Seated Cable Leg Pulls are to work the adductors in the outer thigh. In both cases, keep the tension constant throughout the movement by going slowly. Don't jerk the weights. These can both be done with ankle weights if you don't have access to a wall pulley machine, but, as noted above, the effect is not as great.

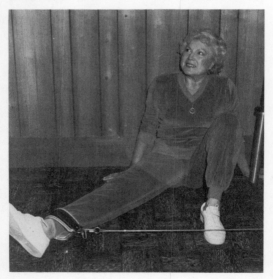

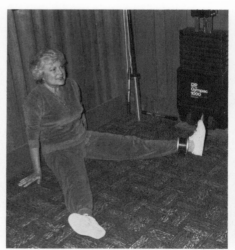

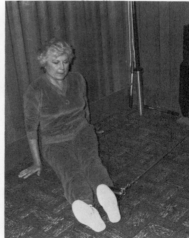

**Muscles worked:** Obliques

**Directions:** Grasp a single dumbbell in your hand and allow it to hang at your side. With your free hand, grasp the back of your head, and slowly bend over to the side where the dumbbell is. Allow the dumbbell to pull you as low as possible before coming back upright and bending to the other side. Repeat for the desired number of repetitions.

**Tips:** You've no doubt seen photos of folks holding two dumbbells at the same time. Yes, you can do them that way, but you won't get nearly the benefits you will from using only one. By using two, the weights counteract each other, and so you won't stretch as far as you will by holding one. The only other trick to these is to keep your torso in line with your hips and legs — don't bend forward, just to the sides.

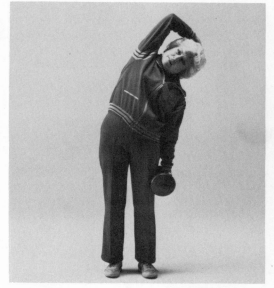

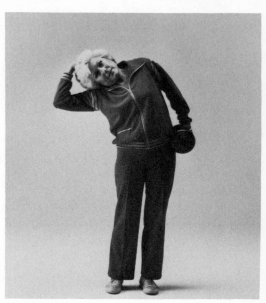

## Slant Board Sit-up

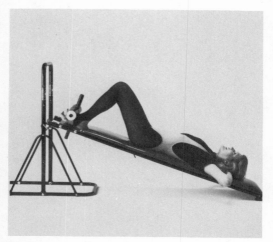

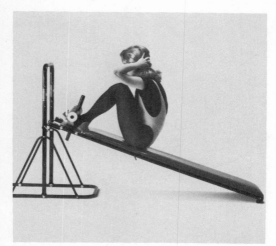

**Muscles worked:** Upper abdominals

**Directions:** Set up the slant board and lie down with your feet at the elevated end, knees bent. Place your hands behind your head and tuck your chin against your chest as you curl your body toward your knees. Keep your knees bent throughout the movement and try not to jerk yourself upward, but to curl up as if you were rolling up a carpet. Lower yourself slowly back to the bottom and repeat.

**Tips:** Because your lower body is higher than your upper body, these will seem much harder than regular sit-ups on the floor. This is because you've increased the resistance by changing the angle. The higher you raise your feet, the more difficult, of course, these will become. If you include these in your workouts, increase the angle every week or so until you're able to do them at the top position. Then, if you still feel the need of further resistance, hold a light barbell plate behind your head.

**Variations:** Twisting Slant Board Sit-ups are done in precisely the same manner, with the exception that just prior to reaching your knees, you twist your upper body to either the right or the left before you lower yourself back to the start. Or, if you're feeling Rocky-like, twist to both sides and then lower yourself. This twisting action works the oblique muscles along the sides of the abdomen, as well as the upper abdominals.

**Muscles worked:** Lower abdominals

**Directions:** Lie on the slant board so that your head is at the elevated end and your hands are behind you, grasping the board for support. Slightly bend the knees and raise the legs from the board until they are at roughly an 90-degree angle with your torso. Slowly, lower the legs until they are about 2 inches from the board and then reverse the movement to raise them again. Do not go all the way back to the board on each repetition because this releases the stomach tension.

**Tips:** Some slant boards made for home use will simply be too short to allow you to do these. Don't despair. Doing leg raises on a flat bench is almost as effective, but if you don't mind the extra trouble, you can elevate one of the ends of your bench-press bench.

**Variations:** Slant Board Kicks can be done by assuming the leg raise position, feet off the board by several inches, and then raising and lowering the legs one at a time as if you were doing the flutter kick. You don't need to raise the legs very high to feel the abdominal muscles begin to tense. If you try these, do them in fairly high reps, at least 25 per leg for best effect. Slant Board Leg Scissors are another variation that work the lower abdominal sheath in yet another manner. Raise the legs from the board and spread both legs as far out to the sides as possible. Then, bring the legs together, allowing the left leg to cross over the top of the right. Spread the legs back to the wide position, and this time bring them together with the right leg crossing over the left. Besides working the lower abdomen, these also work the inner and outer thigh muscles, making them a good exercise for women. Finally, all three of these can be made more intense by adding ankle weights to provide extra resistance.

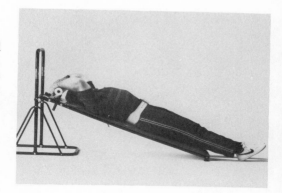

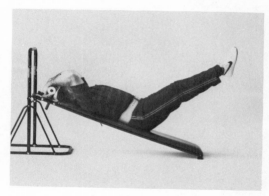

## Slant Board Knee-in

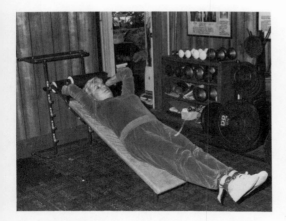

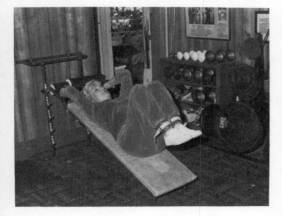

**Muscles worked:** Lower abdominals

**Directions:** Lie on the slant board with your head at the elevated end, your hands behind you, grasping the board for support. Extend your legs, toes pointed, slightly above the board and then draw your knees toward your chest as far as possible. Straighten the legs, keeping them just above the slant board, and repeat for the desired repetitions.

**Tips:** Pull your knees as close to your chest as possible without raising your hips from the slant board. "Curling" your hips off the bench by bringing your knees close to your face doesn't work your abdominals. Only the first part of the movement — while the hips are still flat — works the abs. The raising of the hips primarily involves the hip flexors, so just pull your legs till they're roughly perpendicular to your trunk and then repeat. Also, the higher the board is raised the more difficult knee-ins will be, so start out at a low position, and as your abdominal strength improves, increase the angle.

**Variations:** Knee-ins are an excellent exercise for using ankle weights. The extra weight added to the angle of the slant board transforms what's normally an "easy" abdominal exercise into an extremely effective waist whittler. Just make sure you've gotten your abdominal muscles in good shape before you start adding extra resistance. For further variety, try pulling in one leg at a time, as if you were riding a bicycle. And, instead of pointing your toes for all your repetitions, do some *heels first* for yet another ever-so-slight variation in the muscles involved.

# 19 / Training at a Commercial Gym

WE'VE designed this book primarily as an aid for people who either no longer have competitive urges to fulfill or who never did — people who just want to achieve and maintain a certain level of fitness as they go through their life. It's our belief that this can be done very successfully by training at home with a relatively small investment of money and, in fact, with a fairly small investment of time as well. But, there will no doubt be some of you who, for a variety of reasons, may not wish to set up a home gym for your workouts or who, due to limitations of space, won't be able to set one up. If this describes your circumstances you'll have to find a gym or health spa for your workout. Also, there will be some of you who, having trained at home for a while, will want to know more about what it might be like training at a "real" gym.

Training at a health club or gym *is* different from training at home. It has advantages — such as more equipment to use, readily available spotters, and a group of people to whom you can talk about training. But gyms also have disadvantages — travel time to and from the gym, waiting in line for equipment, membership costs, and the distraction of fellow gym members who want to socialize rather than work out.

And gyms vary. Where you choose to train will to a large extent determine how successful you are with your training. **Jan:** "I really believe that part of my early resistance to weight training came from the fact that for the first six months or so I worked out, we trained in a tiny room in the basement of the basketball arena at Mercer University. It had only one small window near the ceiling. It was dark, smelled of mildew, and all the bars and plates were so rusty from the high Macon humidity that every time I went to the gym I knew I'd return not just tired, but dirty and depressed. Later, when we found a men's gym that would agree to let me train, I found my interest in the weights soaring.

"Even though I was the only woman training there, the guys were always supportive. They helped out when I needed a spotter, gave me tips on how to do certain exercises, and the gym itself "felt" good. It was clean and light and you felt healthy just being there. And watching the guys train hard made me push myself. It was, I see now, the best thing that could have happened.

"I was lucky. I was able to train at Powerbuilders, a club filled with serious trainers and run by a man, Wayne Montgomery, who knew a great deal about weight training himself. Having been a lifter, Wayne understood what serious trainers needed, not just in equipment but in atmosphere. When a new member joined, Wayne would spend hours explaining how to train and why. In the summer when the young boys came in to get stronger for high-school football, he'd be on the gym floor all day showing them the right way to lift. His care and concern instilled in all of us a seriousness of purpose that pervaded the gym. But people had a good time, too. They laughed and joked and teased but when someone was training for a powerlifting contest or a bodybuilding show, and was putting all their efforts into their workouts, everyone did what they could to support those efforts — shouting encouragement, helping to spot, offering advice. But then most of the members also did the same thing for the businessmen who came at lunch or after work and did a short workout. It was an atmosphere of support, and it was largely the result of a dedicated, well-informed gym owner who wanted people to have a good training environment. I've been in a lot of gyms since my days at Powerbuilders and some of those gyms seem to have the same environment, but many don't. As you begin to search for a training facility, don't overlook this crucial aspect of a spa or club."

No plethora of equipment, no shiny mirrors, sauna, or swimming pool will ever do for your training what that indefinable atmosphere will, and all gyms have different atmospheres. There are currently six different "types" of gyms that dominate the health-field industry: health spas, Nautilus centers, figure salons, YMCA's, gyms, and racquet club–multisport facilities. Each of these six types of facilities has its pros and cons and each offers a slightly different type of atmosphere. If you live in a large metropolitan area you should be able to pick and choose from a variety of such places, but if you live in a small town, or in a rural setting, your choices will, of course, be limited. Yet even if there's just one health club in your town, *don't* jump in and join right away until you take a good hard look at what you'll be getting for your money.

Before we analyze the individual types of clubs, let's talk about reasons for choosing a commercial gym. First of all, if you've got to drive for more than 30 minutes to get to your barbells, forget it. Though you're now brimful of the very best resolve, the chances are you wouldn't go regularly — simply because of the time you'd lose traveling both ways. And with that hour and your own equipment at home you could be finished with your workout and using your extra time to catch up on your reading. Another consideration for city dwellers is parking. We've heard more than one friend lament, "Oh, I know I should go but it's always so hard to get a parking place downtown." What you need is a place you can get to without a lot of hassles. Otherwise you'll be wasting your money, and you'd have been better off with home equipment.

Before you start "shopping" for a training facility, talk with your friends. We'll bet that someone you know belongs to a health club in your area. What do they think about their gym? What are its advantages and disadvantages? Would they recommend it? Another place to investigate before you enter the commercial marketplace is your local high school, recreational center, or university. Many schools (and almost all universities) now have weight training equipment that may or may not be available for public use. It never hurts to check, and even if it's not "public" the odds are that you might be able to get access.

Even if your friends do have a strong recommendation for a club or a public facility, before you decide to do anything, go to the training facility and take a long look at what you're getting into. Whenever you go to look over a health spa or gym, promise to give yourself *at least 30 minutes* at the place. Remember, gyms and spas make their money by selling memberships. Those sleek, bright-eyed young "instructors" are primarily there to sell those memberships. So when you go for a visit, let them take you through the place and give you their best sales pitch, but then ask them a few questions as well. Don't forget, you're going to be paying money to belong to this club. You'll spend several hours every week there, so you have every right to ask. First of all, find out if the club is owned by a private individual or by a large corporate chain. Generally, private clubs where the boss comes in every day to look things over and make sure the place is being kept clean are better places for serious trainers. Chains are generally more interested in the sale of memberships than in the long-term continuance of those memberships. That's why you'll often see "two-for-one" specials in the paper. Health-spa chains and salons advertise heavily because they know a large percentage of the people who buy memberships will never use them after their first visit. So they concentrate their energies on selling memberships that are often 100 percent profit for the gym owner. In short, watch out for the hard sell on your first visit and evaluate the spa on the basis of its equipment, not its ad campaign.

You should also find out whether or not the spa is open to both men and women all the time or if there are certain days for men and certain days for women. It's been a great pleasure for the two of us to train together these past ten years. We've helped to motivate each other, we assist each other during the workouts, and we can travel to and from the gym together. If you would like to train with a person of the opposite sex, find out if you'll be able to do so. Sometimes even though men and women can train on the same days, they have to work on separate "sides." Is this what you want? Or do you want to be together? And, if you're a woman, does the women's "side" have the equipment you need? Be sure to check: often women's "sides" contain mostly machines and light dumbbells — no regular barbells or racks of any kind. And, many spas won't let women have access to the barbells and free weights on the men's side, even if there are no men training that day.

The next thing to inquire about are the hours during the day when the gym or spa is available for weight training. We know this last statement sounds a bit strange, but with the increase in aerobic dance and group exercise classes, many spas now spend a large portion of their days teaching "classes" on the floor of the gym where you and many others would prefer to be doing your weight work.

Having found out about the schedule, the owner, and what it costs (and remember that paying $300 a year to be able to train on Monday, Wednesday, and Friday from 2:00 to 4:00 P.M. and from 8:00 to 10:00 P.M. is not the same as paying $300 a year to train seven days a week at all "open" hours), tell the instructor to leave you alone for a few minutes so you can sit in the exercise area and watch what's going on. The instructor may try to stay with you, but *insist* on being left alone so you can observe what really happens at this gym. And be sure to plan your visit to a prospective gym or spa at approximately the time during the day when you'd be training there. If you work and will be stopping by the gym on the way home, stop by to visit the gym at the same time. Visiting a spa or gym in the morning when there are generally few trainers and visiting the same spa at 5:30 P.M. will leave you with two vastly different impressions.

As you sit there, look around. Are people standing in line to use the equipment because the spa has sold more memberships than they can adequately handle? What kind of folks are training there? Do you see other people your age? Are there women? Men? Children? Are the people really exercising or are they mainly talking? Some gyms and spas have gotten reputations as great "singles" meeting places. This is not in itself bad — but if that's the primary motivation of the other gym members, will you feel comfortable there? Or to consider another possible problem, is there so much screamimg and shouting as some behemoth in the back of the gym tries to lift the building that you feel intimidated? Don't be ashamed, most people do. Being in a gym of hard-core fanatics can be extremely unpleasant for some people over time. Don't forget, if you've never trained in a gym before, it will look and seem strange — and perhaps even frightening. But don't give up hope. Remember that over 90 percent of the spa users have never entered any sort of organized weight-related competition. They're just regular folks — like you — who want to lead fuller, longer, healthier lives.

If you can screw up the courage, go over to one of the gym members and explain your situation. Ask them how they like the place. Do they feel as if they've gotten their money's worth? Is the place always this crowded? This empty? How have the staff people seemed to them? Are they helpful? Do they know anything about training theory? Most people will be glad to give you some advice, and their opinion of the place could be valuable to you in making your decision.

And remember, while you're sitting there watching the interplay of the trainers, try to take in as much as you can of the "environment" of the gym. Is there music on? If so, how loud is it? Does it bother you? Is the place clean? Does the air conditioning work? The heat? Are the showers and restrooms adequate? And finally, what are the "instructors" doing? Are they out on the floor giving advice and helping to spot or are they back at their desk talking on the phone? Sadly, most spa personnel are not hired for their knowledge of exercise and physiology but for their appearance. This is especially true among the thousands of young women who work in spas all over the country and whose "physiques," displayed so fetchingly in leotards and leg warmers, are less a result of weight work and a knowledge of diet than of being twenty years old and having a handsome set of parents. Still, some spa personnel *do* know their stuff, but if you've read all the way through this book, the odds are good that you know more than they do. So, although they can make a difference in your success with the weights, you can't depend on their being able to give sound advice. Generally, the serious trainers in a gym, who read the muscle mags and keep up with the sport, will be better informed.

Here are a few other observations about the various types of weight-training facilities that might prove helpful to you as you shop for the right place to exercise.

**YMCA / YWCA:** For some reason many people overlook these fine old institutions when they begin to think about weight training. This is especially true of women who don't realize that even the YMCA's have allowed women to use their facilities for years. Almost every major city "Y" has a weight-training room, many of them stocked with first-rate equipment. Y memberships generally cost less than traditional health-spa memberships but then they don't offer some of the extras that spas do — saunas, steam rooms, and jacuzzis. But on the plus side, most large Y's have swimming pools that you can really swim in, and many have indoor running tracks and basketball courts, all definite advantages if you want to include some pure cardiovascular work in your training. Another advantage of Y memberships is that there are often enough things going on to entertain the whole family. While you do your weight work, for instance, the kids can go for a swim or take a gymnastics class. The primary drawback to Y memberships is the heavy use made of the facilities. Last fall, while we were in New York City, we trained several times at one of the large Manhattan YMCA's. Although it was fine for a morning workout, the next day we went in the afternoon and found people standing five and six deep to get to the equipment. Again, visit the Y in your area at the time of day you'll be using it.

**Figure Salons,** or women's "fitness" centers, should get a long critical look. We are frankly reluctant to recommend that you join one. Most "salons" are run by large chains whose primary goal, as stated earlier, is to decrease the size of your wallet rather than your hips and thighs. Many salons have little or no weight-training equipment; often they have only a few machines and some vibrators and rollers of various kinds. Remember, unless there are some barbells and dumbbells that can be adjusted to different weights, you'd be better to spend your time and money elsewhere. Salons and other sorts of women's centers are set up to hold "classes," generally consisting of stretching and light calisthenics often done to music, and while we're not at all opposed to the basic principles of aerobic dance and/or calisthenics, we are opposed to having that as the *only* form of exercise a person does. The other aspect of some "salons" that bothers us is their inability to resist offering such gimmicks as bodywraps for cellulite, mudpacks for the skin, and "circulation" and massage in place of exercise. The mind-set in most salons still seems to be that hard work and sweat are unfeminine, so unless they are the only option in your town, look elsewhere.

**Health spas,** or health clubs, form the backbone of the fitness industry. Most are well-run, orderly places with more than enough equipment to allow you to do the exercises we've outlined. Besides good equipment, most also offer saunas and whirlpools; some even have swimming pools. Vic Tanny helped to conceptualize the "health spa" as we know it, and with his Vic Tanny Spas in the forties, fifties, and sixties, he set a standard of elegance and style that most spas still strive to maintain. Because of these pretentions to elegance, many spas are even today filled with chrome-plated equipment, mirrors, plush carpets, and glittering machines, all of which help to project an image of sophisticated chic. In the past, most spas had no Olympic-style weights or squat and power racks, though now most do — even if they're in a separate room at the back where they're out of sight. But *where* the weights are in the spa doesn't matter. What matters is being able to use them, so if there's a good spa in your town that has the equipment you need at a price you can afford to pay, you'll probably want to seriously consider joining.

**Gyms:** It used to be easy to differentiate between gyms and spas because gyms were for guys who wanted to lift heavy weights and spas were for women and businessmen. But now that women want to lift heavy weights too, and businessmen have discovered their bodies respond best to hard work, the difference is less distinct. The main difference these days seems not to be in the people at the gyms but in the equipment and extras. Most gyms are designed with "serious" trainers in mind who want weights and lots of them. Accordingly, the equipment is basic and solidly built. Most gyms have the basic machines but the standard equipment is free weights, heavily built benches and racks, and, often, wooden platforms for solid footing. Some gyms also have saunas but they seldom come with pools and ja-cuzzis, nor will you find the thick carpets and the chrome plates. Not surprisingly, because they offer few extras, gym memberships generally cost less.

The great advantage gyms offer the beginning trainer is that they are often run by people who have been lifters or bodybuilders and who, because of their long-term interest in weight training, have read a lot on the subject. And, since they are owned by one person, who's generally there every day to run the place, most gyms take on the personality of the owner — good owner, good gym; bad owner, bad gym. If he's like most gym owners we know, who depend on people staying members for years and years, he'll do everything he can to help you with your training and to make sure that you want to stay a member. One potential disadvantage to gyms is that some cater only to serious bodybuilders or serious powerlifters. In these gyms most of the members compete at one sport or the other, and in such an environment you might feel out of place with your more moderate program and aspirations. Conversely, such an atmosphere may help you train harder and get better gains *because* of the company you're keeping. Hard to say. But a privately run gym with a good owner would probably be our own first choice of a place to train.

**Racquet Clubs / Multisport Facilities** are generally run by people who are experts in areas other than weight training. Many racquet clubs, however, do have weight rooms as part of their package and if you feel confident about training without supervision — which you should feel after having read this book — there is absolutely no reason not to take out a membership if you also want to take advantage of the excellent sport of racquetball. Most racquet clubs will not have the variety of equipment offered by a large commercial gym, but they generally will have some free weights and often a multistation Universal machine that will allow you to do a lot of the exercises we've included in this book. Again, there are trade-offs to be considered. Just make sure before you sign at *any* club that you investigate all the possibilities.

**Nautilus Centers:** Many health spas, gyms, schools, and even some Y's now have Nautilus equipment — the most well-known exercise machines. While the primary use of Nautilus machines (and all other exercise machines for that matter) is made by people who use them for auxiliary work, there are a growing number of people who exercise their entire bodies by using only Nautilus. To assist these folks, Nautilus centers have sprung up throughout the country. There, a person can use all the different exercise machines now manufactured by Nautilus, machines that, according to their inventor, Arthur Jones, are more efficient and result-producing than traditional barbells. While the majority of exercise physiologists would disagree with Jones, there's no denying that the machines are well engineered, sturdily constructed, and that they will produce results. The primary reservation we have about training solely on Nautilus equipment has to do with Arthur Jones's notion of the *way* one should use the machines. The Nautilus system as explained by Jones, and by Ellington Darden, Ph.D., in *The Nautilus Book*, involves doing only *one* set of 8 to 12 repetitions per exercise at each workout. Each set should be a set to failure — meaning that you couldn't, for instance, do even one more rep with the weight. The resistance on the machines is increased only when you can do at least 12 reps. Then, you increase the weight on the next workout day and work again to failure, and so on. Darden further recommends only 4 to 6 exercises for the lower body and 6 to 8 for the upper body, with a maximum of 12 exercises per workout. According to Darden, athletes should rest no more than one minute between any two exercises, and the goal should be to do the entire workout in as short a time as possible.

Says Darden, "It is entirely possible to go through an entire workout of 12 Nautilus exercises in less than 15 minutes." This high-intensity training is not without its drawbacks, as Darden himself admits in *The Nautilus Book:* "Perhaps an individual can push himself to a 100 percent effort occasionally, or on two or three Nautilus exercises, but experience proves that this is virtually impossible to do consistently. Nautilus high-intensity exercise is not easy. Properly performed, it is very demanding, and it is not surprising that few people can do it on their own initiative. An instructor is needed to supervise and urge most trainees to work at the required level of intensity."

This is the crux of the Nautilus problem. While it is indeed possible to get good results by doing one set to failure of each exercise in a workout that would last less than 30 minutes, the odds of *your* being that highly motivated individual who can train with gung-ho intensity week after week, even year after year on your own are, not surprisingly, slim. And the odds that the instructor at your local Nautilus center will be the sort of individual who could instill such an attitude in you — let alone maintain it — are even slimmer. If you could work under the personal supervision of Arthur Jones, things might be different. He is an intense, driven man with the capacity to instill belief, and perhaps he could motivate you sufficiently to train at the required level over time. But, quite honestly, it's tough to face a workout, every training day, that may result in a feeling of active nausea. Our personal feeling is that the Nautilus machines might produce better results if a periodization approach were used, as with barbells and dumbbells.

In a recent research study done at Auburn, using only barbells, the "train to failure" concept was tested against the periodization approach that we outlined in Chapter 13. What we found was that the test group that was asked to go "all out" on one set — to push or pull until they could do no more — not only did not increase in strength in the same manner as the periodization group but also began to dread and lose interest in their workouts. While the train to failure group did make some initial strength gains, by the end of the study they were significantly behind the other group, which had used a standard cycle or periodization approach, the sort we recommend. Simple common sense would indicate the likelihood of his happening. What would happen with a periodization approach to Nautilus we can't say. To our knowledge it has not so far been tested. But some day soon someone will do a research project on the use of Nautilus machines for multiple sets using a standard periodization approach, and then we may need to reassess our position.

In any case, if there *is* a Nautilus center in your neighborhood it might be worth your time to stop by and visit and see what goes on there. Most Nautilus machines are well designed, they are effective, and you may find, as thousands of other Americans certainly have, that the scientific look and feel of the machines appeals to you and to your notions of training.

## Gym Equipment

While some of these observations will, we hope, be helpful to you in your choice of facilities, your primary consideration in choosing a gym should be the equipment that's there for you to use. Here's a check list of basic equipment every good gym should have:

1. Several Olympic-style barbell sets with enough Olympic plates to load each barbell to at least 300 pounds, plus a pair of collars for each bar
2. At least two pairs of squat racks
3. At least one — perhaps two or more — power rack for partial movements
4. At least one heavy-duty lat machine with cable attachments for seated rowing as well as for regular pulldowns
5. Dumbbells — in 5-pound increments from 5 to over 100 pounds
6. At least one leg-curl/leg-extension machine
7. Several sturdy benches for bench presses and at least two incline benches, one of which should be adjustable
8. Heavy-duty leg-press machine
9. Dipping station
10. Chinning bar
11. Wall pulleys for doing various sorts of cable work
12. Incline boards for abdominal work
13. Several curl bars
14. Hyperextension machine
15. Calf machine
16. Mirrors
17. Clean shower and dressing area
18. Physician's scale
19. Enough floor space so that all the equipment can be housed without the gym members feeling claustrophobic each time they enter the gym

## Your First Visit

Once you've decided where to join, the first day you go to your new training facility you'll be asked to do two things. First you'll be asked to take out a membership, and the pressure will probably be put on you to sign up for at least a year. Resist the pressure. Most clubs offer daily, weekly, monthly, yearly, and lifetime memberships, and while it's certainly true that the longer you sign up for the less you'll pay per visit, it's also true that a $300 yearly membership at a club you come to hate is a lot more money lost than a $30 one-month membership. Allow yourself a trial run. Give yourself at least a month to get used to the place and the whole process of weight training in a commercial setting. Then, if you still feel awkward and uncomfortable, try to find another gym or buy yourself some extra equipment to use at home. Some people *never* feel comfortable in health clubs or gyms and that, of course, is why so much exercise equipment is manufactured for home use. (We suspect that in the future, many, perhaps most, people will equip their dens or a special room with exercise equipment as a matter of course. As more and more people learn how to train, they'll opt for the home fitness-center approach because of the savings in both time and money.)

The second thing you'll be asked to do that first day will be to begin the club's program. If you are a woman, this will be an important first step, for many clubs will pressure you to not lift the barbells but to use the machines and take the "classes" instead. You need to explain from the beginning that you have your own routine. When we were working on the sedentary women's study, we spent a lot of time at the local spa in town, watching what happened to women who trained there regularly and to the new women who joined. With new members the pattern was always the same (and we've seen this repeated in countless other spas around the country). The woman would come in and have her height and weight recorded by the attendant, who then gave her a card explaining the spa's "routine." Then the attendant would lead her from machine to machine and tell her that the workout would consist of one or two sets of 8 to 10 repetitions for each exercise. It would be stressed that they should always be careful to not strain themselves by trying to do "too much." There was little talk of warming up and no explanation of how to increase the weights, just the briefest introduction about how to do the machine movements and the admonition to not do "too much." With no understanding of the value of increased resistance, most of the women were still using nearly the same weights 10 weeks later that they used on their first day. And, as you probably guessed, most of them didn't notice a lot of change in their bodies, either. Interestingly, when we would take our group of middle-aged women to the back, where the barbell and benches were kept, we'd often find that the other women gym members would come back to watch what was going on. And as the program ran its course and our women began to look trimmer and the regular spa members continued to look more or less the same, we began to get questions from some of the regular spa members about our "research." While we always did our best to answer the women's questions, we could tell that even though most of the other women could see the benefits our group had gotten from the study, they could still not make the psychological break from what they considered "feminine." And the young women who worked at the spa did little, even in the face of the evidence, to make any changes in the way they instructed new members.

In fact, at the end of the study several of our subjects decided to continue their weight work at the spa and took out a membership. Again, they were almost immediately faced with the same "don't do too much" philosophy. As one of the women told us later, "After you left, we decided to keep training and just started in on our regular routine, doing the sets of ten again. The first day nobody said anything about it, but the next day one of the instructors came over and started asking me if I wasn't afraid I'd get big muscles from lifting all those heavy weights." I really laughed. 'I don't know about the muscles,' I told her, 'they haven't shown up yet. But the one thing I *do* know is that I feel a whole lot better doing this than I did when I used to only do an aerobics class. And my friends tell me I look better, too.' She made me mad. You'd think she'd have learned something by watching us work out during that ten weeks but she didn't know any more at the end of our program than she did at the beginning."

So, our advice to you on your first visit is to take a look at what they recommend for you, and be gracious, but then tell them straight out that you've already gotten a program that you want to try and that you'd like to have their help with it — but that you will be responsible for your own training. You've got to remember that part of what goes through a gym instructor's (generally gym owner's) mind is that he does not want his members to be injured. Injuries mean he may lose them as members, and there's always the possibility that someone will decide to sue. So, most spa programs are conservative, and women are especially urged to use light weights. But our basic program is conservative, too. No less than the cost-conscious gym owner, we want you to be injury free. But we also want you to reach your maximum potential in terms of fitness, and, to do that, research project after research project indicate that you need to train hard, do multiple sets, and vary the resistance as outlined in Chapter 13.

## Gym Training — Dos and Don'ts

Although we've tried to point out a few of the pitfalls that accompany training in health spas and clubs, don't misunderstand. We're not opposed to them, not at all, but we want you to be able to spend your money and use your training time to the best possible advantage. And there's no denying that the variety of equipment offered by gyms and spas can make training more interesting and, often, more area specific.

For best results, watch the amount of time you spend socializing or waiting in line to use the next piece of equipment. While it's fun to talk, you lose most of the cardiovascular effect of weight work if you wait too long between your sets. To avoid this problem — and to make your transition to gym training more natural — here are a couple of other observations on gym etiquette.

**1.** Never be afraid to ask another gym member to give you a "spot" when you're squatting, benching, or doing any exercise that requires careful watching. No one minds spotting because at some time or other they too will need help; don't suffer in silence or stay with weights lighter than you feel capable of using because of your shyness. Likewise, if you're asked to spot someone else, lend a hand. As a matter of fact, it's not a bad idea, if you see someone benching alone, to ask them if they'd like a little help.

**2.** Always unload your bars and replace the plates in the racks after you've finished with an exercise. There's nothing more maddening than to come along behind some guy who finished up his squats with 800 pounds and then headed for the shower too weak to unload the bar. That sort of behavior shows nothing but contempt for your fellow trainers.

**3.** When someone is performing a lift, even if it's with a light weight and he's handling it easily, don't talk to him until he has placed the bar back on the floor or the rack. You'll make a lot of new friends at the gym, and one of the nicest parts of gym training is the talk in between the sets; but when it comes time to lift the weights, allow others a chance to concentrate on what they're doing, just as you should demand a chance to focus on what you're doing when it's your time to lift. There will be occasions, when someone is attempting a near max lift, when it would be appropriate to shout some encouragement to the lifter — if he desires it. But don't expect someone to continue discussing interest rates and property taxes while they're doing their bench presses.

**4.** Don't be afraid to ask for advice from your fellow gym members as to whether or not you're doing a lift properly. If you've never trained before and your sole introduction to weight training has been this book, you would be well served to ask some experienced lifter if you feel at all uncertain about any lift. Again, try to find someone who knows what he or she is talking about. Almost all gyms have serious trainers, and they're almost always willing to help out beginners.

**5.** If, say, you've finished your squats and want to do some leg presses but some other guy is working on the machine and taking fairly long breaks between his sets, don't be afraid to go over and ask him if you can "work in." This is commonly done, and unless you get in the habit of "working in," you may find yourself never finishing your workouts. No one minds letting someone share equipment as long as you help to load and unload the bar or machine each time if you're using different weights. Try your best to not hold the other person back, naturally, but don't feel reluctant to ask. (The one exception to this rule would involve high-level bodybuilders who do set after set after set with virtually no rest between sets. If you see some huge hulk on a bench or machine who's taking only fifteen-second rests, you'd probably be better off to wait till he's finished so that you can have the equipment to yourself and train at your own pace. Don't hesitate, however, to ask how many more sets he has on the equipment. If he has ten, you might want to rearrange the order of your workout slightly so that you don't cool down too much.)

**6.** There are certain exercises such as squats, deadlifts, high pulls, etc., that require a great deal of concentration and a clear field of vision. Nothing is more distracting to a person with a heavy deadlift in his hands than to see some gym rat walk right in front of him. So, if the local Hercules is performing miracles in the back and you want to stop your training for a second and watch, fine. But don't stand directly in front of the guy. And, if you don't really care to watch but need to get to the other side of the gym, try to find a way to walk that won't interrupt his field of vision, or else wait for a few seconds till he's done. It's a matter of simple courtesy, we know, but it means a lot to the men and women lifting the heavy weights.

## Gym Training — Where to Start

For the person who's trained at home with only the very basic equipment we outlined in Chapter 17, walking into a fully equipped gym for your first workout is not unlike being a kid in the proverbial candy store. Not only will you not know where to start, but you're not even going to know what a lot of things are. In the exercise section that accompanies this chapter we've tried to go into as much detail as possible about the numerous exercises one can do at a gym on the basic machines usually found there. But there is no way we can describe all the machines or all the exercises. For one thing, we don't have the space, and for another, equipment varies considerably from gym to gym. Much equipment is manufactured by small, one-man companies, and, because of this, machines vary considerably in design. So, we've stuck with the basic pieces of equipment outlined on page 233 with a few exceptions. Don't hesitate to ask the gym manager or one of the gym members how to use a machine properly.

If you are a beginner — have done no home training — and will be starting your first workouts at a gym, you should still follow the basic routine we outlined in Chapter 17. Don't forget, the first twelve-week cycle you do is moderate in nature because most of you will not have done any form of regular exercise in some time. Obviously, if you've already been training and have simply decided to join a gym, then you can probably start on a more advanced routine while still applying the periodization approach to an expanded workout. But for those of you who'll be starting out in a gym environment, we'd like to caution you again to not do too much *if you have not already been involved in some form of regular exercise.* The temptation to try all the different machines and exercises will be great, but resist the temptation. You'll get the best results by sticking to a routine throughout an entire cycle and then, at the completion of the cycle, by adding or deleting any exercises you wish. Just remember your goals to develop a level of fitness that will allow you to enjoy life more, improve your health, and extend the active years of your life. We believe this can be done by fairly simple, relatively pain-free training that leaves you feeling neither utterly fatigued nor injured.

Injuries are largely the result either of ignorance of proper form in a lift or of overtraining. Don't be a victim of your own lack of restraint. Before you hop onto that Nautilus machine to see how it "feels," just remember how long it took to get your body into the shape it's in today. Was it twenty years? Thirty? Is twelve weeks too long to ask you to work toward getting it back in shape before you start experimenting? Play it safe, and smart. Do the basic routine for the first twelve weeks as explained in Chapter 17 and then, as we explain in Part Four, add or delete exercises on each cycle as you handcraft a series of programs that will produce results and prevent boredom.

**Muscles worked:** Pectorals, deltoids

**Directions:** Lie on the decline bench with your feet secured so that you won't slip on the bench as you do your repetitions. Take the bar from the rack with the help of your spotter — be very careful when doing this exercise, as the head down position *is* dangerous. From the straight arm position, lower the bar to the chest and then push it back to arms' length by pushing slightly upward and away from the face, to counter the angle of the bench.

**Tips:** Decline presses work the lower part of the pectoral, making them a good exercise for women to include in their training programs. The only difficulty with decline presses is in getting the bar to the starting position. A good gym should have a decline bench with a rack attached to it; but, if it doesn't, have someone hand the bar to you for your repetitions and then hand the bar back when the set is done. Another suggestion would be to set the decline bench up in front of a power rack so that you could take the bar off the pins as if it were a regular bench rack. Two other reminders for best results in the exercise: The greater the angle of the decline bench, the more the stress will be placed on the lower pectoral and the more you will have to push "away" from your face as well as upward to compensate for the changed angle. Decline presses are not "finished" over the face — the bar should be over the chest or even the upper abdomen at completion. And, if your decline bench does not have an attached bar under which to lock your feet, try bracing them by wrapping them around the bench legs, or, cross your ankles and keep your calves tightly against the edge of the bench to hold yourself in place.

**Variations:** Dumbbell Decline Presses are done by grasping a pair of dumbbells in the hands while sitting at the end of a decline bench, and then lying down to get the dumbbells in the proper position. Do your repetitions as if you were using a barbell, keeping the dumbbells in a horizontal line throughout the movement. With heavy weights, we advise you to have a spotter hand you the dumbbells after you've assumed your position on the bench.

*The model through the end of this chapter is fifty-three-year-old Bill Pearl.*

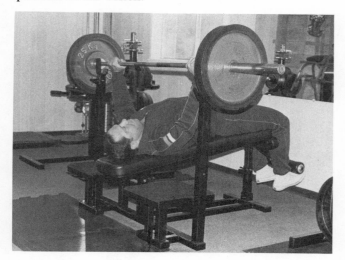
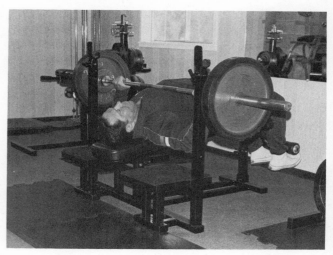

## Decline Dumbbell Fly

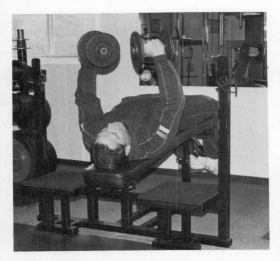

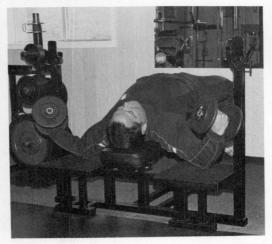

**Muscles worked:** Pectorals and front deltoids

**Directions:** Grasping a pair of light dumbbells, secure your feet at the high end of the decline bench and lie back, extending the arms over the chest with the palms of your hands facing one another. Slightly "cock" the wrists and, keeping the arms almost straight, lower both dumbbells in a semicircular pattern to the sides of the body until the arms are slightly lower than shoulder height and you feel a stretching sensation in the pectoral-deltoid region. Reverse the movement, keeping the wrists cocked and the elbows slightly bent, to return the dumbbells to the top. Repeat for the desired number of repetitions.

**Tips:** Again, the decline puts greater stress on the lower pectoral region, and the sharper the angle, the more the lower pec is isolated. **Jan:** "I have used this exercise a lot during the past several years and I prefer a fairly moderate angle, generally around 30 degrees. At that angle, I feel the lower pectoral is stressed, but the whole pec is still fully worked."

**Variations:** Incline Dumbbell Flies are done on an incline bench, again using light to moderate weights. Clean a pair of dumbbells and lie back on the bench to perform your repetitions. Incline flies, like incline presses, work the upper pectorals, so one suggestion would be to employ both incline and decline flies in a "superset" for maximal pectoral development.

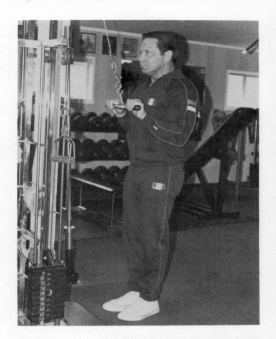

**Muscles worked:** Triceps

**Directions:** Stand in front of the lat machine and grasp the straight bar with an overhand grip, hands about 8 inches apart. Lock the elbows against the sides of the body and slowly push the bar downward, straightening the arms until the elbows lock. Then, *very* slowly unlock the elbows and allow the bar to return to midchest level before pushing it downward again. Be sure to concentrate on the triceps muscle while doing the exercise and to maintain a constant tension while moving the bar up and down.

**Tips:** Triceps Pressdowns are one of the best exercises you can do for the triceps if you do them properly. Properly, in this case, means slowly, with the elbows always against the sides of the trunk and with only the triceps muscles moving the weight. While doing these, don't bend the upper body forward to use your body weight to help lower the bar. Keep the shoulders squared. Likewise, don't use your legs to dip down and pull the weight. Proper form is important in these, so choose a weight you can handle without sacrificing the technique of the lift.

**Variations:** Reverse Triceps Pressdowns can be done by taking an underhand grip on the straight bar, hands about 8 inches apart. Again, lock the elbows against the sides of the torso and use only the triceps muscles to raise and lower the weight.

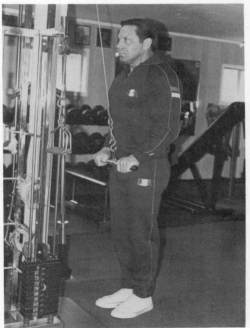

# Hyperextension

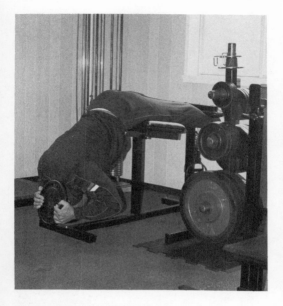

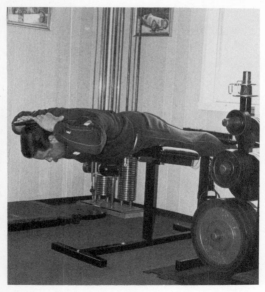

**Muscles worked:** Lumbars

**Directions:** Situate yourself on the hyperextension bench, as shown in the photograph, with your feet secured under the foot pad, your hips and thighs supported by the main pad so that your upper body is free to bend at the waist. To start the exercise, bend at the waist until your upper body forms a right angle with your lower body and place your hands behind your neck as if you were doing a sit-up. Then, raise (don't swing) your upper body until your body is once again straight, your upper body parallel to the floor. Do not arch your body at the top. Come to parallel and then reverse the motion, controlling your downward movement as you return to the start.

**Tips:** Don't be surprised if the first time or two that you do these you get dizzy. If you do, stop, allow the blood to return to your trunk, and try another set. Don't continue with these if you feel uncomfortable about the exercise. For two reasons, we personally don't recommend arching backward at the top of the hyperextension movement. First of all, very little additional work is gained once the body is past parallel, and, secondly, there is a danger of injuring the spinal column by that sort of backward contraction. Actually, they shouldn't even be called *hyper* extensions. One final word: make sure that your feet are secure. If you feel as if you might slip, get someone to help hold your feet.

**Variations:** Once you've included these in your program for several weeks, you may want to try Weighted Hyperextensions to provide some additional resistance. Simply hold a barbell plate behind your head as you do your repetitions, or use a loaded barbell and continue to do your repetitions as usual. Twisting Hyperextensions can also be done either with or without additional weight. Simply rise to the parallel position and then twist to either side before returning to the bottom. The twisting motion will work the obliques as well as the lumbars as you do your repetitions. And, finally, if you have difficulty raising your body to parallel, cross your arms on your chest and try your repetitions. This lessens the difficulty of the exercise and is a good way for beginners to start out. But, as soon as you can do them properly, place your hands behind your head.

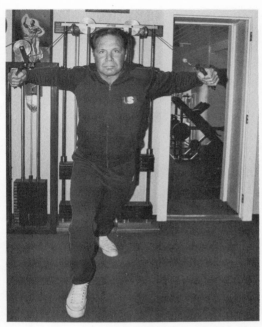

**Muscles worked:** Inner Pectorals

**Directions:** You will need a wall pulley machine with two handles for this exercise. Stand with your face away from the pulleys, grasping the handles with your palms facing each other. Step away from the machine until the cables are tight and then extend your arms to the side as if you were in the bottom position for dumbbell flies. Lean slightly forward and, keeping the elbows slightly bent, bring your hands together in front of your chest at shoulder height. Slowly return the arms to the sides, and repeat.

**Tips:** Make sure to get far enough away from the wall pulley so that you have tension throughout the movement, even on the way back to the starting position. Try to concentrate on the way the pectoral muscles feel as you do these and remember to keep your legs and back stationary so that only the pectoral muscles are being worked. Also, when you reach the center, contract the pectoral muscles fully by pausing for just a second before you allow the arms to return to the sides.

**Variations:** Single-Arm Chest Laterals can be done from two positions. They can be done with your back toward the wall pulleys exactly as we described above, but the more common variation is to stand with your side toward the pulleys, holding a single cable handle with that hand. These are generally called Pectoral Crossovers, as maximum benefit is gained by bringing the arm from the starting position all the way across the front of the chest so that your arm is fully extended, your hand at the level of your opposite shoulder. Concentrate on the inner pectorals as you do these, stop for just a second, and fully contract the pec at the top before you allow the arm to go back to the starting position. As with other single arm exercises, do all your repetitions for one side before you turn and work the opposite arm in the same manner to complete the set.

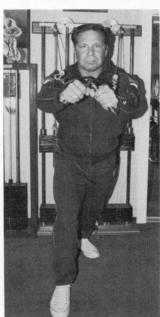

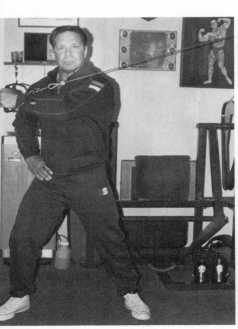

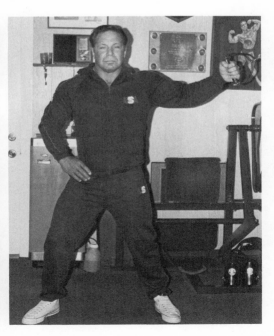

# Dip

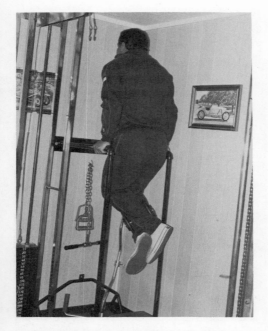

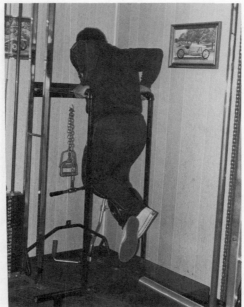

**Muscles worked:** Pectorals, front deltoids, and triceps

**Directions:** Most gyms will have a dipping station or a set of parallel bars, such as gymnasts use, for this exercise. To position yourself for the start, grasp the dipping bars at the end and jump upward until your body is supported by your locked arms. Your feet should not touch the floor at any point during the performance of the exercise. If the bars are not high enough, bend your knees and cross your ankles to keep yourself from kicking off the floor. To lower yourself, keep the elbows close to the sides of the body and allow your upper body to bend forward slightly. Then, slowly unlock your elbows and descend until your elbows are well bent, your forearms and biceps touching each other. Stop for just a second to get the full stretch and then press yourself upward, locking the elbows at the top to get a full triceps contraction. Repeat for the desired number of repetitions.

**Tips:** These are one of the most popular and result-producing upper-body exercises. However, they require a fair degree of strength. Women may find them difficult, and so we would suggest two ways to build sufficient strength to do them properly. The first way would be doing dips between benches as explained in the *Variations* below. The second method would be to do "negative" dips. Negative dips are done by lowering yourself as usual, but then having someone assist you with your return to the starting position by lifting you at the waist. Or, you can place a small stool under your feet, lower yourself to the stool, and then assume the starting position again by pushing upward from the stool.

**Variations:** Dips between Benches are done using two flat exercise benches. If possible, have one slightly higher than the other. Place your feet on the taller bench and sit on the lower bench with your hands at the sides of your buttocks, fingers pointing toward your feet. Allow your hips to slide off the side of the bench so that you're supported solely by your straight arms and your feet, as shown in the photo. Lower yourself by bending the elbows until your upper arms are almost parallel to the floor; keep your legs straight and your head up throughout the movement. Reverse and repeat for the desired number of repetitions. When these become easy, have your training partner place a barbell plate in your lap to provide added resistance. Some of you will also develop sufficient triceps strength to do regular Weighted Dips. You will need a dipping belt for these, which most gyms will provide for their members. Place the belt around your waist and attach a barbell plate to the harness, then perform your repetitions as usual. If your gym has no harness, you can also put a dumbbell between your calves, bending your knees and crossing your ankles to hold the dumbbell in place.

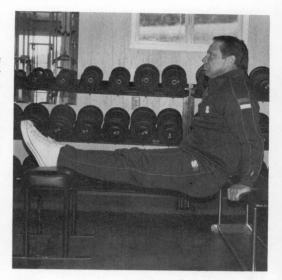

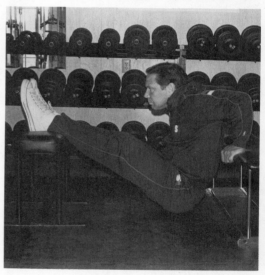

## Standing Press in Power Rack

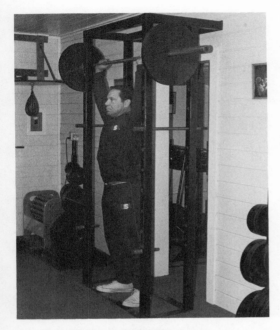

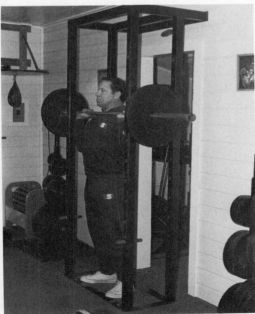

**Muscles worked:** Front and outer deltoids

**Directions:** Set the pins on the power rack so that the barbell will be at shoulder height. Then, with your hands shoulder-width apart, press the bar overhead as you did for standing presses. Remember to keep your knees locked and your back straight.

**Tips:** The only advantage of doing standing presses in the power rack is that you don't have to clean the weight to the shoulders to do the lift. Otherwise, the lift is identical.

**Variations:** Standing Presses against the Rack are done in exactly the same manner only the barbell is moved upward while riding up the sides of the power rack. This ensures that you keep the bar in a straight line, though a lot of gym owners will frown at having their paint scratched away. A more profitable variation would be to vary the height at which you set the pins. Putting the bar at different heights can make the same weight very light or very heavy as there are "sticking" points during the performance of many lifts when you are biomechanically "weaker." These Partial Rack Presses are done by many Olympic lifters who want greater overhead strength for the clean and jerk. Just make sure you keep your back and legs straight and push the bar overhead — don't jerk it.

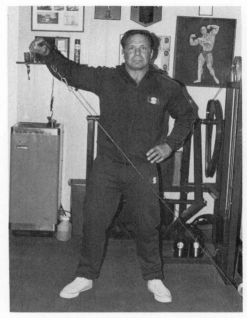

**Muscles worked:** Outer deltoids

**Directions:** Using a wall pulley that has handles at the bottom, stand with one side facing the pulley, holding in your opposite hand a single cable handle. Back away from the machine until the cable is tight and then raise the cable from the bottom position, as shown in the photograph, to shoulder height on the side away from the machine. Keep the elbow slightly bent throughout the exercise and move the hand through a semicircular motion from the hip to shoulder level, keeping constant tension on the cable. At the top position, your arm will be basically straight, the elbow only slightly bent, and you should feel a pulling sensation in the shoulder area. Then, lower the arm to hip level and repeat, keeping constant tension on the cable. Do all your repetitions for one side before working the other to complete the set.

**Tips:** Use a light enough weight so that you can do these with good form, getting a full extension of the weighted arm at the top.

**Variations:** You can shift the workload from the outer deltoids to the rear deltoids by bending at the waist, keeping the back flat and the legs slightly bent. Bent-Over Pulley Raises start with the hand near the calves and are finished when the arm is fully extended out to the side, parallel to the floor. To maintain the flat-backed position, brace yourself with your free hand by placing it against your thigh or a bench.

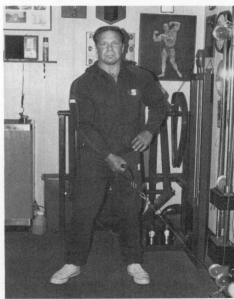

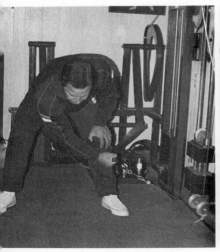

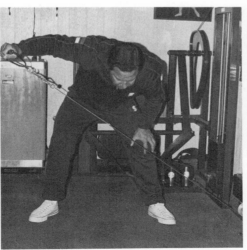

## Preacher Bench Curl

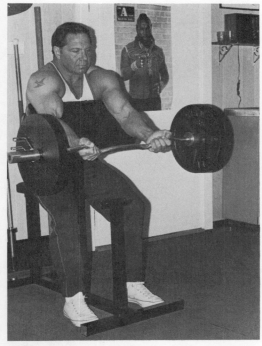

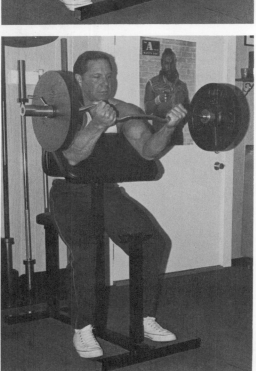

**Muscles worked:** Biceps

**Directions:** Preacher benches (sometimes called Scott benches after bodybuilder Larry Scott, who helped popularize their use back in the sixties) consist of a large padded surface attached to a stand that may or may not also include a seat. Using a curl bar, either sit or stand behind the bench and place the upper arms against the pad. Then, keeping the elbows and upper arms stationary, perform curls; raise and lower the curl bar just as if you were doing standing curls.

**Tips:** The preacher bench was designed to isolate the biceps, so make sure you choose an appropriately light weight when doing these. Always remember that when only one muscle is being worked — not a group — a lighter weight will generally have to be used. Otherwise, proceed as for regular curls.

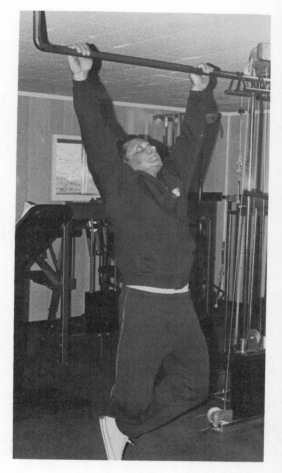

**Muscles worked:** Latissimus dorsi and biceps

**Directions:** Grasp the chinning bar with an overhand grip just slightly wider than your shoulders. Pull yourself upward until your chin is parallel with the bar and then lower yourself slowly to arms' length. Make sure that your feet don't touch the floor — let all the pulling come from the large muscles of your upper back. Make sure you completely straighten the arms before you begin your next repetition.

**Tips:** Many people, especially women, have trouble learning to do chins because, as with dips, a relatively high level of strength is required for the movement. So, if you can't do a full set, or even one, do negative chins, using a small stool or a training partner to get yourself in the proper position, and then lower yourself down for each "rep." Make sure that you lower yourself very slowly, as the longer you take to get to the bottom the more the muscles are being stressed.

**Variations:** While the overhand grip is best biomechanically — it works the lat muscles most fully — you can also use an underhand grip, which allows the biceps of the arms to carry more of the load. Several women with whom we've worked first learned to do negative chins, then moved to underhand chins, and then, finally, developed the strength to do overhand chins. Another thing to consider is that the wider the hand-grip you use, the more the pull comes from the lat muscles alone and less from the lats plus the arms. Later, as you've gained sufficient strength, attach extra weight to yourself as we described for dips.

# Neck Exercise with Head Strap

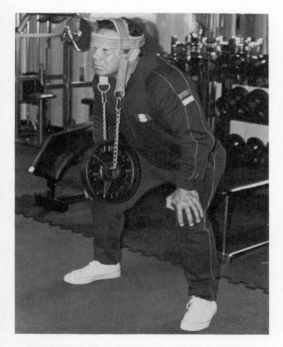

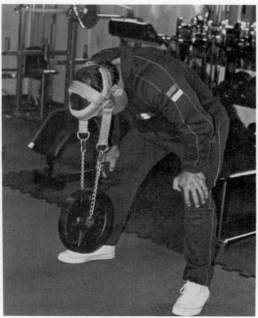

**Muscles worked:** Side and rear neck muscles

**Directions:** Most gyms will have a head strap or head harness that's made so a barbell plate can be attached to provide resistance. Put on the harness, with the added plate, and either sit on the end of a bench or stand, bending the knees slightly and bracing both hands against your upper thighs. Lower your head as far forward as you can, then reverse the motion and roll it as far backward as possible. After you've done your front to back repetitions, bend the head to the right side as far as possible, then all the way to the left side, and continue until all the reps scheduled have been completed.

**Tips:** Some of you may wonder why we would bother to include neck exercises in a book aimed at older adults. While the young generally do neck work to help themselves with such sports as wrestling and football, older adults need to keep the muscles in their neck strong to help their posture, their circulation, and to minimize injuries to the spine and back from falls and other unforeseen jarring motions to the head. Also, keeping the muscles in the neck firm and full will help to keep the skin tighter, lending the appearance of youthfulness. Obviously, you don't need to do a lot of neck work, and the other exercises such as high pulls and overhead presses will work the neck muscles some, but after you've gotten into your training for a cycle or two, we suggest you give it a try. Just remember, as you're looking for reasons to justify the time, that not only will you be helping to protect your back and your brain, you'll also be getting closer to the Greek notion of the ideal physical form, which, for those of you who aren't classically grounded, stated that the neck should be the same size as the calf and biceps.

**Variations:** Many gyms will have neck machines that you can also try but if there are no neck machines, and no head strap available, you can still get a good neck workout by using a single barbell plate. Simply lie face down on a bench and hold the plate on the top of the back of your head. Then, keeping the plate secure with your hands, lower your head as far down as possible over the edge of the bench and then reverse, pulling the head upward as far as possible by arching the neck backwrd. This is an especially good exercise for the rear neck muscles. To work the front of the neck, lie face upward, hold the plate against your forehead (you may wish to place a towel over your face), and raise and lower your head as far as possible. You should feel a contraction in the neck at the upward position and a stretching sensation in the bottom position.

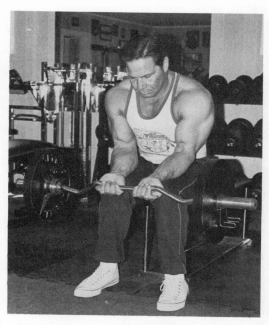

**Muscles worked:** Flexors of the forearm

**Directions:** Load a curl bar and place it on the floor at the end of a flat bench. Grasp it with an underhand grip on the closest hand spacing and lift the bar to your thighs so that as you sit on the end of the bench, your forearms are resting on your thighs and your hands, holding the curl bar, extend just past your knees. Then, lower the hands by bending the wrist backward until a definite stretch sensation is felt. Reverse, raising the bar up past the starting position until the wrists are fully contracted and you feel a tightness in the forearms. Hold this position for a second before you lower the bar to the bottom and repeat for the next repetition.

**Tips:** Besides helping to keep the forearms full, these help to maintain gripping strength, which you'll not only need in daily life but to assist you with some of these exercises. The advantage the curl bar has over the straight bar, as described in Chapter 17, is that the angulated hand spacings are often more comfortable to use.

**Variations:** Reverse Wrist Curls with the Curl Bar are done using an overhand grip while the wrists are moved upward and downward, the forearms resting on the thighs. You may need to try a slightly wider grip with these so that they're comfortable.

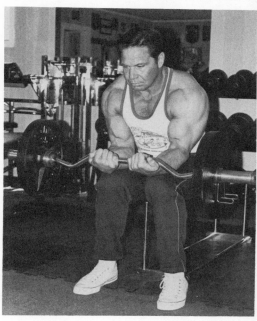

# Dumbbell Wrist Curl

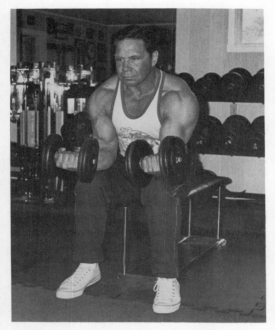

**Muscles worked:** Flexors of the forearm

**Directions:** Grasp a pair of moderately heavy dumbbells with an underhand grip and sit on the end of an exercise bench, your forearms resting against your thighs. Lower the dumbbells, by bending the wrists backward, and allow them to roll down into the fingers of the hand. Then, roll the dumbbells back to the palms and continue rolling the hands upward until the wrists are fully cocked at the top position and a tight sensation is felt in the forearms. Hold the contraction for just a second before doing the next repetition.

**Tips:** Be careful in rolling the dumbbells down into your fingertips that you don't drop them on your toes. Allowing them to roll into the fingers works more of the muscles in the hands and allows you to stretch the wrist back further because the dumbbells are in a lower position. If you feel any sharp pains in the wrist as you do these, however, back off and don't try to go as low.

**Variations:** Reverse Curls with Dumbbells are exactly what the name implies. Use an overhand grip, but don't try to let the dumbbells roll down into your fingers. Also, both regular and reverse curls can be worked by using only one dumbbell at a time. Many bodybuilders work only one arm at a time so they can "concentrate" on the muscles doing the exercise. Suit yourself, but you'll save time by working them as a pair.

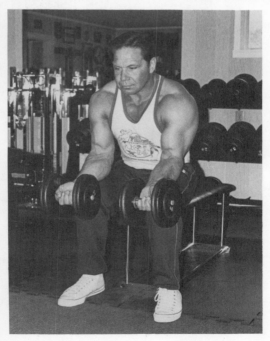

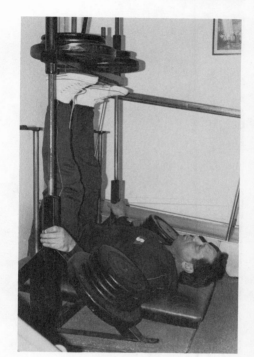

**Muscles worked:** Quadriceps and related thigh muscles

**Directions:** Traditional leg-press machines contain a padded cushion on the floor and a footpad overhead. However, there are now a number of leg-press machines on the market that call for the body to be either seated or partly lying-partly seated. If your gym does not have a standard wall-type leg-press machine, as pictured, ask the gym manager or one of the other trainers how to use what they have for best results. To do standard leg presses, lie on the floor pad and place your feet against the footrest with your *hips directly below* the footpad and weights. Push the weight upward until the knees lock and then move the pins so that you can lower the weight all the way down to do your repetitions. Unlock your knees and lower the weight until your thighs are almost touching your chest. Then, push it upward, locking your knees at the top for a second until you do your next repetition.

**Tips:** These are a great leg developer, and many people who have back problems have found that they can greatly increase their leg strength by doing these while not running the risk of further back injuries. You'll note that we didn't specify foot spacing on these. Like many other exercises we've already discussed, varying the feet will effect the way leg presses develop the thighs. To stress the outer thighs keep the feet close together, almost touching each other. To work the inner thigh, place the feet quite wide and turn the toes outward. Or, choose an in-between position, which places more of the stress on the front and upper thighs. If you feel any discomfort in the lower back while doing these, place your hands up under your hips, palms downward, to slightly elevate the pelvis. Otherwise, we like to keep our hands on the pins so that we can swing them back into place should we fatigue quickly.

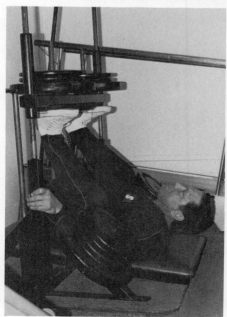

# Hack Squat

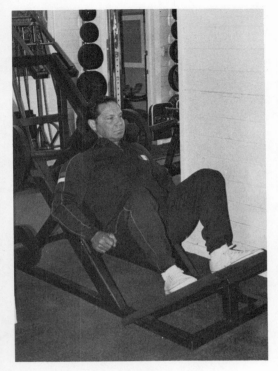

**Muscles worked:** Quadriceps and gluteus maximus

**Directions:** Situate yourself on the hack squat machine, facing outward with your feet placed shoulder-width apart on the slanted footboard and your shoulders against the pads. Push upward (and slightly backward) until the knees are locked and then, if the machine has them, release the pins so that you'll be able to do your repetitions all the way down. Keeping the back straight and the head up, lower the tops of the thighs until they are in the same position that you assume for a parallel squat done on the floor. Return to the locked knee position and repeat for the desired number of repetitions.

**Tips:** Hack squats are generally done following regular squats or leg presses to provide auxiliary thigh development. You can experiment with your foot spacing here as well. Putting the feet close together will once again stress the outer thighs, and putting the feet past shoulder width, with the toes turned outward, will work the inner thigh. If hack squats feel awkward, try placing your feet closer to the top edge of the footboard so that you will be closer to a true squat position.

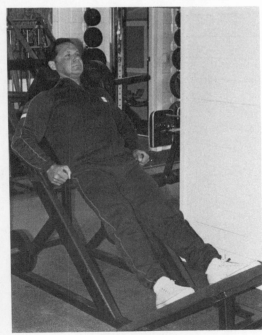

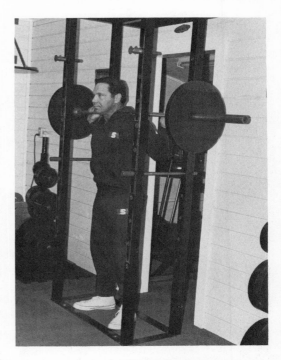

**Muscles worked:** Quadriceps, gluteus maximus, lumbars

**Directions:** Set the pins on the power rack so that the bar will be about 3 inches above your waistline. Place the bar on the pins and get your training partner to check and see if, when you assume the squat position with the bar across your shoulders, the legs form a 90 degree angle at the knee, when the bar is resting on the pins. Push upward from this position, keeping the back flat and the head up until the knees are locked. Slowly return the bar to the pins and repeat.

**Tips:** To start this lift properly, you need to assume your regular squat stance as if you were halfway up with the bar. This is very important. Set your feet at the same width, point your toes as you normally would, place your hands the same distance apart on the bar, and place the bar at the regular spot on your upper back. Partial squats (in this case what would be called half squats) are used to help you gain strength for the regular squat, and every effort should be made to keep the body in its usual squatting form. We prefer to do these after our regular squats, and since the bar is moving a much shorter distance, you can use greater weights in this exercise than you can with regular squats. The main trick in doing these is to break the inertia of the bar resting on the pins. Before you begin to push, make sure that you've flattened out your back and that your feet are in line with your shoulders. Then, push slowly upward, maintaining your pressure for several seconds until the bar breaks free of the pins, at which point it will move more easily. Remember to keep the bar in the center of the rack: don't try to slide it up and down the pins, as this increases the resistance because of the friction.

**Variations:** Quarter squats are done by setting the bar at an even higher pin position, so that you move it through only a fourth of the total squat range of motion. Greater weights can again be used because of the shorter movements, and it's sometimes fun to use such big weights; besides they make you stronger. As with partial or half squats, however, make sure you flatten your back before you begin to push upward.

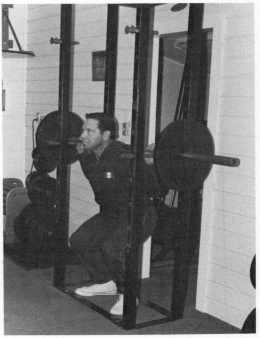

## Partial Deadlift in Power Rack

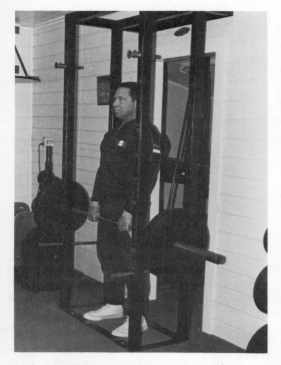

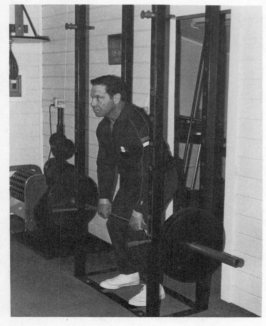

**Muscles worked:** Lumbars, trapezius, latissimus dorsi

**Directions:** Set the pins on the power rack so that the bar will rest just below your knees. Assume the flat-backed deadlift stance described earlier, using an alternating grip or an overhand grip with hand straps, and pull the weight from the pins until you're erect, shoulders back, with the bar resting against your thighs. Slowly lower the bar back to the pins, *reset your back,* and repeat for the desired number of repetitions.

**Tips:** Since most people find the upper part of the deadlift most difficult, partial movements such as these have been used to add greater strength to the back muscles. If you wish to add these to your routine, do them on a different day than you would normally do your deadlifts from the floor. We have recommended to our lifters that they add them on their heavy squat day, following their squat workout. In our opinion, two types of deadlift on the same day are too much. As with the partial squats, you'll need to pull for several seconds before the bar will move from the pins when you use heavy weights. Once you've broken the inertia, however, perform these as if they were regular deadlifts. And, don't allow the bar to bounce on the pins. Make sure your back is properly aligned for each repetition to avoid injury.

**Variations:** Setting the bar at different heights will allow you to work different parts of the deadlift and your back. Setting the bar above the knees allows you to work the trapezius and upper-back muscles, placing it further down the shin stresses the lumbars and *then* the upper back. Again, the shorter the movement of the bar, the more weight you can and should lift for maximum results.

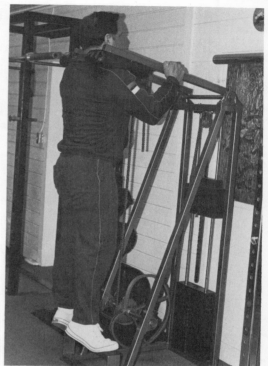

**Muscles worked:** Gastrocnemius and related calf muscles

**Directions:** Place the shoulder pads of the standing calf machine against your shoulders and rise on your toes until you feel a tight sensation in the calf muscles. Then, lower yourself, allowing the heels to go below the level of the footpad, until the muscles are fully stretched. Reverse and repeat for the desired number of repetitions.

**Tips:** Most gyms will have a standing calf machine, but if they don't you can still do calf work by lying under the leg-press machine, by facing the hack-squat machine with your shoulders under the shoulder pads, by using a Universal leg-press station, or by using the good old barbell, your calf block, and the power rack. To do this latter version, set the bar on the pins at shoulder height, put your toes up on the calf block and work the calves by pushing the bar up and down against the sides of the power rack. By sliding the bar against the power rack, it's much easier to keep your balance, and you can use greater weights than if you were standing free with the bar across your shoulders. You can even do what are called "donkey" calf raises by placing your toes up on the calf block, supporting your upper body against a bench of waist height, and then having your training partner sit across your hips to provide the resistance. In other words, just about any movement in which you rise onto your toes and then come back down below parallel will work the calves. Some gyms will also have seated calf machines that work on the same principles we described for seated barbell calf raises (see page 159). Just remember, your calves respond best to high repetition training, so work them in sets of 15 to 20 repetitions — not tens and fives — and stretch as far upward and downward as possible.

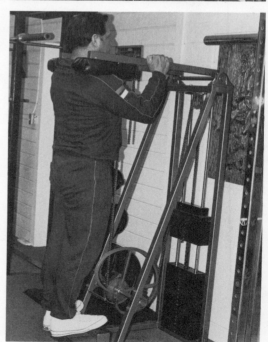

We realize that there are fewer leg and lower-body exercises included in this section than there are upper-body exercises. There are two reasons for this. The first is that we have already described most of the standard leg and hip exercises in Chapters 17 and 18. The second is that the sort of auxiliary exercise done on machines varies a great deal from gym to gym, based on the available equipment. While many gyms include a multistation Universal machine that would allow you to do seated leg presses and seated calf extensions (as well as leg curls and leg extensions) many other gyms do not. And the Nautilus, Polaris, Cam II, Iron Company, Hydra-Gym, and other assorted machines vary greatly in design and effectiveness. The Nautilus people have a fuller line of leg and hip machines, ranging all the way from a hip and low-back machine that works a number of lower-body muscles at once, to their adductor machine, which is able to isolate that one particular muscle. And our recommendation, if your gym contains a number of Nautilus machines, is to buy Ellington Darden's *The Nautilus Book* to learn the Nautilus-recommended method of training on each of the machines. Where the various seats, footpads, arm pads, etc., are set, does make a difference in the effectiveness of the exercise, just as a wider stance in the leg press creates a different stress for the thigh muscles than a close foot stance would. For the other makes of machines, ask the manager before trying any of them so you can get them set properly. But above all, don't neglect your barbells totally for machines. Squats and high pulls are good, result-producing exercises that work a number of muscles at one time as well as helping to increase your cardiovascular efficiency. And, use a periodization approach to your machine exercises, just as we recommend for your barbell training.

# Abdominal Exercises

**Muscles worked:** Lower abdomen

**Directions:** Grasp a chinning bar with an overhand, shoulder-width grip and hang straight down, toes pointed. Bend your knees and pull your thighs to your chest. Lower the legs and repeat for the desired number of repetitions.

**Tips:** These are great, but sometimes your grip will go before your abdomen fatigues. To avoid this, stand on a small stool and strap yourself to the bar with your hand straps. Then have your training partner remove the stool and proceed as usual. One problem many beginners face is that they try to do these so rapidly they begin swinging and can't continue with the exercise. To correct this, have someone brace you from behind, or simply slow down and stop just for a second at the bottom of each repetition before you begin to pull your knees upward again.

**Variations:** Frog Kicks are done in exactly the same manner, although at the top, the knees are flared out to the sides of the trunk, allowing the pelvis to tip further forward. Again, avoid swinging and concentrate on how the lower abdomen feels as you hold the contraction at the top for a second. Another good exercise to do on the chinning bar is the Hanging Leg Raise. To do these, raise your legs with the knees kept almost straight and the toes pointed until they are parallel to the floor. Then, slowly lower them back to the straight downward position and repeat.

Many gyms will have a special piece of equipment that allows leg raises and knee-ups to be done by supporting your body on your elbows and forearms as they rest on padded parallel bars. Most of these abdominal machines will have a large pad for your back to prevent swinging and a step to let you position yourself easily. Whether you're doing leg raises or knee-ups, make sure to keep your back pressed firmly against the pad and keep your head up as you do your repetitions. If you feel any discomfort in your shoulders or elbows from supporting your body weight, go back to the chinning bar.

## Hanging Knee-up

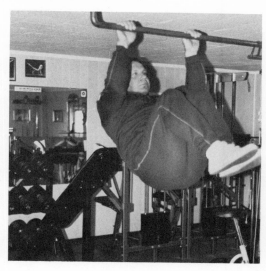

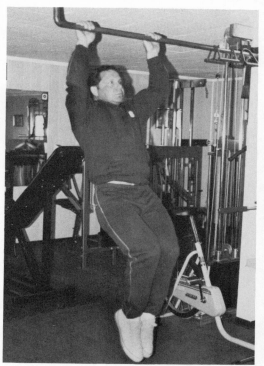

# 20 / Aerobics and Weight Training

ALTHOUGH research has shown that weight training *alone* produces cardiovascular benefits, we nevertheless recommend that you include some aerobic exercise either at the end of your workouts or on your "off" days. Aerobic exercise, as we mentioned in Part Two, is any regular, repetitive activity that elevates the pulse — swimming, jogging, cross-country skiing, cycling, walking, etc. To achieve an aerobic effect, and thereby improve your cardiovascular fitness, your pulse must be elevated to within 80 percent of 220 minus your age and be maintained at that level for at least 15 minutes, three or more times a week. Three times a week seems to be the minimum number of workouts for aerobic fitness. Studies have shown that training twice a week will produce increased strength and other parameters of fitness such as altering body-fat levels, but unless aerobic exercise is engaged in three times a week, there's still little change in such standard tests of aerobic fitness as maximum oxygen uptake levels.

Since the pulse levels attainable with advancing age *decrease,* it's important that you learn to check your pulse periodically during both your weight training and your aerobic workouts. Exercise that's too vigorous can strain the heart and lungs, so periodically stop during your workouts, place your fingers on the large carotid artery that runs up the side of your neck, and count the number of heartbeats that occur during 15 seconds, then multiply by four. You can also take the pulse at the wrist by placing your fingers just below the base of the thumb, but the carotid artery is generally easier to find and, since the pulse is stronger there, easier to count.

As you determine your pulse rate during or after exercise, you'll know if you are within the proper range. For example, a fifty-year-old person would first determine maximum pulse rate by subtracting 50 from 220 — 170. Then he or she would multiply 170 by .80 to get 136 beats per minute, a figure the physiologist call the *target heart rate.* This 136 beats per minute is the pulse rate you want to achieve — and maintain — for at least 15 minutes. Make sure to check your pulse as soon as you stop exercising, since it will rapidly slow down. If you're walking, and your pulse registers only 90 after you've been going for 10 minutes, step up the pace until you're at your target pulse rate and then *maintain that pulse rate for a full 15 minutes.* Likewise, if you've been cycling over hilly country and discover that your pulse is up to 155 when your target rate is 130, allow yourself a minute or so to return to the 130 level before you start out again.

As for how best to consistently match and maintain your target heart rate, there are two forms of aerobic exercise that we feel are superior to all others for convenient aerobic conditioning in older individuals. These two forms are cycling and a type of rapid walking called "powerwalking." We chose these two because (1) they are likely to create the least injuries in those who do them regularly, (2) they require little equipment (a good pair of walking shoes and/or a bicycle), and (3) to do them, most of us don't have to go anywhere except right outside our doors — if that. You don't have to wait for the pool to open, schedule your racquetball court three days in advance, or pray for snow so that you can go cross-country skiing. All you've got to do is either go outside to walk or ride or get on your stationary bike and get to work.

## Walk — Don't Run

Podiatrists and orthopedic surgeons have loved the jogging boom. As tens of thousands of individuals took to the streets and tracks to improve their cardiovascular fitness, the incidence of knee, hip, foot, back, and leg injuries soared dramatically. In fact, some doctors have been able to create entire medical practices based on treating injured joggers. Don't misunderstand us. Jogging can be wonderful aerobic exercise, but the increasingly high incidence of foot and knee injuries that are turning up in doctor's waiting rooms across the country suggests that compared to walking or cycling it is not a particularly "safe" activity — especially not for those over thirty-five. Though both powerwalking and cycling will elevate your pulse to target level more slowly, they are equally as result-producing aerobic activities as jogging. Many doctors have been recommending cycling and walking for their older patients for years, and we've found that by walking rapidly, perhaps with added weights, or by cycling, excellent aerobic benefits will result.

## Powerwalking

Steve Reeves, legendary bodybuilder and star of the *Hercules* films of the fifties and sixties, coined the term "powerwalking" several years ago to describe a type of walking he began doing some years after his retirement from the screen. Now in his late fifties, Steve lives on a large ranch in California where he raises and trains Morgan horses, horses that, he says, were responsible for his discovery of "powerwalking." As he tells the story in his book, *Powerwalking,* he was on a trail ride with some greenhorns and decided, since he knew how sore they would get without a little walking to

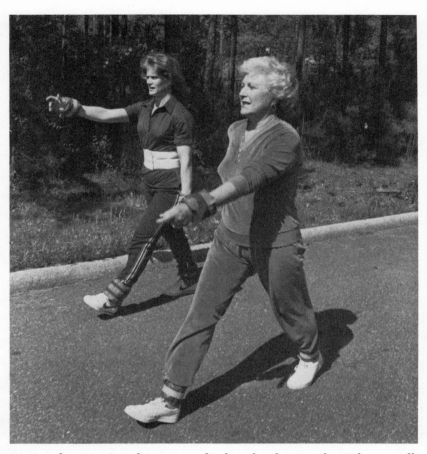

*Wearing extra weights on their ankles, wrists, and around their waists, Eleanor Curry and Jan step out for a session of "powerwalking."*

stretch their muscles, to give them periodic breaks during the ride to walk beside their horses. Steve's horse, however, was an especially fast walker, and so Steve really had to pick up his own pace.

He says, "I learned that by lengthening my stride and picking up my pace, while swinging my arms in rhythm with my stride and taking in deeper breaths, I was able to keep up with my horse. I also observed that at the end of the ten-minute walk, my horse and I had left the other riders and their mounts far behind. As I stood there waiting for the others to catch up, I reviewed in my mind what I had experienced in that ten-minute walk. I had been breathing more deeply, thus increasing my oxygen intake, and my heartbeat had quickened considerably and remained accelerated. It was a great aerobic exercise."

And so it was. But for powerwalking to have an effect on your cardiovascular system, it must be done *rapidly* and you must do it for at least fifteen minutes at a stretch. After you've developed a good fitness base, try adding extra resistance with ankle weights, wrist weights, and a weight belt to make the walking harder and to help you cut more calories while you're doing it. You may actually need the extra weight to cause your pulse to elevate to the target level.

**Terry:** "For a while after Jan started powerwalking, I heard about little else from her. Naturally, she quickly started using added weights — a total of 36 pounds made up of a 20-pound weight belt, two 3-pound wrist weights and two 5-pound ankle weights — and to add even more 'fun' to her program she began climbing the stairs in the stadium, for 30 minutes straight. I keep trying to explain to her that since I weigh, already, significantly more than she does, even with her 36 pounds, that when I walk with her I'm actually doing far more work than she is, but she hasn't seemed to take me very seriously."

Both of us will attest, however, despite our different levels of training, that Steve's technique really does increase aerobic fitness and decrease body fat. But, it's got to be done as he describes, with a long, arm-swinging gait, and with added weight as soon as you're able to walk rapidly for 20 minutes or so without reaching your target heart rate. Rapid powerwalking uses about 900 calories an hour, according to Reeves, and is approximately the equivalent of running 10 miles in an hour or swimming 2 miles in the same time. This figure is based on being able to powerwalk (without added weights) 5 miles in an hour — a very rapid pace. Don't worry if you can't match this pace initially. Few of us start out being able to run 6-minute miles either. Just work progressively at your walking — try to go a little further or a little faster each time you do an aerobic workout — and the progress will come, we promise.

## Cycling

This is probably our favorite aerobic activity — when we get to do it outdoors — because you can see so many things. We're lucky to have often lived outside one small town or another where there were still lots of beautiful country roads with few cars and good clean air. Now that we're more city-bound, in Austin, we do more indoor cycling since it's not only safer but you inhale less carbon monoxide. But we go to the country when we can. There's something about being out on the back roads on a bicycle that makes us feel young. Maybe it's because bikes played such a big part in both of our childhoods, or maybe it's simply the wind in what's left of our hair. Whatever, it's hard not to feel fine when you're rolling along looking at the cattle and the farms.

If you decide to give it a try, remember that good used bicycles can be found in many bike shops, and while ten speeds are nice, they aren't necessary for good cardiovascular work. However, if you live in a hilly area, we recommend that you get at least a five-speed bicycle, until you build up a high level of leg strength, so you won't end up walking half the hills. But if the area where you'll be cycling is flat, a one-speed bike will cost you a good deal less and still give you good results.

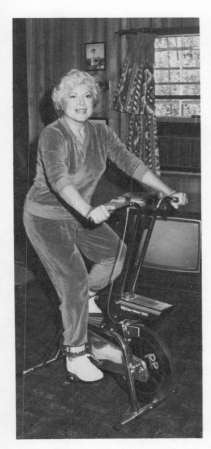

*One of the most convenient and efficient forms of cardiovascular exercise is the regular use of an exercise bicycle such as the one ridden here by sixty-year-old Eleanor Curry.*

As for "technique," there's little you need to be concerned with in cycling except getting the seat set to the right height and not tumbling over once you get rolling. Set the seat so that when you sit, your knees will be slightly bent at the bottom position. Make sure that you measure this with the ball of your foot — not the toes. If you are at all unsure setting your seat height, have a bike shop set it for you.

There are several things you may want to acquire. If we're riding in a subdivision or area where there are likely to be many dogs, we often carry a water pistol loaded with ammonia to discourage those incautious canines who think our calves look inviting. It's also a good idea to invest in lights for both the front and back of your bike, as well as in a heavy chain and padlock. And if you'll be riding in traffic a good bit, we'd also recommend a protective helmet. Even though many cities now have bike lanes set aside, far too many motorists are disdainful of cyclists and in a bicycle-car collision you'll lose every time. And finally, wear something bright, especially if you'll be out after dark. Most bike shops sell fluorescent trouser clips, jackets, and tape that can be applied to your clothes and bike, and that will greatly increase your safety after dark.

On the other hand, be reminded that cyclists are subject to the same stop signs, traffic lights, and common courtesies that motorized vehicles should extend to one another. Even in daylight, it's often difficult to see a cyclist, so be extra careful when you cross intersections or merge into traffic.

If you'll be using a stationary bike, make sure that you get one that has an adjustment on it so you can vary the tension at which the pedals revolve. This allows you to simulate "hills" by increasing the tension and then decreasing it after you've stood it as long as you can. It's a good idea to change the intensity as you ride indoors; otherwise there's a tendency to make it too easy on yourself. Remember that you need to keep your pulse rate up to 80 percent of your maximum heart rate for your cycling to do you the most good. At that level of activity — you should be perspiring fairly vigorously — by the time you've ridden for fifteen minutes, you'll really "feel" your legs.

If you have an exercise bike that adjusts easily, you can also vary the seat height from time to time to work the muscles of the legs in slightly different ways. Lowering the seat will involve the hip and thigh muscles more. Raising the seat way up puts more strain on the calves. In any case, whether you decide to cycle indoors or out or to powerwalk is a decision we'll leave up to you. What we do recommend in the strongest possible way is that you choose to do *some sort* of cardiovascular work. Remember, all the sleek, youthful muscles in the world won't be much help to you as you age if you develop heart trouble or cardiovascular disease. And why have either, since both can be combatted by a *regular* program of aerobic training?

PART FOUR

# Keeping It Up

IN many ways, being a weight trainer is a lot like being an architect. Both of you begin with an image — an ideal — then draw up a set of plans before finally beginning "construction." While the architect draws up a blueprint, of course, you'll be drawing up workout routines, routines that — just like the architect's blueprint — should logically lead you toward the realization of your original image. And when you begin construction, instead of saws, hammers, and nails, the "tools" you'll use will be barbells, dumbbells, and the machines you have accessible for training. Your building "materials" will be not wood or concrete but your body and the food, rest, and exercise you'll give it over the course of your training/construction cycle. And just as an architect will never see his high-tech skyscraper completed if his construction crew goes on strike, so will your plans for physical improvement go for naught if you're not diligent and regular about your training.

Regularity, as we've said before, is *vital* if you plan to attain your goals. As you begin to plan the workouts that will follow your first Basic cycle, make sure you're realistic about the amount of time you can allocate to training. Training only twice a week, regularly, even if you only do the Big Three exercises each time, is a lot better for you than training five days one week and only one the next.

In the three preceding exercise sections, we've done our best to tell you as much as we possibly could about each exercise so that when you began designing your own workouts, you'd have more than a brief description and a photo to help you make choices. And if you're ready now to begin your second or third training cycle, we urge you to go back and carefully reread each exercise description, and the Tips and Variations, before you begin preparing your next routine. We included, for each exercise, the same hints and explanations we would normally give our training partners, and we also did our best to indicate which exercises we've found to be especially beneficial. We have also indicated, for each exercise, which muscles are primarily benefited by that exercise, and though we don't expect you to become a physiologist, it's important that you not only check to see which muscles are being worked by which exercise but that you check the muscles listed against the muscle chart on page 305 to see exactly where those muscles are located on your own body.

As for how to create a personalized routine, we want to be perfectly clear that all of the material that follows is to be considered as a series of *suggestions* on how you should proceed with your training after your first Basic cycle. Unfortunately, there is absolutely no way, having never met you, for us to make any rigid, absolute suggestions as to how you, individually, should train. There is no way for us to know how old you are, what sort of physical shape you're in, whether you're a man or a woman, obese or thin, new to weights or a veteran, or how much time and money you feel willing to invest in weight training. Only you know the answers to those questions and only you know how you want to change your body through weight training so that it approaches the image you have in your mind. Therefore, what we have tried to do is provide you with three things: (1) some generalized suggestions about how to proceed after your first cycle, (2) some guidelines for selecting and ordering exercises for your workouts, and (3) some sample routines.

So, to begin, here are some guidelines to keep in mind when planning your new workouts.

**1.** Always include at least 10 minutes of stretching and warm-up exercises at the beginning of each workout and, if you have time, include stretching at the end of your workout to relax the muscles, reduce soreness, and to increase your flexibility.

**2.** If you plan to follow a two- or three-day schedule, choose *at least one* "multiple-muscle exercise" for each of the following divisions of the body: (1) legs, hips, and low back, (2) chest, arms, and shoulders, (3) upper back. You can easily tell which exercises are "multiple-muscle exercises." For example, a description of a squat will say: "Works the gluteus maximus, quadriceps, spinal erectors, and hamstrings," as opposed to the description of an exercise such as a curl, which will say only: "Works the biceps." Whether you plan to use a two-day or a three-day schedule, at least three multiple-muscle exercises would be done in each workout, one for each of the three major body divisions.

**3.** Always do your multiple-muscle exercises before doing the assistance work for that body part. For example, first do squats, then do other exercises, such as leg curls and leg extensions, that isolate individual muscles in the thigh. Likewise, do bench presses first and then triceps presses to isolate individual muscles in the upper arm.

**4.** Though you should be able to tell which exercises are multiple-muscle exercises from the exercise descriptions, we've listed below our favorites for your reference.

*Legs, Hips, and Low Back:* Squat, High Pull, Deadlift, Leg Press, Lunge
*Chest, Arms, and Shoulders:* Bench Press, Incline Press, Standing or Military Press, Press behind Neck, Dip
*Upper Back:* Rowing Motion (dumbbell or barbell), Wide-Grip Lat Pulldown, Seated Cable Pull, Partial Deadlift, Chin

**5.** Choose your additional or "assistance" exercises according to your own personal needs and desires. Don't do a routine just because someone else is doing it. Tailor your routine to your desire for bigger arms, firmer hips, a better golf swing, or more control in tennis. Read the Tips on each exercise for more information on each exercise's effect.

**6.** Don't try to choose too many exercises for one workout. Keep in mind that you'll be doing five sets of most exercises, which quickly become a lot of work even with just two or three exercises. Choose one, maybe two assistance exercises for your three multiple-muscle exercises, but no more than that for your second cycle, unless you were training with weights before. If you feel you're ready for more than two assistance exercises, read the section on Split Routines on pages 278–283 and be advised by it.

**7.** Make sure to include abdominal exercises.

**8.** Don't neglect your aerobic work.

**9.** Keep a training diary.

**10.** In writing your schedule, try to project some end-of-the-training-cycle goal poundages for yourself as well as what weights you'd need to lift in each workout along the way to your goal. For instance, if you finished your first cycle with 3 sets of 3 reps at 125 pounds in the squat, and you'd like to hit 155 for 3 reps on your second cycle, figure out what sort of incremental increases you'd need to make to get you there. If your goal weight is 65 pounds for your first squat workout in the hypertrophy stage, for instance, then making a 10-pound gain each week would let you come pretty close. This takes a little work, but setting goals is important. But make sure to be realistic about your goals, and if you can't do all 3 sets with a goal weight, don't increase on your next heavy day.

## A Word to Beginners

Those of you who've been uninvolved in any sort of regular exercise program prior to the purchase of this book will need to increase the frequency of your training and the number of exercises done in a workout session more slowly than those who've already done some weight training or who have been regular athletes in a fairly vigorous sport. Our blanket suggestion for novices is to do the *expanded* version (see page 182) of the basic workout for your *second* cycle, and then, after your body has achieved a higher base fitness level, tailor a routine that really suits you. For those of you who had no troubles adjusting to the basic workload and feel as if you'd like to spend more time exercising each week or for those of you who've been involved in an exercise program prior to your basic cycle, we'd suggest a three-day-per-week program rather than the two days per week of your first cycle. Please note, however, that there's nothing at all wrong with continuing to train only twice a week as long as you stick to periodization and really work on the days you train. Most weight trainers, however, find they make more rapid progress by working out three or more days a week. If you *do* decide to try a three-day program, work on Monday-Wednesday-Friday or Tuesday-Thursday-Saturday to give your body ample rest between workouts. *Do not train on consecutive days* unless you're using a split routine.

# 21 / Three-Day Training

I F you train three days per week, you have two recommended options. You can either use the same routine all three days, or you can do the same workout twice a week and a different routine on the other day. We prefer the latter. We do *not* recommend that you do three completely different workouts. Research has shown that best progress is made by using a light-day/heavy-day approach, which is not possible if all three workouts are different. If you choose to use a different routine for one day, make that day a moderately hard day, but not a real killer. Below you'll find several three-day-a-week routines. Here is an example of how to schedule the expanded basic routine for a three-day-a-week routine, using the same exercises each day.

**Routine A**

**Monday**
Stretching
Squat — Heavy
Lunge — Heavy
Bench Press — Light (80% of heavy day's weight)
Press behind Neck — Light
Bent-Forward Rowing Motion — Light
Bent-Leg Sit-up

**Wednesday**
Stretching
Squat — Light (80% of heavy day's weight)
Lunge — Light
Bench Press — Heavy
Press behind Neck — Heavy
Bent-Forward Rowing Motion — Heavy
Bent-Leg Sit-up

**Friday**
Stretching
Squat — Medium Heavy (90% of heavy day's weight)
Lunge — Medium Heavy
Bench Press — Medium Heavy
Press behind Neck — Medium Heavy
Bent-Forward Rowing Motion — Medium Heavy
Bent-Leg Sit-up

**Routine B**   Make sure that Friday's workout is only 85 percent as heavy as Monday's workout. Note that the Expanded Basic Workout is done on Monday and Friday with a different routine on Wednesday.

| Monday and Friday | Wednesday |
| --- | --- |
| Stretching | Stretching |
| Squat | High Pull |
| Lunge | Military Press |
| Bench Press | Triceps Press |
| Press behind Neck | Chin |
| Bent-Forward Rowing Motion | Seated Cable Pull |
| Lat Pulldown | Crunch |
| Hanging Leg Raise | Twist |
| Sit-up | |

**Routine C**   **The Sedentary Women's Study Routine**

The women in the study we described in Chapter 11 were divided into two groups because of equipment availability and time considerations at the health spa where the group met. They did identical routines, with the exception that one group did heavy squats on Mondays and heavy high pulls on Fridays while the other group did heavy high pulls on Monday and heavy squats on Friday. The Wednesday workouts were identical for both groups. This was group A's schedule.

| Monday | Wednesday | Friday |
| --- | --- | --- |
| Stretching | Stretching | Stretching |
| Partial Squat — Heavy | Full Squat | High Pull — Heavy |
| High Pull — Light | Leg Press | Partial Squat — Light |
| Lunge — Heavy | Incline Press | Lunge — Light |
| Leg Extension — Heavy | Dumbbell Fly | Leg Extension — Light |
| Leg Curl — Heavy | Dumbbell Row | Leg Curl — Light |
| Bench Press — Light | Sit-up | Bench Press — Heavy |
| Lat Pulldown — Light | Side bend | Lat Pulldown — Heavy |
| Sit-up | | Sit-up |
| Side bend | | Side bend |

There are several interesting things we want to point out about this routine. First, note that we changed the order of the first two exercises on Mondays and Fridays. This was done so that the women would be as fresh as possible for their heaviest exercise on any given day. The second thing to notice is the large number of leg exercises the women did. There were two reasons for this, the first being the women's desire to tone and firm their legs and the second being our desire to see them increase their leg and back power. Finally, we should mention that partial squats were chosen for the Monday and Friday workouts instead of regular squats because we wanted, as much as possible, to have the women's routine be similar to the men's. Partial squats and high pulls were the foundation exercises used in the men's study and so we used them with the women as well. Though several of the women were initially resistant to the partial squat, we found, after several weeks, that they preferred it to the deeper squats that were done on Wednesday because they felt safer working inside the power rack.

## The Sedentary Men's Study Routine

**Routine D**

As you can see, the men did fewer exercises than the women. There were two reasons for this. The first was that the men were doing exercises that involved many pulling movements. Heavy high pulls and power cleans work nearly all the muscles in the body, so it seemed unnecessary for the men to do too much assistance work. The second consideration was time. The men trained during their working day — usually at lunchtime — and they couldn't afford the time to do a lot of assistance work. As with the women, the men's program varied the intensity of the Monday and Friday workouts, and the men made increases on their Wednesday exercises as they could. This is a good example of a workout that can be done in a relatively short period of time and yet produces excellent results.

**Monday and Friday**
Stretching
High Pull (Done off of blocks so that the bar is at a height just above the knees)
Squat
Bench Press
Leg Extension
Leg Curl
Sit-up

**Wednesday**
Stretching
High Pull (Below knees — on blocks)
Power Clean
Press behind Neck
Curl
Sit-up

## Case Histories

Below are some case histories that we hope will provide you with some further clues on how to proceed with devising your individualized routine.

**Case History 1**    "Mary Smith" is a forty-year-old mother of three who started working again three months ago. She's of average height, a bit above average in weight — twenty pounds more than she'd like to be carrying. Between her new job and caring for her family, Mary figures she can invest five hours a week in training and has decided to exercise at home. She is especially concerned with the appearance of her hips and legs, which are too large in proportion to the rest of her body. For the past several years she has jogged three times a week, and though she's dropped ten pounds since she started jogging, she's still a long way from her goal weight.

Since Mary has been jogging on a regular basis, and has already completed one basic cycle, she's ready to begin serious work on reshaping her physique. Knowing this, she purchased not only a bench and weights but also a machine that allows her to do cable work for her hips and legs. While little weight loss will occur if she doesn't follow our nutritional suggestions in Chapter 9, the following routine will give her a good start on reshaping her lower body and improving her general level of fitness. Mary's five hours per week include her aerobic workouts, so she would need to do each day's weight workout within seventy minutes.

**Monday and Friday**
Stretching
Bench Press
Dumbbell Fly
Squat
Lunge
Cable Leg Pull (Inner and outer thigh)
Dumbbell Rowing Motion
Seated Cable Pull
Bent-Leg Sit-up
Leg Raise
Powerwalking — 30 minutes

**Wednesday**
Stretching
Incline Press
Leg Press
Leg Extension
Leg Curl
Barbell Rowing Motion
Crunch
Side bend
Powerwalking — 30 minutes

**Case History 2**    "John Smith" is Mary's older brother, a CPA for a large corporation. Though not overweight, John's concerned about the way his body is beginning to age. There seems to be less width to his shoulders than there once was, and so, besides improving his general fitness, he'd like to regain some of his lost upper-body size. John and his family belong to the Y, which has a well-equipped weight room, but because of his busy schedule, he can only train three days a week, for no more than an hour and a half at a time. The following routine would be our suggestion for John, who is forty-five, fairly tall, and of average weight.

**Monday and Friday**
Stretching
Squat
Bench Press
Press behind Neck
Triceps Press
Lat Pulldown
Dumbbell Rowing Motion
Curl
Sit-up
Exercise Bicycle — 30 minutes

**Wednesday**
Stretching
High Pull
Chin
Leg Curl
Leg Extension
Incline Press
Dumbbell Fly
Dumbbell Front Raise
Sit-up
Exercise Bicycle — 30 minutes

"Becky Edwards" is a thirty-year-old professional who is single. She is tall and tends to put weight on her waist rather than her hips and legs, both of which are a bit too small for the rest of her body. She realizes the value of a good appearance to her work and the value of exercise for general good health but her time is limited. She feels she can devote three hours a week to exercise at a local, well-equipped gym. She has completed one cycle of the basic program. (In this case we've scheduled the stationary cycling immediately after the squats in order to maximize the aerobic effect the squats have begun.)

**Case History 3**

**Monday and Friday**
Stretching
Incline Dumbbell Press
One-Hand Dumbbell Rowing
   Motion
Squat (Wide stance)
Squat (Narrow stance with heels
   raised on board)
Stationary Bicycle (Heavy resist-
   ance — 20 minutes)
Bent-Leg Sit-up — Twisting
Leg Raise
Standing Twist

**Wednesday**
Stretching
Leg Press
Lunge
Stationary Bicycle (Heavy resis-
   tance — 20 minutes)
Bent-Leg Sit-up — twisting
Leg Raise
Standing Twist

**Case History 4**    "Joe Williams" is thirty-five years old, of average height, and works in a factory. Even though he is on his feet most of the day, he is at least fifty pounds overweight. He is worried about his health and has decided to do what it takes to get back in shape again. The only sport he's spent much time with since high school has been softball. He has gone to a doctor, who encouraged him to begin a program of exercise and diet. The doctor gave him the go-ahead to train much harder than he had done during the ten weeks he spent on the basic program. Joe just bought enough equipment to fully equip his basement as a home gym.

| **Monday and Friday** | **Tuesday and Saturday** | **Wednesday** |
|---|---|---|
| Stretching | Stretching | Stretching |
| High Pull | Powerwalking or Cycling for 1 hour | Dumbbell Row |
| Squat | Abdominal work as on the other days. | Wide-Grip Pulldown |
| Lunge | | Close-Grip Pulldown |
| Leg Press | | Incline Press |
| Leg Curl | | Dumbbell Press (Seated) |
| Bent-Leg Sit-up | | Curl Bar Triceps Press |
| Crunch | | Dumbbell Curl |
| Leg Raise | | Crunch |
| | | Leg Raise |
| | | Powerwalking or Stationary Cycling for 30 minutes, depending on the weather |

**Case History 5**    "Martin Stevens" is a sixty-five-year-old former insurance salesman who lives in a typical suburb. Since his retirement three months ago, Martin has been able to more actively pursue his old love, golf. He's discovered, however, that his drives aren't nearly as long — nor as straight — as they were in years past, and he feels that his poor physical condition is responsible. Over the past twenty years, he's taken no regular exercise, playing golf only on warmer Sundays. Overweight, and a former smoker, he is also concerned about his cardiovascular condition. His doctor has given him permission to train but has encouraged him to take things slowly. He's completed one basic cycle, though he has not done as much aerobic training as his doctor would recommend. He'll be training at a health club. He has unlimited time for training, and has decided this time around to help not just his golf game, but to listen to his doctor's advice about the aerobics. Naturally, he will build up to this full program very gradually.

**Monday and Friday**
Stretching
Leg Press
Leg Extension
Wide-Grip Lat Pulldown
Bench Press
Triceps Pressdown
Crunch
Leg Raise
Stationary Cycling or
    Powerwalking — 30 min-
    utes

**Sunday**
Powerwalking — 30 min-
    utes

**Wednesday**
Stretching
Squats
Dumbbell Rowing Motion
Seated Cable Pull
Incline Press
Wrist Curl
Curl-Bar Curl
Knee-in
Standing Twist
Stationary Cycling or
    Powerwalking — 30 min-
    utes

# 22 / Split Routines and Circuit Training

THERE are two main reasons people choose to split their routines. Some do it to cut down on training time — preferring to do fewer exercises per day than a total body workout involves. (Note: many who choose this first option also want to allow more time and energy each day for cardiovascular work.) The second and opposite reason is to allow *more* time to work out with weights. This is actually the more common reason among serious weight trainers, and, as you become more acquainted with the wide variety of exercises possible, you too may find yourself wanting to split your workouts to include several assistance exercises for each body part so that you can really concentrate on a particular area.

The most common split is to do four workouts a week — two upper-body workouts and two lower-body workouts — with abdominal work done all four days. Generally these are done on Monday-Tuesday and Thursday-Friday with Wednesday, Saturday, and Sunday off; but some people prefer Tuesday-Thursday and Saturday-Sunday so they'll have more time on the weekends for longer workouts. Lower-body workouts alternate with upper-body workouts to allow proper recovery.

Some long-term trainers break their workouts down even further — using a six-day schedule that allows, for instance, two chest, shoulders, and triceps workouts, two upper back and biceps workouts, and two leg and hip workouts. This intense schedule is generally done only by experienced trainers who have reached a high level of fitness that allows them to both recover and benefit from workouts such as these.

**Jan:** "I trained on a six-day schedule during my final competitive years and during the eighteen months of my weight loss. But when I first started training, back in 1974, I trained only twice a week and moved to three days only after I'd gone through several cycles. I moved to six days mainly because, when we were at Auburn University, we coached both men and women powerlifters and I was in the gym on a daily basis. I liked training that way, actually, and I made good gains, but after I dropped my body weight and leveled off, I cut back to a four-day routine simply because of time. Now, I train Monday-Wednesday, Friday-Saturday, and do aerobic work on the other three days."

If you've adapted well to the basic program and have the time and the intestinal fortitude, give split routines a try. Just remember that you don't want to train your legs every day — give them at least one and preferably two days to rest before you stress them with weights again. Since split routines grew out of the desire for greater diversity, you'll note in some of the samples that while both workouts for the lower body, for instance, are similar, they are not necessarily exactly the same. Many trainers make some substitutions in their split routines in order to work the muscles in as many ways as possible. Also, most lifters find that certain particularly exhausting exercises — especially the deadlift — can't be borne more than once a week. Again, look at all the sample routines that follow, study the patterns, and review the Tips for each exercise before committing yourself.

## Split Routine A

This introductory four-day split routine should follow completion of the basic cycle and the expanded basic cycle. If an exercise is indicated as being "heavy" on Monday, then it would be "light" (85%) on Thursday, etc. This applies to both the upper- and lower-body days.

**Mondays and Thursdays — Upper Body**
Stretching
Wide-Grip Lat Pulldown — Heavy
Dumbbell Rowing Motion — Heavy
Bench Press — Light
Dumbbell Fly — Light
Triceps Press — Light
Curl — Light
Sit-up
Leg Raises

**Tuesdays and Fridays — Lower Body**
High Pull — Heavy
Squat — Light
Leg Extension — Light
Leg Curl — Light
Calf Raise — Light
Seated Twist
Side bend

## Split Routine B

**Jan:** "This is my four-day-per-week routine that I've been doing since our move to Texas. Since my body weight has stabilized and I'm not training for a powerlifting competition, this could, I suppose, be called a 'maintenance' program. One of the things I'm trying to 'maintain' is some extra size in my upper body so that my proportions are better. That's why there's so much emphasis on upper-body work. Please remember that this would have to be considered an *advanced* routine. Don't try to do this many exercises in one workout until you've trained for quite a while, if you work close to your limit as we recommend. Note that I deadlift only once a week, doing high pulls on the other leg and hip day. I also have some slight variations in my upper-body work."

**Monday**
Stretching
Bench Press — Heavy
Incline Dumbbell Press — Heavy
Incline Dumbbell Fly — Heavy
Press behind Neck — Heavy
Close-Grip Bench Press — Heavy
Dip
Triceps Pressdown — Heavy
Wide-Grip Lat Pulldown — Light
Close-Grip Lat Pulldown — Light
Dumbbell Rowing Motion — Light
Curl — Light
Sit-up
Leg Raise

**Wednesday**
Stretching
Deadlift — Heavy
Squat — Light
Lunge — Light
Leg Press — Light
Leg Extention — Light
Jackknife
Standing Twist

**Friday**
Stretching
Wide-Grip Lat Pulldown — Heavy
Close-Grip Lat Pulldown — Heavy
Dumbbell Rowing Motion — Heavy
Bench Press — Light
Incline Barbell Press — Light
Decline Dumbbell Fly — Light
Press behind Neck — Light
Close-Grip Bench Press — Light
Triceps Pressdown — Light
Curl — Heavy
Sit-up
Leg Raise

**Saturday**
Stretching
Squat — Heavy
High Pull
Lunge — Light
Leg Extension — Light
Leg Curl — Light
Sit-up
Side bend

This is a six-day-per-week routine for *advanced* trainers.

**Monday-Friday**
(*Make Monday heavy and Friday light*)
Stretching
Chin
Wide-Grip Lat Pulldown
Close-Grip Lat Pulldown
Curl-Bar Curl
Concentration Curl
Bent-Leg Sit-up
Hanging Knee-in

**Tuesday-Saturday**
(*Make Tuesday light and Saturday heavy*)
Stretching
Bench Press
Incline Press
Seated Dumbbell Press
Front Raise with Dumbbell
Curl-Bar Triceps Press
Triceps Pressdown
Seated Twist
Side bend
Crunch

**Thursday**
Stretching
Stiff-Leg Deadlift
Power Snatch
Leg Press — Light
Lunge
Leg Curl — Light
Leg Extension — Light
Bent-Leg Sit-up

**Sunday**
Stretching
Squat — Heavy
Leg Press — Heavy
Leg Extension — Heavy
Leg Curl — Heavy
Calf Raise
Hyperextension
Crunch
Seated Twist

**Jan:** "This is the six-day-per-week routine that I used to train for the 1983 Women's Nationals, at which I weighed 146 pounds and made a world-record deadlift. It is the hardest workout routine I've ever done in my many years of training. Some exercises are grouped together to indicate that they were done in what are called 'supersets,' meaning that one exercise was done immediately after another exercise had been completed. Then after both (or more) exercise sets had been completed, I took a short rest before proceeding to the next superset. This routine is exceptionally long — I would never recommend that anyone do this many exercises at a time. I did it because I wanted to create rapid changes as I lost my body weight and because, once I got started on this high-level training, I got hooked. I liked the way all the upper-body work helped my figure become more proportional and how much larger my bust measurement got, even though I was losing weight, not to mention how strong I was getting everywhere. During this cycle I also did a lot of powerwalking, with added weight, and rode my bicycle at least three times a week. However, as I got close to the contest, I cut back drastically on my cycling and powerwalking to save my energies for my workouts. After the meet was over, I went right back to my aerobics and started another cycle.''

**Monday-Friday**
(*Monday light and Friday heavy*)
Stretching
Chin
Wide-Grip Lat Pulldown ⎤
Close-Grip Lat Pulldown ⎦ Superset
Seated Cable Pull
Dumbbell Rowing Motion
Curl-Bar Curl ⎤
Concentration Curl ⎦ Superset
Abdominal Work

**Tuesday-Saturday**
(*Tuesday light and Saturday heavy*)
Bench Press
Incline Dumbbell Press
Decline Dumbbell Press ⎤
Decline Dumbbell fly ⎦ Superset
Press behind Neck ⎤
Dumbbell Press ⎦ Superset
Front Raise with Dumbbell
Side Lateral ⎤
Rear-Deltoid Raise ⎦ Superset
Triceps Press
Triceps Pressdown
Abdominal Work

**Thursday**
Stretching
Deadlift
Squat — Lift
Leg Press — Light
Lunge — Light
Leg Curl — Light ⎤
Leg Extension — Light ⎦ Superset
Abdominal Work

**Sunday**
Stretching
Squat — Heavy
Partial Squat
Partial Deadlift below Knee
Leg Press — Heavy
Lunge — Heavy
Leg Curl — Heavy ⎤
Leg Extension — Heavy ⎦ Superset
Abdominal Work

Throughout this book we have encouraged you to train as rapidly as possible in order to get maximum aerobic benefit from your weight workouts. If your time is very limited, however, and you want to try to really squeeze a lot of aerobic benefit from your weight workouts, you might want to give circuit training a try. Popular with many coaches because it is an efficient way to put large groups of people through a workout and because it builds endurance as well as some muscular strength, circuit training is still not a method used much by those who train outside of institutional settings. Who knows why? Perhaps because it doesn't build strength and muscle as well as standard training; or perhaps because you don't get that feeling of a good, tight pump, since your blood is rushing hither and yon over your entire body instead of engorging one particular area at a time, or perhaps because it's a tough routine to follow on a regular basis.

To do circuit training you need either a multistation weight-training machine or enough equipment at your home or gym to set up five or six different exercises so you are able to move from one to another without stopping. This is often tough in many gyms because you have to share equipment and sometimes wait in lines. However, with two bars and some dumbbells, you can easily do circuit training at home. Simply set up a pattern of exercises such as this: squat, bench press, lat pulldown, lunge, curl, triceps press, squat, bench press, etc. Continue moving from exercise to exercise until five sets of each exercise have been done and follow the principles of periodization as much as possible. Circuit training works well during the Hypertrophy stage of periodization, though we would not recommend it during Power. For that phase you need to take more time, concentrate on increasing your poundages, and do activities such as cycling and power-walking for your aerobics.

But if you want cardiovascular improvement to the max, research has shown that circuit training does produce marked aerobic benefits. In fact, in a study done by Drs. Paul Ward, Larry Gettman, and R. D. Hagan, it was found that a group of men doing only circuit training made just as much aerobic improvement as another group who did circuit training *and* jogging.

The trick to aerobic improvement from circuit training is to keep your pulse elevated for long periods of time. This is great if you've got the stamina for it, though we admit we've found it a hard way to train for more than a few weeks at a time.

If you do want to give circuit training a try, alternate lower-body and upper-body exercises. Here are two sample routines, which could be used on alternate workout days. Make sure to stretch before beginning your weight work.

**Sample Circuit 1**
Squat
Bench Press
Lunge
Overhead Dumbbell Press
Leg Curl
Curl-Bar Curl
Bent-Leg Sit-up

**Sample Circuit 2**
High Pull
Incline Press
Leg Press
Bench Press
Lunge
Triceps Pressdown
Bent-Leg Sit-up

# 23 / Maintenance

THIS section is not going to tell you how to clean your gym or repair your equipment. It *will* give you some further hints on how to make weight training a part of your life from now on. Though it may seem as if you have an awfully long way to go physically, there will come a day — if you apply yourself — when most of you will look down, smile at what you've accomplished, and say, "This I can live with. What I want to do now is try and stay more or less the way I am without killing myself." Some of you, however, may never reach that point either because you don't have the willpower to change your eating habits, or because you enjoy experimenting with your physique, trying various new exercises for your chest, trying front squats for a different workout on the thighs, or trying to see how strong you can be at some particular age and so on.

**Terry:** "Jan and I typify two different philosophies of training. After eleven years of training, she's still eager to experiment and try new training methods. She's always been very goal oriented and has continued to train that way, even though she's supposedly retired as a competitor, a decision I'm still suspicious of. As for me, though, I see the weights these days as a way to maintain what I achieved years ago. I no longer train for maximum strength gains, nor am I trying to cut up and be a bodybuilder. As I said in the beginning of this book, my workouts take very little time and are geared toward keeping my body weight and strength at levels that are acceptable to me. I still use periodization though I don't work very close to my full strength, even in the few exercises I use."

**Jan:** "Unlike most of us, Terry gains muscle exceptionally rapidly. He's found that if he trains very hard with weights that really tax him, he immediately starts getting larger all over. So, since a 52-inch chest, a 20-inch arm, and a 30-inch thigh are as large as he wants them to be, he uses weights that are about 70 to 90 percent of what his real limit would be. He never uses heavy weights for his legs anymore as his legs really grow quickly and he has enough trouble buying clothes as it is. Even so, he has to watch himself, and if he feels himself getting too big, he cuts back on his eating and on his poundages. His other variation on our periodization model is that he doesn't do a Power phase. He stays with tens and fives, working only to maintain his considerable muscle size and strength. He was as strong as anyone around during his prime and I guess that satisfied him. Usually, after he's done an eight-week cycle — four weeks of tens and four weeks of fives — he takes a couple weeks or so off and then starts again.

"One thing many people don't realize is that it takes far less work to maintain muscle than to build it. So, if you find yourself satisfied with your physical condition and/or extremely busy, try a maintenance cycle. See how you like it. Terry trains only twice a week or even twice every eight or nine days. His workouts take less than an hour, and on two or three other days of the week he'll either play squash, tennis, or, if he's really pushed for time, he'll ride the stationary cycle.

"Here's his normal maintenance routine, one day 'heavy,' one light:
>Stretching
>High Pull
>Squat
>Dumbbell Row
>Incline Press
>Dumbbell Press
>Crunch

"When he gets in a hurry, he does only three exercises:
>High Pull
>Squat
>Incline Press"

If *you* go on a maintenance routine, be as regular about your workouts as you were on a normal periodization program. Do all five sets for each exercise and have a heavy day and a light day. And if you find that you aren't maintaining as much strength and muscle as you'd like, add an exercise or two and up the poundage a bit. Fine tune it.

Any combination of exercises can be considered a "maintenance routine," but if you do plan to cut back significantly on time and intensity, make sure to concentrate on multiple-muscle exercises.

## Maintenance over Time

Maintenance of a more important sort, of course, is the maintenance of your commitment to the regularity of your exercise program, from now on out. We hope you do find a way, as we have done, to make training an integral part of your life, because we're convinced it will make the rest of your life better than it otherwise would be, and we're not ashamed to say we'd be pleased to think our work contributed to the sum of human satisfaction. Somehow, the two of us stopped worrying a long while back about whether we'll continue to train; we'd be as unlikely now to stop bathing or brushing our teeth as we would to stop exercising. And we know our own lives are the richer for that. As yours can be if you can manage to keep it up.

# 24 / The Curry Family

Through the years, our friendship with Bill and Eleanor Curry and their family has meant a lot to us. Not only were the Currys our neighbors in Opelika, Alabama, but they were often our training partners and dinner companions in the evenings. Besides all that, though, they were our soulmates and even our role models, having been in the iron game long before either of us knew a barbell from a bassinet. And the fact that both of them — as well as their children — always seemed so brimful of health gave us extra support and confidence as we did the reading, research, and writing that went into this book. If books had godparents, the Currys would be this book's.

**Bill Curry**
When Bill Curry first began training with barbells in 1936, he had a dream. That dream was to become a member of the most exclusive club in weightlifting — the York Barbell 300-Pound Club — sponsored by the York Barbell Company, publishers, even then, of the widely read magazine *Strength and Health.* For young Bill Curry, in Athens, Georgia, far from the mainstream of barbell culture, the dream seemed at first remote. "When I graduated from high school I weighed 142 pounds," he recalls, "and my senior year I'd played tackle and guard on the school football team. There were no weights at the YMCA then, and, in fact, we all thought weights would be bad for us. But then the Y hired L. H. Cunningham to be the physical director for the club in Athens, and that changed everything."

Under Cunningham's direction, young Bill did become the first man south of the Mason-Dixon line to join the 300-Pound Club and today, at age sixty-seven he's shooting for *another* exclusive club — one that also revolves around 300 pounds. Bill, whose sixty-fifth birthday fell on December 3, 1982, is determined to break the 300-pound barrier in the bench press, which would not only be a national record for his age and weight group, but would be more than he has ever lifted before — a personal best. "In the old days, everyone trained in the Olympic lifts. We didn't have benches or racks or machines or even very many dumbbells to use, and so almost everyone back then did the basic Olympic movements: press, snatch, and clean and jerk. Training then was very unscientific. Now, most lifters train in cycles and "peak" for a meet. I suppose that part of my fascination for this new periodization training I'm doing on the bench is that I'm still able to make physical gains."

Bill's competitive career flourished during the late thirties, and in early 1940 he began training for the 1940 Olympic trials, which were scheduled for Madison Square Garden. Two men from each weight division were expected to be taken on the squad, but as Bill remembers, "Several weeks away from the Olympic trials, we got word that the Olympic Games had been canceled due to the war and it took the heart right out of my training. Later that fall, I had the best meet of my life, making lifts that would have guaranteed me that trip to the games."

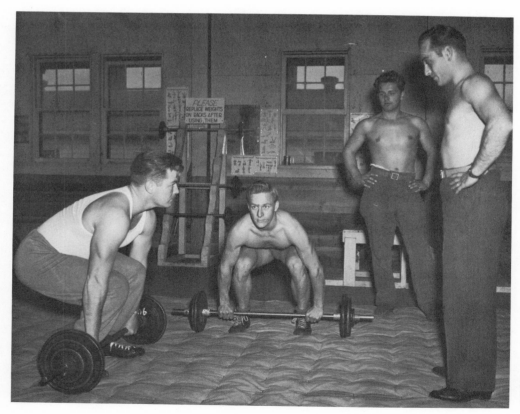

*Bill Curry, on the left, as he instructs recruits during World War II.*

In 1941, having graduated from the University of Georgia, Bill was hired by the Georgia Military Academy to work as a physical education teacher. He got married that year as well and though he continued to train, he didn't compete that winter, concentrating instead on coaching the various teams at GMA. In 1942 he entered the service as a lieutenant and was stationed at Fort McClellan. It didn't take long for word of Bill's strength and weightlifting abilities to spread, and soon he was assigned to a special group that traveled around entertaining the troops. "I was the strongman," he laughs. "I'd fooled around with strength stunts some in my early training and so I knew a little about what I was getting into, but I didn't realize how hard it would be to perform and lift heavy every night. One of the things I did was the human bridge; I'd get down in sort of a backbend, only with my arms down straight and not back over my head. On top of the 'bridge' they'd set an upright piano, and we'd have one guy playing it and one or two others sitting on top. L. H. Cunningham taught me how to do the bridge, and one night during a show, I did not only the piano, but three men as well, and while the one man played I even sang a little bit. Well, it was a big hit, and a photograph of it got picked up by the AP wireservice and sent all over the country."

During the war years, Bill spent the major part of his time working as a physical trainer for the army. Following his stint as a strongman for the service, he was put in charge of whipping into shape an entire battalion of men who had been classified 1-B (not fit for active duty) by the army's physicians. "They were a real mess," Bill recalls. "Some of them had been injured and been sent back to the States, but most were just rundown and out of shape from never having done any exercise.

"I had thirteen weeks to work with these men and so I immediately put them to work building equipment. We got pipe and #10 tin cans that we filled with concrete, and made up 50 'barbells' for the guys to use. There were 800 men to a battalion, so I had to work them in groups of 50, which meant we went through all our exercises as a group. It was quite a sight to see them all lined up, going through their paces with their tin-can barbells made of pipe and concrete. But at the end of the thirteen weeks, I had more than 25 percent of the men reclassified to 1-A, which was an unusually high success rate, and shortly after the end of the program they promoted me to captain and put me in charge of the physical training for the entire camp."

When the war ended, Bill returned to the Georgia Military Academy as a physical education instructor and founded what was probably one of the first high-school weight-lifting teams in the United States at GMA. He also coached boxing and gymnastics and helped with the physical conditioning of the swim team. "I had all the teams I coached train with weights. The boxers showed remarkable improvements after they started their weight work, and I had six all-American swimmers during my five years at GMA and all six of them trained with weights."

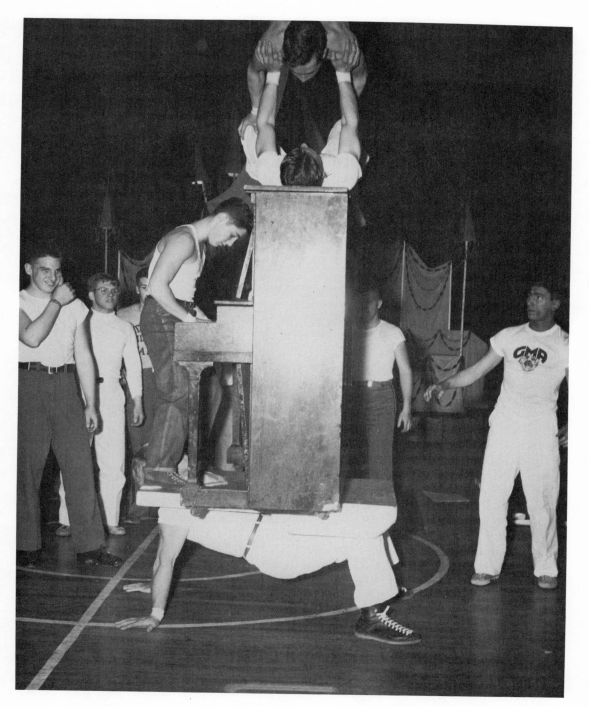

*Bill performing his spectacular "Human Bridge" at the Georgia Military Academy just after the war.*

In 1951, Bill was offered a job by Rich's Department Stores in Atlanta and he soon became head buyer of sporting goods for all their stores. But his training suffered. "Without the boys to coach, I found myself slipping away from the weights," he remembers. But like many other Americans, Bill got on the jogging bandwagon when Kenneth Cooper's book *Aerobics* came out in 1968. "I started running after that, and for about nine years I'd get up every morning and run my one to two miles, but something was missing. Having done the weights, I knew how it felt to have my body in good total shape. The running was fine for my heart and lungs, but it did little for the overall appearance of my body or for my strength. I wanted to look good outside, not just be healthy inside. And once I started training with weights again, regularly, I could tell the difference at once. My arms and shoulders filled back out and I had that spring in my step again."

In 1974, Bill retired from Rich's and took a job as a marketing executive in Opelika, Alabama, with Diversified Products, the largest manufacturer of

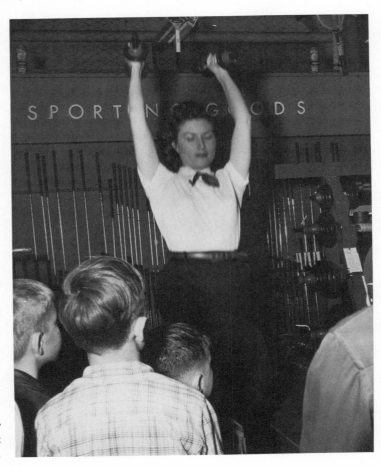

*Eleanor Curry often helped out in the 1950s at the many exhibitions Bill gave at sporting-goods stores in Georgia.*

barbells in the world. He wasted no time in outfitting a gym in the den of his new home, where he, his wife, Eleanor, and a varying number of neighborhood kids and friends congregate to train. Part of the joy in Bill Curry's rediscovery of the weights is the way it has made him feel about himself again. "When I look around a room at the people who are my age, I see very, very few I'd trade places with. I've been told a lot of times that I don't look my age, though I'm not really sure how my 'age' is supposed to look. What I do know is that I don't really feel much different than when I was thirty. I really mean that. I have energy, I'm stronger in my arms and shoulders now than ever, and I'm within a pound or two of my same body weight. I never trained to build a great body in the sense of a bodybuilder's body — only a strong, healthy body fit to do the jobs I asked of it. That's all I still ask."

In the course of his work for Diversified Products, Bill sets up and emcees many strength and fitness exhibitions in sporting-goods stores around the United States, and often, during a lull when one of the featured athletes is taking a rest, Bill will step in and do a bit of bench pressing. Many is the time during these exhibitions when we've seen him exceed the current world records for his age group, yet the lifting is done in shirt-sleeves, dress slacks, and with the same casual joy a teenage boy might display in a strange weight room, showing off a bit. "I guess the bench has really gotten to be sort of an ego trip for me," Bill will say with a laugh. "It's the one exercise that I never did when I was younger and in which I can really try to

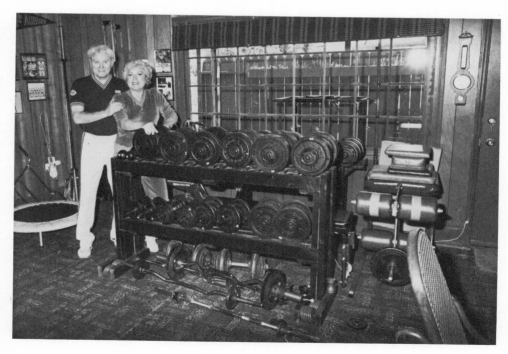

*The Currys proudly pose by their rack of dumbbells.*

continue to see my strength grow. Though I train my total body, I really concentrate on my bench work."

Curry is convincing as he explains his commonsensical approach to nutrition — his brown eyes clear, his white hair thick and full, his complexion rosy with health. He is, indeed, a vigorous man. At sixty-seven he is the wonder of his fellow executives, going to work at 7:00 each morning, working through lunch while drinking a homemade shake and eating a piece of fruit, and then going home at five to his gym to meet six or eight or ten neighbors — young and old — for a two-hour workout. A member of the President's Council on Physical Fitness, he often speaks to local, state, and national groups about the benefit of progressive resistance exercise, and it's hard to imagine how anyone could better physically personify the truth of his words. And, as the following pages will explain, he bred true.

## Bill Curry — The Son

Bill Curry — the son — recently turned forty. During that forty years he has seen and done a great many things. He played baseball as a boy — played it well, too — but it was as a football player that he found a means for the full expression of his best self. He was an outstanding player in high school, and, although many high-school stars set as they enter college, he also became an all-American at Georgia Tech. Then, although many all-Americans fail to even play a single down in the NFL, Bill not only started but starred again, playing for eleven years, during four of which he made all-pro. And, as a coach, one who played under such legends as Vince Lombardi and George Allen, he has quickly risen from a position as offensive line coach for the Green Bay Packers to that of being the head coach at his alma mater, Georgia Tech.

Predictably, he has succeeded even in the enormously difficult job of reestablishing a successful major college program at a school whose entrance and academic standards are among the highest in the country. His intelligence and character have been central to the success not only of the Georgia Tech football team of late but also of two of George Plimpton's most insightful sports books — *Paper Lion* and *One More July*. In *One More July*, a description of his last training camp, Curry's decency and perception — the very traits that have made him so respected by the players and fans at Georgia Tech — are everywhere evident. And, like any honest son who is at all analytical, he credits much of his success to his parents.

"I realize how lucky I am to have had the parents I had," he said recently. "They blessed me with a sound, healthy body, although," he laughed, "I did get my father's skinny legs. And my parents showed me by example how to work hard. The earliest memories I have are of going to the gym with my father and watching him train with weights, watching him work *hard*. I still remember the intensity and the regularity of his training."

However, as happens with many other bright youngsters whose fathers try to show them The Way, Bill Jr. rejected the medium, if not the message.

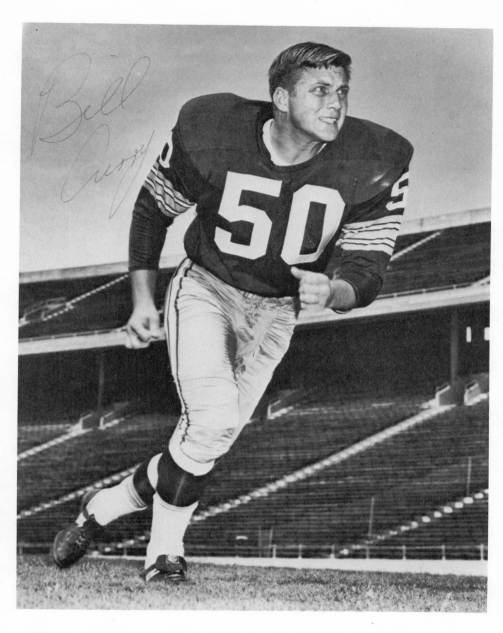

*Bill Curry, Jr.,*
*during his all-America year*
*at Georgia Tech.*

In Bill's case, he internalized the message of iron-willed dedication to the achievement of a goal through work and effort, but he rejected the medium of the barbell. "I know how much Dad wanted to help me and he knew that if I trained with weights when I was young it would give me a big edge," Bill remembers, "but I just wouldn't do it. I'd sometimes go through the motions but I didn't really try and he knew it. And he resented it. It was a battle of wills and once I got up to Little League age I had the coaches on my side. They all told me not to ever lift weights because it would slow me up and make me muscle-bound and so my Dad backed off, bless him. But I was still burning with the need to do well in sports.

"I went on into high school and I played football but I wasn't really outstanding. But in my junior year my dad came to me one day and asked me if I wanted to go to college. He said he thought I could get a scholarship in football if I'd listen to him and do what he said in the weight room. He told me he couldn't pay all my college bills and that I'd either have to get a scholarship or a job. So, I began to train again — really hard training with lots of squats and cleans and presses — and I began to grow. I was a skinny kid when I started but I really filled out fast. I gained size and strength and speed and in my senior year I played well enough to get a full scholarship to Georgia Tech. But then I quit lifting, because we had no lifting program at Tech.

"Later, after my sophomore season, when I'd been fourth string, here came Dad again. He told me that if I wanted to start I'd have to go back on the weights during the off-season and really lift. And so once again I started to work out and once again I gained weight and strength and played better football. I wound up my college days by having a good year and getting drafted to play pro ball. I trained with weights under Dad's direction all during the summer after graduation and gained 20 pounds and was able to make the team with Green Bay."

During the ten years Bill played pro ball — 1965 to 1975 — he saw the league change from one whose line play was dominated by players who did not train with weights to one dominated by players who did. "It was a drastic change," he says. "It was unusual to find a lineman who trained hard with weights when I came up, yet when I left, it was unusual to find one who didn't. We used to have a lot of linemen who were quite fat, but that's rare now because of all the lifting. The guys are even bigger now, but most of it's muscle."

As a coach, Bill has used his hindsight to create a training program in which weights play a central role. "We really push our weight program," he says, "because we know we may not be getting men whose natural size and ability is on a par with some of the schools whose academic standards aren't what ours are. Our only chance to even this size and strength gap is by adding as much as we can to the tools the boy brings to Tech. So we train year-round at Tech, in season and out, and we train hard. Like my dad did."

As for his own training, now that he has emerged from the trenches of the NFL, it has been quite different. His weight, for one thing, which usually stayed around 240 during his playing days, has dropped to 200, which is not much for a man so tall and big-framed. He became interested in running after he quit, and he used it to gradually lower his body weight and maintain his level of cardiovascular fitness. He took no other exercise, so as he ran, the heavy muscle structure he had built through all his years of foot-

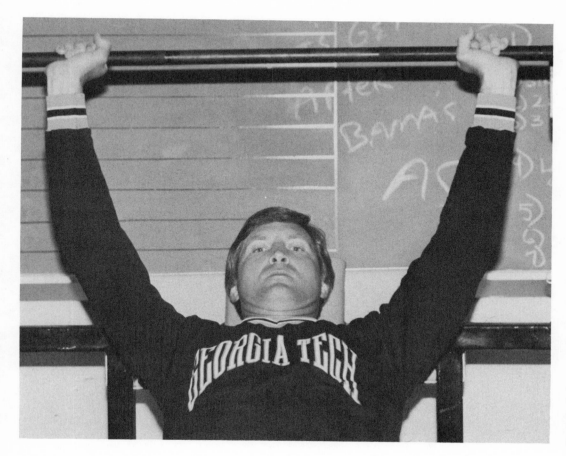

*Now the coach at Georgia Tech, Bill still finds time to squeeze in a little lifting.*

ball and weight training began to disappear. At first, the lightness he felt was truly liberating.

"It's hard to describe how free I felt with that forty to fifty pounds of weight off my body. I felt like a young antelope, able to spring and to bound and to run almost tirelessly. It was wonderful. And it was wonderful to have people compliment me on my appearance. I'd be dishonest if I failed to mention that."

But even with the feeling of freedom and the many compliments on his appearance, Bill felt as if something was missing. He felt that although his weight was where he wanted it and he had good cardiovascular fitness, his overall muscle tone left a lot to be desired. "I remember the thing that triggered it," he said recently, laughing. "I was at the beach in Florida with my family and my eleven-year-old son said, 'Dad, your boobs are flabby.' Well, you can imagine how that made me feel.

"Here I was thinking I was so trim and sleek and my own son points out to me the thing I knew was wrong — I wasn't getting enough all-around exercise. So, although I was awhile getting around to it, I called Dad and he sent me a new wall unit that lets you do most weight-training exercises fast. It's got a weight stack and this makes it easy to change the resistance. I put it in my den and it saves a lot of time for me, and time is precious now. I have to make my exercise sessions short and intense, and even then I don't do as much as I want to do. I also train at school occasionally, on the free weights, but for the most part I train at home.

"But I can already feel a big difference in my body. It's tightening up again and I like that sensation. I've missed it. I still like to run but I don't want *only* to run. I'm going to get ready for the beach next summer."

## Linda Curry

As can be seen on the cover of this book, Linda Curry, at thirty-eight, looks more than anything else like a lioness. There is about her an aura of animalistic power and health. She glides as she walks, shoulders back, stomach flat, and head high, sleek muscles rippling under glowing skin. Even her slightly hoarse voice is leonine, somewhere between a purr and a growl. This is what all women could be.

The mother of two children, aged thirteen and twelve, Linda grew up in Atlanta, Georgia, and as the daughter of Bill Curry and the younger sister of a football star, it was almost impossible for her not to train a bit with weights. She laughed recently, as she recalled her years in high school. "From the time I can remember, Dad had a gym in the house somewhere. In high school, I played on the basketball team, and Dad convinced me that weights would make me play better. He had me do lots of lunges and squats for my legs and bench presses and flys for my upper body. Naturally, I was the only player who did any weight training.

"When basketball season was over, I'd generally slack off until early spring. That's when all the big dances were, and it became sort of a joke in our house that I'd have to 'train' for the prom. Sounds silly, I know, but Dad had it in his head that I'd look a lot better in my formal if I was all trim and muscular again, and before you knew it, back I'd be in the basement, getting back my muscle tone. I knew he was right about it, and so I never really minded when he'd encourage me to start back again. Friends, of course, teased me a lot."

Linda's friends aren't laughing now. Recently, at a major department store in Atlanta, Linda, several other women bodybuilders, and several top-level powerlifters were involved in an exhibition and clinic about strength training and bodybuilding, and at the end of the session, a short, graying woman who was about forty pounds overweight approached Linda holding a ten-year-old boy by the hand. "Linda, do you remember me?" she asked, with a somewhat nervous smile. "I can't believe you look so good," the woman continued, before Linda had a chance to reply. "You still look exactly like you did in high school. Better. I wish I could say the same for me." The woman, it turned out, was one of Linda's teammates from that high-school basketball team, and, as often happens, the children and the many thoughtless meals had taken their toll.

As they talked and as Linda encouraged the woman to seek out some sort of program, one of the young men involved in the show turned to us and said quietly, "Gee, she looks old enough to be Linda's mother, doesn't she?" Indeed she did, for while her face was furrowed here and there, it was mainly the posture of her body that made her look so old, so defeated by time. The droop of her shoulders, the thickness through the stomach and hips, and the paunches on the upper thighs, visible through her stretch slacks, all gave vivid testimony to inactivity and lack of concern for her body.

"I remember her well from high school," Linda said afterward, "and she was so cute it used to make me sick. While I always felt big and sort of gangly, she was petite and adorable. All the guys were crazy about her."

Totally unlike her friend, Linda trains every day; in fact she opens the doors each morning to one of her two health studios in Atlanta. Her first club, Linda Curry's Studio, has been open for four years now, and what started as an experiment has turned into a rousing success for motivated women. "It's my feeling that weight training, as well as any other sort of exercise program, should be fun. I've done a lot of running through the years, especially at times when I was away at college and wasn't training with weights, but even if I try to run in different places and at different times, it still gets boring to me. What we do in the studio is to combine the use of free weights with music so that the workouts that we teach as classes take on more of the character of a dance session. We have a weight room as well, where we take traditional sorts of weight workouts, but in our classes we use ankle weights, dumbbells, and exercise bars and go through a total body workout to music.

Unlike many health-spa employees, Linda does have some real knowledge when it comes to training and health, even though it took her several years to return to the teachings of her father. Following high school and college she worked for Delta airlines, got married, had her first child, and then decided that she wanted to do something more physical with her life. "I started by taking yoga, then went to slimnastics, aerobic dance, and prenatal-postnatal exercises, and I loved it all. During this period I also worked up to the point where I was running between thirty to fifty miles each week, but I still didn't find any time for the weights."

"Linda really had the running bug back then," her father recalls, "and she thought running would be the answer to all her dreams of physical beauty. But to be honest, her legs and hips were still quite soft and she had lost most of her bust. I told her that she ought to begin doing some hard work with the weights again, just like she'd done in high school. So she began to train, and train hard. Within a year she had literally reshaped her hips and thighs and built up her bustline wonderfully. She dropped from a

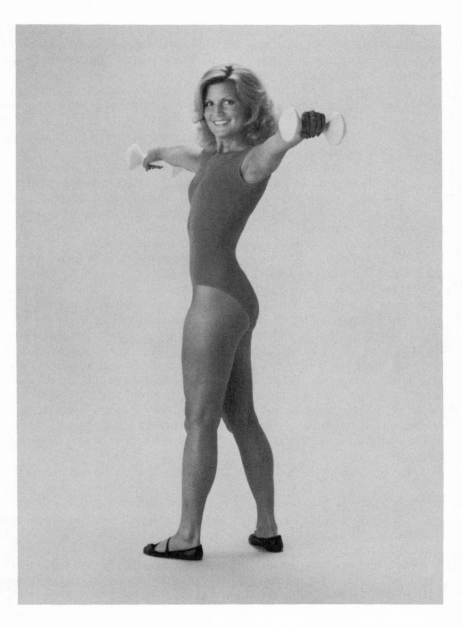

*Thirty-eight-year-young
Linda Curry as she begins
a set of twists.*

size ten-eleven to a size eight-nine in her pants, and yet she gained ten to twelve pounds.''

    Linda admits to the remarkable changes the weights made in her life. ''I guess I figured that my flabby hips and sagging bustline were just part of the price I had to pay for being over thirty, so you can imagine how excited I was to see the differences in my body. I could hardly believe it. I got so many compliments on my changed appearance, and I know I must sound too evangelical, but I really did feel a need to share what I learned with other women. And since my studio opened I've had even more time to concentrate on my weight training. I've gone down at least two more dress sizes, yet I've only lost five pounds or so. I'm trimmer now than I was in high school, when I wore a size ten. I measure thirty-eight in the bust now, which means that in clothes, I give the appearance of having a big difference between my bust and waist even though most of it comes from muscle, not bust.

"Even though I've trained for a long time, I still feel like I'm making progress. I plan to look better at forty than I do today and even better when I'm fifty. I've done a lot of different sorts of exercise — the running, yoga, straight slimnastics — and all of it has not been as beneficial to me as the weight training has been. What makes people look good is that their bodies are firm and full. That's what the weights do. When I think about all the women across the USA who go three times a week to an 'exercise class,' go through a thirty-minute routine, and then feel frustrated because they see no change, it makes me feel really sad. If they only knew what to do, and how to go about it, they could see such dramatic changes in their bodies. I know, because I've done it all, and I've seen dozens of women come in these doors and go out three months later looking ten years younger. Some people change really fast and some change more slowly, but changes do come, if you're willing to spend the time, do the work, and stick to a sound diet. I'm proud of the way I look, and I know anyone will be proud of the changes they can make if they'll use a good weight program. I keep thinking of that friend of mine from the basketball team, and I know how easily our lives could have been reversed. I just thank God for my dad and for how he brought me back to the weights after all those years."

**Eleanor Curry**

Half of the genetic heritage and attitude inherited by both Bill and Linda Curry came from a vivacious, warmhearted woman — Eleanor Barnes Curry — who was born in 1922 and whose beauty and zest for life are so overwhelming that her contemporaries are not merely awed, they're jealous. "Why on earth should I be 'old'?" she asked us recently as we sat in the den turned weight room that's part of her home in Opelika, Alabama. "Just because I've reached sixty doesn't mean that I have to give up all the things that are fun for me to do and 'start acting my age.' What hogwash. You should see me up at Linda's studio in Atlanta. I go once a week to do her class, and she turns the music way up so you can hear it pounding in your head as you go through the exercises, using the dumbbells and ankle weights. A lot of the girls in the classes are a third my age, but I can keep up with all of them, except for Linda. Every now and then some new girl will join who'll give me a look as if to say, 'What's this old gray-headed lady doing here?' But by the time class is over and she's dying and I'm still going strong, she begins to understand why I'm there and that I've *been* there."

At 5 feet 6 inches, and 139 pounds, there is a leanness and tightness to Eleanor's body that belies her age. "I have some problem areas that I keep a pretty close eye on, and it's harder for me now to keep my body as I want it than it used to be, but if I didn't do the weight work, things would be a disaster. I'm one of these women who gain weight on their torsos rather than on their hips and legs, so I do a lot of toning exercises aimed at what Bill calls my 'bloopies' — those little fat deposits so many women have on their backs right above the tops of their bras."

.It was after Eleanor and Bill married and he began his job at the Georgia Military Academy that Eleanor began her first weight training. During these early years, and again when Bill returned from World War II and resumed his duties at the academy, Eleanor began to be more involved with demonstrations and exhibitions involving the use of weights. "For a while, Bill and one of his friends were building barbells in the garage and selling them. We'd go to department stores and give demonstrations in our street clothes — the idea being that you could come home from work, do a few exercises in your work clothes with minimal hassle, and develop strength and fitness. I'd always help out, and later, when Bill had all the boys at the academy doing strength exhibitions, I'd generally do a few light things with dumbbells just to show that it was okay for women to use weights, too. During those years I trained pretty regularly, in between the babies and the housework."

When Bill left the academy to join Rich's Department Store, Eleanor made the transition with Bill to training at home all the time. "My periods of weight training pretty much paralleled Bill's" she recalls, "but I let the weights go for a while, until I woke up one morning, took a good look at myself, and said this has got to change. Now that I've started back and have become regular at the weight work, I can maintain my body where I want it."

With her renewed interest in weight training, Eleanor also began to explore other avenues for health. "About five or six years ago, Bill and I started noticing that a lot of our friends were dying. We went through one of those times when several close friends died either through cancer or heart disease and it scared both of us. I decided that I was going to read and learn everything I could about both conditions, and it wasn't long before that led me to more in-depth studies of nutrition. We've always been concerned about what we and the kids ate, and I'll never forget the time Bill came home from school as a little boy and asked me why he had to have brown bread in his lunchbox when all the other kids had white bread. He was about nine, then, and I gave him a fairly simple answer about brown bread being more healthy for us. But then he told me that he'd been wondering because the other kids had said it was because we were too poor to afford white bread, the 'store bought' kind. I'd say he seems to have come out of it okay, but at the time it gave me quite a laugh. Although we were careful about what our kids ate, we weren't fanatics. We didn't let them drink Cokes or soft drinks till their teens and we watched the number of sweets they ate, but for the most part we fed them regular food, but a lot more vegetables and fruit than most families."

Yet lately, as she has read and learned about the connections between nutrition, aging, and health, certain eating patterns have changed for the Currys. "We eat our big meal at night — generally broiled fish or chicken, plus a salad and vegetable. We also take vitamin supplements every day, usually C, E, B-Complex, lecithin, and a multivitamin. Both of us can really tell the difference in how we feel.

"It's too much of a cliché to say that you're as old as you feel, but I think we've trapped too many Americans into believing that physical life is over at forty or fifty or sixty, or seventy, and *really* over after retirement. I think too many people begin to feel changes in their body and instead of fighting back, they give up. Well, they shouldn't give up . . . there's lots they can do to change the way they feel. If I can start back with my weight work at age fifty-five, then so can anyone. The best way to cure a disease, I've learned, is to prevent it. And the best way to prevent disease is by exercising and eating properly. And it's not really so hard, once you get started."

When one looks at the richness of the lives the Currys lead, one can't help but wonder at their youth and vigor, their good looks and good health. They are, after all, a fairly typical American family — middle class, white, the only difference from our standard being their long-term interest in resistance training and nutrition. When one sees Eleanor Curry at work on her hands and knees in her flower beds, or with her shovel and hoe in her organic vegetable garden, or dressed for church on Sunday, or striding around her suburban neighborhood in the predawn hours for her three-mile daily walk with weights, one forgets she is sixty — or fifty — and instead sees a lovely woman in the fullness of her health and life. She is, as we would all hope to be at her age, straight of back and square of shoulder, able to work and to run and to play, just as the young do.

**Good Luck and Good Training**

# Appendices

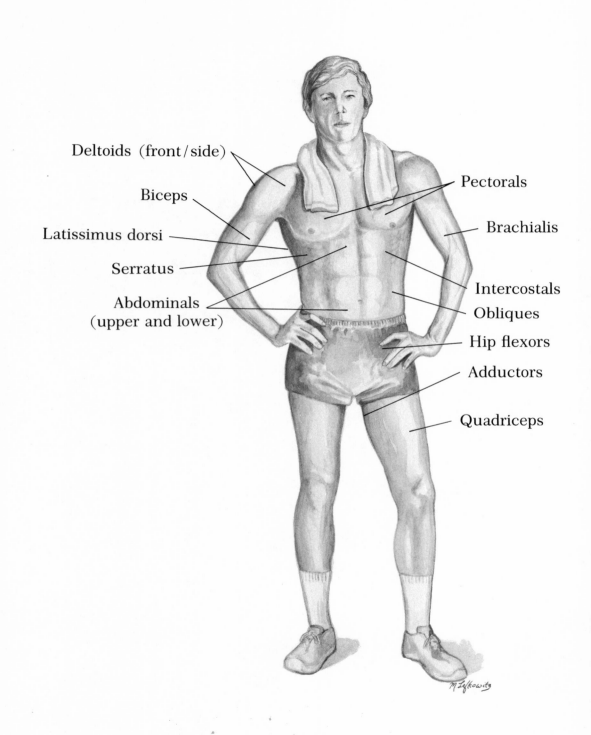

Deltoids (front/side)

Biceps

Latissimus dorsi

Serratus

Abdominals
(upper and lower)

Pectorals

Brachialis

Intercostals

Obliques

Hip flexors

Adductors

Quadriceps

# Muscle Chart

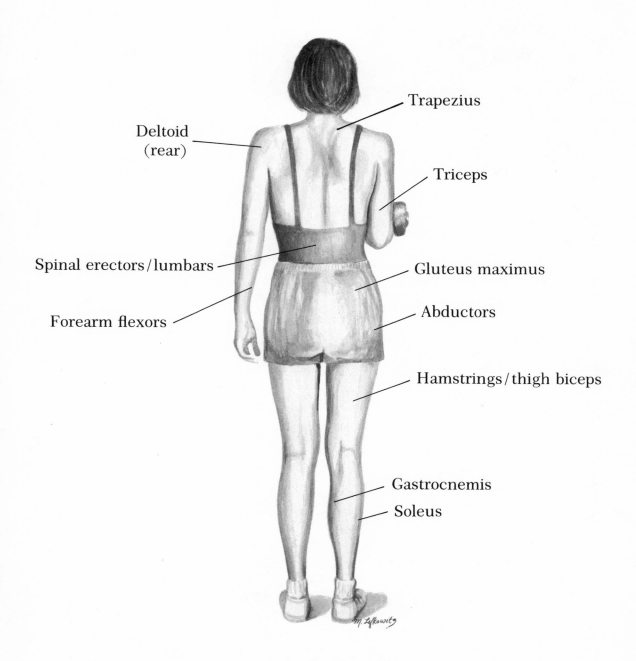

Trapezius

Deltoid
(rear)

Triceps

Spinal erectors/lumbars

Gluteus maximus

Forearm flexors

Abductors

Hamstrings/thigh biceps

Gastrocnemis

Soleus

M. Lefkowitz

# Theories of Aging

Really, you have seen the old age of the eagle, as the saying is.
(Terence)

WE have always searched for the "old age of the eagle," an old age full of vigor, strength, and joy. Ponce de León, for instance, was sure that a fountain of youth existed, but though he combed the steamy wilds of Florida, he found only an arrow that hastened him toward death. Yet his deep fascination with longevity lived on beyond him in the lives of the countless physicians, alchemists, philosophers, and priests who for centuries have profited from man's desire for eternal youth. And, of course, we're still searching, still dreaming, that science or magic or faith will unlock that final door.

Even in many Eastern cultures, where the aged are revered for their wisdom, the desire for longevity *and* physical vigor is well documented. Records from well before the birth of Christ indicate that the Taoists believed that the preservation of the semen would lengthen a man's life. Taoist monks taught a ritualized system of exercises called the "Kung Fu," which was practiced by the old as well as the young. In one handwritten manuscript, in fact, which has come down to us from the second century A.D., Wei Po Yang claimed life could be extended by a combination of general and sexual gymnastics. With luck, perhaps, one could score a double "10."

Western civilization, however, founded upon the writings of the classical Greek period, has always idolized the strength, the beauty, and the vitality of the young. As the Roman dramatist Plautus wrote, "He whom the gods favor dies in youth." But though certainly not "favored," the older men in Greece did continue going to the gymnasia to exercise in order to preserve youth as long as possible. Plato speaks of the "old men in the gymnasia . . . still fond of their exercises," and in the *Politics* Aristotle writes about exercise among older men, apparently not even *considering* that a man wouldn't continue to train up to the time of his death. The fact is, however, that before the Industrial Revolution few men had sufficient wealth to be *free* from some sort of exercise on a regular basis simply because the demands of living in a preindustrial society required lots of walking and lots of work for survival.

**Terry:** "One of the clear memories of my childhood is of the amount of physical work all four of my grandparents did through the years. I was lucky enough to live right next door to one set of grandparents and a mile or so away from the other set. My grandfather Todd was a postman who walked his long route every day before coming home to help my grandmother do the chores around the house and yard. He'd chop firewood for their fireplace, mow his yard with an old push mower, build stone walls, work in his garden, milk, and tend to whatever animals he had at the time. And my grandmother worked right along beside him — grabbing a shovel when it was time to dig up the flower beds, carrying her huge baskets of wet laundry out to the line to dry, walking to the store for her groceries, and cooking up those wonderful meals I still miss. She was tough and strong, just as my grandfather was, and they both used to laugh at my notions of how 'hard' some particular job was. Both of them had become so accustomed to regular, hard work — the bending and stretching and lifting — that they were in a very real way similar to athletes. They were *fit* for hard work."

Consider, on the other hand, the life of the average American apartment dweller. The alarm rings. He or she gets up to go to work. Following a shower, a bowl of cold sugary cereal (still America's most popular breakfast) and coffee are consumed before the drive to work. He or she then parks as close as possible to the workplace, walks in, then sits at a desk till the 10:30 coffee-doughnut break. Lunch comes at a fast-food place, and the day ends at 4:30 or 5:00 with another drive home. He or she now feels "tired," largely as a result of having done nothing physical all day. Back at the apartment there's no grass to cut, no wood to haul, no livestock to worry about, and so on goes the tube, followed by dinner, followed by more tube.

Sound like a rut? It is, a very deadly rut that may well deepen into an early grave. Our parents wanted so much for life to be better for those of us now in our middle years and it is — yet it isn't. Is it better that we have the highest level of coronary heart disease in the world? Is it better that a larger percentage of Americans are overweight than ever before?

**Terry:** "My grandfather Todd was eighty-nine when he finally passed away and my grandmother died only a few years ago at ninety-seven. She kept her own home till the end. No doubt she must have finally worked herself to death. On the other side of the family, my mother's parents both lived into their eighties even though both of them were considered — as were the Todds — to be overweight according to the insurance tables. My grandfather Williams, who was cattleman, had been considered one of the strongest men in Central Texas as a young man and when he finally died in 1978 at the age of eighty-nine he still weighed around 210 pounds. Even at the end of his life he had a big chest, excellent posture, and a surprising amount of strength. The year before he passed away, in fact, my aunt Janice took him to the doctor's for his annual checkup and the doctor — not his old doctor — wanted to check Papa's grip. One way that doctors check the vigor of geriatric patients is by asking them to shake hands as hard as they can. Janice really laughed when she told us how the doctor squalled when Papa turned on the juice."

Were our ancestors healthier than the men and women of today? They took no formal exercise, but the average workday was filled with physical activity and in the jobs and tasks of day to day survival people placed their bodies under stress just as we do in weight training. And their diet consisted of more wholesome foods, without the monosodium glutamate, the sodium nitrates, and the other chemicals we find listed on the outside of our packages today. But most of us no longer live the simple life and eat the simple foods we need to duplicate the effect of that life-style through our own exercise program and diet. Duplicate is the wrong word. We should — and can — improve on it.

Human nature being what it is, however, people often eschewed hard work and looked for shortcuts. One such man was Charles Edouard Brown-Sequard, whom many consider the father of modern gerontology, the study of aging. Brown-Sequard earned this title with an amazing announcement on June 1, 1889, to a meeting of the *Societe' de Biologique* in Paris. Brown-Sequard was convinced along with many other physiologists of his day that a relationship existed between man's waning sexual powers and aging, and he told the society that he had taken one of the testicles of a two-year-old dog; crushed it up in a saline solution; extracted a pinkish, semiclear liquid from the crushed mass; then injected the liquid into his thigh. He also claimed to have received almost immediate rejuvenation from this experiment and reported an increase in his strength when tested on a dynamometer, more energy, and the ability to run up and down stairs again as he had in his youth. No doubt this procedure did have an effect, but not for the reason he thought. Apparently, since testosterone can't be extracted by a saline solution, the injection caused in Brown-Sequard what scientists call a "placebo effect," meaning that because he *wanted* to believe an improvement would occur, it did. Sugar pills, given to patients complaining of pain, will often have the same effect because the patient wants the pain to go away.

But, while some of Brown-Sequard's fellow scientists thought him a bit mad and his wife is reported to have called him a senile old fool, others took note and began experiments of their own. One who followed in his footsteps was the Viennese physiologist Eugen Steinach, who also believed that the testicles and semen played an important role in maintaining vigor in the later years. Steinach developed a surgical technique called Vasoligature, in which the ducts through which the sperm leave the testes and travel to the penis were severed to allow more of "something" (since testosterone was not yet clearly identified) to enter the bloodstream and create vigor. Steinach reported many cases of success with his technique on both rats and humans. Modern vasectomy is essentially the same procedure, though done for different reasons. While there have been a few cited cases of increased vitality following vasectomy there's no clear data to substantiate Steinach's claims.

Perhaps the most tragic story among those of Brown-Sequard's followers is that of Serge Voronoff, who became a millionaire in the 1920s by transplanting the testicles of chimpanzees, gibbons, and orangutans into men. Voronoff charged $5,000 for the procedure, and most medical historians believe he started out fully believing that this outrageous procedure would really work. Though he reported great success stories and was a popular lecturer about his "Fountain of Youth"; what we now know of the difficulties in transplanting human organs from one person to another, let alone primate organs to man, leaves no room for doubt about the utter failure of the procedure. Still, Voronoff did over 2,000 of these operations before public opinion turned against him and he had to close his shop. Besides the dangerous side effects of placing foreign organs in the human body, Voronoff didn't know that some of his animals were infected with syphilis, which was then passed along to his patients when the testicles were transplanted, and so the helping hand struck again.

It was not until the mid-1930s that the next major step was taken on the rocky road to youth and vigor. A German chemist by the name of Adolph Butenandt used injections of by-then-available synthetic testosterone and subcutaneous implantations of testosterone "tablets" to aid his geriatric patients. Real or "natural" testosterone had been discovered in 1933 by Fred Koch, a Chicago researcher who made his first extract from several *tons* of bull testicles that, in the manner of Brown-Sequard, he systematically mashed, pulverized, and placed under pressure until, by using benzene, alcohol, and acetone as solvents, he was able to extract a tiny amount of highly impure male hormone. (Some of the earliest testing of testosterone was done on castrated roosters, called capons, and, given enough of the still highly impure substance, the capons did indeed take over the barnyard, even when other roosters were present. Later experiments on hens found that when *they* were given large doses, they too would peck any rooster into submission.)

It was Leopold Ruzicka, however, a Yugoslavian chemist working in Zurich, Switzerland, who realized that tons of bull testicles couldn't be delivered with enough regularity to do man much good. So, he set about to see, now that the testosterone molecule had been identified, if something could be altered to produce a synthetic form that would have similar properties. He created the first synthetic testosterone in 1935 from cholesterol, and Butenandt, who had also been working on a synthetic form, used Ruzicka's discovery for his first rejuvenation experiments. Pandora's box was opened. From this work in the early part of the twentieth century have arisen dozens of synthetic hormones now used not just by geriatric patients and burn victims, as was originally intended, but by a growing number of athletes who want greater physical speed and strength.

While these early scientists were looking at the relationship of sex and aging, another group of researchers were looking inside the cells with a technique called "cell therapy." Alexis Carrel was a French physiologist who believed that individual cells were immortal and that, furthermore, young cells could have a rejuvenating effect on older tissues. Carrel based his theory on a cell culture he started in 1912, made from the heart of a chicken embryo. He fed the culture regularly with liquid extracts taken from other chicken embryos, and rather than die as most cell cultures do after a period of time, it continued to live until 1946, when, two years after Carrel's death, it was finally "allowed" to die. Carrel was convinced that something in the young embryo extract with which the culture was nourished kept death at bay, and soon other European researchers were also trying Carrel's youth elixir.

One of these was Paul Niehans, who opened a clinic in Vervay, Switzerland, that is still in operation, though Niehans himself died in 1978, having never availed himself of his own therapy. Niehans developed a technique that called for injections of sheep fetus tissues for his patients. He also developed methods to inject adrenal, parathyroid, testicular, ovarian, and pituitary tissues, in the belief that these would cause rejuvenation to these respective areas. Niehans and his clinic prospered, and in 1954 his business received a divine boost when Pope Pius XII came to undergo cell therapy. Niehans had hundreds of celebrities under his care, many of whom spoke favorably about the way they felt following treatment; and today, in Western Europe, there are a number of physicians who still practice cell therapy, though the procedure is not permitted here in the United States. Subsequent retests of Carrel's chicken embryo culture have not proven successful, and the scientific community's view is that a few live cells must have been passed in with the cell embryo extract that Carrel used to feed the culture in order for it to have survived so long. As for the improvement Niehans's patients reported — since he made them rest and took them off cigarettes and alcohol and put them on special diets while they stayed at his clinic — it's quite possible that many of them *did* feel better after treatment. They should have. And then again, don't discount the old placebo effect.

We've come a long way from Taoist sexual gymnastics and Brown-Sequard's no doubt rather disconsolate dog, but there are still enormous gaps in our knowledge of the aging process. It seems to be easy enough to study the effects of certain variables on the lifespan of fruit flies or mice because of their naturally short lives, but it's been almost impossible, so far, to do any long-term, or longitudinal, studies on human beings. Even in the scientific journals, much of the research literature is based on what's called "anecdotal evidence" from individual case histories. Thirty years from now, our hope is that we can rewrite this book and include some longitudinal studies on the value of weight training as it relates to aging. But so far, few researchers have had the time, or the money, to do longitudinal studies on any aspect of aging, let alone the effect of weight training. So, despite all we've learned over the past years, we're still a long way from understanding the physiology and biochemistry of aging. There are, however, a number of theories as to why the body inexorably deteriorates with the passage of time;

our best guess is that a *combination* of several of the causes suggested by those theories accounts for our increasing aches and pains and ultimately our debility and death.

We're now going to look briefly at a few of the more widely accepted theories of aging; but the physiological foundations of aging are technical, so bear with us. Likewise, if you seriously wish to pursue what some gerontologists are now calling "life extension programs," we urge you to do some reading on your own into the nutritional, phychological, and life-style research that is now being done as a growing response to the desire to prolong youth. Check the bibliography for references we've found especially helpful.

## Genetic Theories of Aging

Most of you are probably familiar with the term "planned obsolescence," Detroit's last laugh on the American consumer and perhaps on themselves. Related to this idea are the two primary genetic theories of aging. The Central Clock Theory says that in each of us a time bomb is slowly ticking away that is scheduled to go off at a certain hour, on a certain day, because of the genetically determined failure of one of the body's *organs*. We'll discuss this theory later after we've examined its closely linked neighbor, the Cellular Theory. The Cellular Theory is based on the notion that each *cell* possesses an internal mechanism genetically programmed to stop working after a set number of days. Both these genetic theories, by the way, are supported by the readily observable fact that long-lived parents tend to produce long-lived offspring and from studies on the lifespans of identical twins — who obviously share the same genetic makeup — that have shown that twins live for similar lengths of time. Detractors of the genetic theories will argue, however, that similar life-styles and diets may be a more telling reason for this similarity in lifespan than the supposed genetic codes.

How such a phenomenon would operate within a cell is a point of still further dispute. The Cellular Theory is based on the work of Leonard Hayflick and Paul Moorhead, who, though research done at the Wistar Institute in Philadelphia in the 1960s, discovered that cells found in human tissues were capable of roughly fifty divisions (mitosis) before they could produce no new offspring and subsequently expired. The "Hayflick limit," as it's called, was determined on the basis of cells growing under laboratory conditions in a culture — not within a normal human being, where a number of environmental forces can interfere with mitosis. It was Hayflick's contention that each cell contains a gene, or "program," for longevity just as they contain genes for hair and eye color. And that when the predetermined time limit is up, the cell ceases functioning and the body part where it's located begins to die. Sounds simple enough, except that new research has found that if you alter the environment of the cells, even in the laboratory tissue cultures, they'll grow for longer periods of time. For instance, if you add extra oxygen to the cultures, they'll keep on splitting well past the magical fifty divisions.

DNA stands for deoxyribonucleic acid and it is the part of each cell on which the genetic makeup of that organism is imprinted. DNA molecules consist of two side-by-side chains of genes that are twisted into spirals. These two spirals separate when cell division occurs, and each single spiral then manufactures a new and supposedly duplicate side so that the newly formed cell will contain the full genetic structure just as it was in the parent cell. There are a number of things, however, that are believed to malfunction during the building of the new DNA side as an organism ages. The most easily explained is that the single spiral makes mistakes when replicating itself. These minute errors, made in the numerous divisions that a cell undergoes throughout the space of a person's life, result in slightly mutated cells that slowly but surely change the way the body looks and functions. A photograph of a photograph of a photograph is never as sharp and clear as the original.

**DNA Error Theories**

Another way DNA may make errors is in the formation of new molecules. Say, for example, that an enzyme molecule is being formed. DNA will send a "message" to these new cells as to how they are supposed to look and function. The messenger boy is called RNA (ribonucleic acid), and some theorists on aging have postulated that the transmission of the genetic message from the DNA to the RNA and then on to the assembly point of the new cells is fraught with dangers. This could mean, at times, that the newly formed molecule doesn't function properly.

Similarly, some scientists believe that environmental factors such as radiation, exposure to chemical pollutants, food additives, and so on, also create slight, but, over time, significant changes in cell structure. The fact that radiation can cause cell mutations is well established. Hiroshima taught us that rather well. What's only recently begun to be understood, however, is that radiation (Don't forget that we receive radiation from the sun every day, cloudy or fair) and other factors create what are known as "free radicals" in the environment and inside our bodies. It's now believed that free radicals can disrupt DNA replication and are responsible for an enormous percentage of the other changes in our bodies that we associate with aging.

**Free Radicals**

A "free radical" is an ion, or part of a molecule, that's been separated during a chemical reaction. Because these ions are not bound to another substance (as, say, hydrogen and oxygen are bonded together in a molecule of water), they will attempt to unite with almost any other molecule with which they come in contact — particularly protein molecules. We normally produce thousands of free radicals inside our bodies during the countless chemical exchanges that are needed to keep the body functioning. However, when too many free radicals are on the prowl because the enzyme system that moderates free-radical activity isn't functioning properly, or when we've been exposed to damaging environmental factors, they will attempt to unite with fibrous protein molecules such as DNA and collagen (and other molecules) and form what are known as "cross-links," now believed to be a major cause of problems associated with aging.

Envision again the side spirals of the DNA molecule and imagine that someone has tied a small thread around the two chains, linking them together. This is their cross-link. When the DNA molecule then needs to separate so the cell can undergo mitosis, several things might happen because of the presence of the cross-link. The preferred happening is that the DNA molecule will be able in some way to excise, or cut out, the portion where the cross-link is attached and "heal" itself. An unfortunate alternative, however, is that the two strands will begin to split down to the point of the thread, where they'll stop, forming a Y-shaped monstrosity that's incapable of completing replication and that some physiologists think may be linked to cancer. The third possibility is that the two strands will decide that they can't separate at all, and the cell won't be able to divide. This third possibility is one explanation given for the measurable decrease in the number of viable cells in the human body and for the growing number of improperly functioning cells that accompany aging.

Cross-links, however, are not all evil death dealers. In collagen, which makes up nearly a fourth of the body's total protein, they are desirable — up to a point — for proper maturation. Collagen is found in all the connective tissues — skin, ligaments, blood-vessel walls, cartilage — and is also inside individual cells, where it helps with the transport of nutrients into and waste products out of the cells. It is elastic in nature, and as a child develops, the cross-links that occur naturally in collagen are responsible for much of natural maturation. However, as the formation of cross-links continues and accelerates with our advancing age (due to exposure to free radicals and a less efficient defensive system to fight those free radicals), our skin dries and wrinkles, our blood-vessel walls lose elasticity, high blood pressure (hypertension) develops, and passage of oxygen into and out of the blood-vessel walls is curtailed, we lose flexibility in our joints, and a lot of other embarrassing and saddening changes occur as well. An easily understood example of this process is the tanning of leather. When the tanning chemicals are placed against the previously soft, flexible skins, cross-links are formed that stiffen the texture of the hide.

No matter how careful we are about X rays, our diet, sun exposure, cigarette smoking, and so on, each of us is bombarded by trillions of externally produced free radicals every day — besides being internally exposed to those naturally occurring within our bodies. Ordinary air, on a sunny day, for instance, contains about 1,000,000,000 hydroxyl free radicals in a single quart of air, and air pollution, pesticides, you name it, can, of course, push that figure significantly higher. Since it's not possible to shut ourselves away in a sterile environment, the only thing we can do is to avoid excessive sun exposure and, if we can afford it, take the advice of those longevity experts who say that certain food supplements, especially vitamins C and E, serve as free-radical warriors and help to nullify their bad effects within the body.

We know we've strayed a bit from our genetic aging discussions, but the effects of free radicals and cross-links on the aging process are important to understand for those who want to enjoy an active healthy life for as long as possible. We strongly recommend that you do some further reading about the free-radical theory and how nutrition may play a role in preventing deleterious side effects from free-radical exposure.

Let's go back now to the Central Clock theory which is based on the belief that the failure of a particular organ — the brain, for instance — is the key to the total failure of the body.

## The Central Clock Theory

The endocrine or glandular system of the human body is enormously complicated. Scientists have prayed for years to have laboratories capable of half the chemical functions that the glands and their messenger hormones carry out in the blink of an eye. Thousands of chemical reactions and chemical adjustments are required to keep the body functioning properly, and the glands release hormones into the bloodstream to regulate the chemical processes. Many gerontologists now speculate that the body's "clock" is linked to endocrine function. In particular, they've been closely scrutinizing the pituitary gland, often called the master gland of the body. We now understand, contrary to Brown-Sequard and his brethren, that it is in the pituitary that the activities of all glands are coordinated and that the pituitary's location — in the brain — means that it responds to brain "messages" when it directs the functions of the various glands.

Hormones control almost all body functions in one way or another, but their most important duties are the regulation of blood volume and the cardiovascular system; the productions of fuels for exercise from proteins and fats; the maintenance of blood glucose levels; and their assistance in the production of new protein (muscle) as a response to exercise and reproduction.

The pituitary is located inside the skull just slightly below the main part of the brain. It receives messages from the hypothalamus that instruct it as to which hormones to release and in what quantities. The pituitary's hormones are then carried by the bloodstream to the other glands, such as the thyroid or the testes, where either they cause glandular activity to occur or they are carried by the blood to the organs to moderate their function.

The endocrine system is responsible for the body's homeostasis and it does it with messages from the hypothalamus about sleep and hunger, blood pressure and sexual desires, messages that are passed along by the pituitary gland. The hypothalamus uses both "releasing factors" and "inhibiting factors" to control the pituitary and as these are simply constructed molecules (rather than complex molecules such as those of which pituitary hormones are constructed), a new crop of ambitious biochemists have begun work to manufacture these factors synthetically. Their hope is that these synthetic "releasors" or "inhibitors" may be able to control hormones such as DECO (an acronym not for describing interior design but for decreasing consumption of oxygen), which inhibits the passage of the thyroid hormone thyroxin into the cells. A lack of thyroxin has been associated with graying of the hair, wrinkling of the skin, and other age-associated diseases, including a poor resistance to stress. It's believed that the pituitary releases other blocking hormones besides DECO, and some gerontologists have begun to call these "death hormones," since they inhibit rather than help the normal functioning of the cells.

W. Donner Denckla, an endocrinologist with the National Institute of Health, has been a leading proponent of the Central Clock Theory of aging. Dr. Denckla's belief that the pituitary is the central agent in man's aging is supported by his work on rats, in which he has removed the pituitary glands and found, not the expected breakdown of the organism, but a rejuvenation and increase in longevity. In rats twelve to eighteen months of age (equivalent to a man of thirty-five to sixty years of age), Denckla and his associates have found that when they measured nineteen physiologic and biochemical functions that normally occur in the bodies of "middle-aged rats," all but two of these rats had not only been brought back to "juvenile levels" following the removal of the pituitary gland but, furthermore, had shown no signs of aging or deteriorating with the passage of further time. Among many other beneficial effects, Denckla found that with the pituitary removed the manufacturing of messenger RNA (which is normally inhibited in older people and animals) returned to younger levels and the ability of the body to utilize oxygen, called maximal oxygen uptake and considered one of the single most important components when measuring fitness, was increased markedly.

Denckla is responsible for coining the acronym DECO, for the agent in the pituitary that he believes is responsible for aging. Several other research projects, also done on animals, have lent credence to the idea of "death hormones" or have at least corroborated that "youth hormones" exist. In these projects the circulatory systems of young animals were connected to those of older animals, making them into Siamese twins. When this was done, and blood from the young animals circulated into the old, and vice-versa, the older animals not only became "younger" in appearance and function but the younger animals aged more rapidly. Exactly why this occurred is not really clear. DECO, however, is thought to be involved, though there is also some belief that the joining of the two systems also allows for a diminution of toxins in the older bodies and may mean that more viable red blood cells are available for oxygen transport. A new technique, currently still in experimental stages as a rejuvenating tool, is plasmapheresis, or cleaning of the blood. Norman Orantreich, a leading proponent of this new system, has bemoaned the fact that so little research attention and research money has been directed toward plasmapheresis. He's stated modestly on more than one occasion that he thinks it has the potential to double human lifespans. The process, which has been used to detoxify drug abusers, involves removing the blood, filtering out the red blood cells, and discarding the plasma or fluid. The red blood cells are then returned to the body in a sterile solution that causes several noticeable changes. Cell production speeds up, blood cholesterol levels are lowered, and waste products or toxin levels are lowered. While plasmapheresis is not readily available, some researchers suggest that donating blood once a month should have a similar effect. Perhaps leech futures would be a sound investment.

In any event, most physiologists agree that hormone production is the biggest piece in the puzzle of aging. Whether the decrease in human capacity that accompanies aging is imprinted on our genes from the time of fertilization as a "program" to shut down such organs as the pituitary, or whether it's the result of a slowdown in our immune system, a reduced blood supply to the brain, simple free-radical damage, or some combination of these and other factors, the role of the endocrine system in coordinating all other body functions is vital to the aging process.

## The Autoimmune Theory of Aging

The body's natural defense to disease is controlled by our immune system. It works in several different ways, though primarily in the bloodstream, where it forms antibodies to fight off "foreign invaders," such as viruses and bacteria. Some of these antibodies, having rousted the enemy, will then (in some cases) remain in the bloodstream throughout the rest of a person's life so that having had the measles once, we won't be very likely to get them again. The immune system provides us with white blood cells, called lymphocytes, which either circulate through the bloodstream or reside in the lymphatic tissues, ready to go into combat at the first sign of an intruder or antigen. There are trillions of these lymphocytes within our bodies and they are manufactured by the bone marrow. When they leave the marrow, some of them travel to the thymus gland, where they become designated as "T" cells, while others finish their maturation in the bloodstream and become known as "B" cells. The "T" cells act as sentries in the bloodstream. When an antigen or foreign body is discovered trying to sneak in, they send a message to the "B" cells, which soon arrive at the scene and destroy the invader by the formation of antibodies. Sometimes, as noted, the antibodies will then remain to prevent the reoccurrence of that particular disease.

During adolescence and early adulthood, this is an extremely efficient system. Over time, though, "T" cells, in some cases, lose ability to distinguish a foreign cell from a naturally occurring cell within the body, and immunological errors begin to occur. When this happens, the lymphocytes are summoned to attack good tissue, and the health of the organism suffers. Also, over time, the "T" cells lose their ability to recognize foreign antigens so that when a flu "bug" gets into the bloodstream of a seventy-five-year-old, it has a much better chance of actually causing the flu than it does in the bloodstream of an eighteen-year-old. These "T" cell failures are caused by several factors. First, the thymus gland begins to diminish in size and function during early adulthood so that fewer new "T" cells are produced, and the instructions that the thymus constantly relays to the working "T" cells become more confused. (Recent research has indicated that nutritional supplements of vitamins A, C, and E, plus cystine, selenium, and zinc, may help rejuvenate thymus function.)

The second cause of immune-system failures is believed to be free-radical damage. When free radicals attach themselves to such fibrous protein molecules as collagen, it's believed that the cross-links "disguise" the protein cells enough so that the increasingly inept "T" cells, unable to identify them, order an attack, and the body goes to battle against itself. Many researchers now believe that rheumatoid arthritis, one of the greatest problems in older men and women, is caused by free-radical changes in the joints, which the immune system mistakenly attacks.

Clearly, all the problems of aging can't be attributed to immune-system failure, though the combination of immunological breakdown in identifying natural body protein and a lowered resistance to disease caused by its failure is one of the major causes of death among the elderly. Far too many older individuals die of such ailments as the flu, when forty years earlier they would have been saved by their then-vigilant lymphocytes on patrol in the bloodstream. Clearly, more research needs to be done into the decline in the size of the thymus gland and the nutritional factors that may help to offset such an apparently inevitable occurrence.

## Wear and Tear and Debris Theories

There are two final theories we should briefly mention, though their names cause them to need little other explanation. According to the Wear and Tear theory, the body wears out as joints, blood vessels, bones and muscles become frayed and fragile, worn away, and torn through repeated use until, like that 1957 Chevy you nursed along for years, something really major happens — you can't get a replacement part — and it goes up on the blocks. While there's a certain wonderful logic to this particular argument, it doesn't take into account the body's ability to form new cells in the case of some body tissues and the fact that within individual cells, there is a constant rebuilding process that keeps them functioning.

The Debris theory is supported by a good bit of clinical evidence that both calcium and a certain pigment called lipofuscin accumulate within individual cells with the passage of time. Whether they act as a cause of aging or merely as a side effect of it is not clear. Anna Aslan, who has advocated the use of a novacaine-type substance called procaine as a life extension tool, believes that the accumulation of calcium, at least, is quite serious. Procaine is widely used in Europe, though it is only legal here in the state of Nevada. It has been found that procaine will release this unwanted form of calcium from the cells, which allows the cells to function more efficiently. Aslan discovered the rejuvenating effects of procaine indirectly. In her search for a drug to help offset some of the crippling effects that occurred in her arthritis patients, she tried procaine and found that besides making immediate flexibility differences in the stiffened joints, her patients felt better, their memories improved, they became unconsciously more active, and many of them had lower blood-pressure readings on subsequent visits. Since Dr. Aslan's first use of procaine back in 1951, well over three hundred research papers have been written, many of them showing favorable results from its use. Several research papers have also documented the presence of lipofuscin within the cells, particularly in the muscles of the heart. The pigment has a high fat content, leading researchers to think that it's formed by the peroxidation of lipid/fat mixtures. There is almost no lipofuscin present in the heart muscles of children, although B. L. Strehler found that by the time a man reached age ninety, 6 to 7 percent of the individual cell's volume would be occupied by the pigment. So far, no research has indicated that lipofuscin impairs the functioning of the muscles, though its presence is hardly looked upon as a positive. One avenue that needs further investigation is the relationship of unsaturated fats, such as many Americans use in vegetable oils, and lipofuscin. Doctors, with their warnings of cholesterol and heart attacks, encouraged us to avoid butter and instead use vegetable oils that are "polyunsaturated." Yet these unsaturated fats in large quantities lead to the formation of ceroid, a type of lipofuscin, which can accumulate in atherosclotic plaque. Sometimes it seems as if the only really safe advice is to exercise regularly.

# Equipment Sources

**Diversified Products,** the inventors of the vinyl-covered barbell plates described in Chapter 17, Training at Home with the Basics, now offers a full range of home use equipment — Olympic weights, exercise weights, stationary bicycles, pulley machines, etc. Their products are available in most major sporting goods and department stores. For further information write: Diversified Products, 309 Williamson Ave., Opelika, Alabama 36802.

**Iron Man Equipment Company,** run by Peary and Mabel Rader, sells some of the best heavy-duty exercise machines in the country. Each issue of *Iron Man* magazine carries eight to ten pages describing the various benches, squat stands, pulley machines, etc. The Raders also have the exclusive U.S. rights to market Eleiko Olympic sets, the crème de la crème of barbells. For further details write: Iron Man Equipment Company, P.O. Box 10, Alliance, Nebraska 69301.

**Jubinville Equipment Company,** run by Ed Jubinville, is a good East Coast source of heavy-duty benches, Olympic-style weights, lat machines, and other equipment suitable for serious home gyms. For catalogue and price list write: Jubinville Equipment Company, P.O. Box 662, Holyoke, Massachusetts 01041.

**Pat's Power Products,** located in West Lafayette, Indiana, is run by Pat Malone. Pat offers good, heavy-duty benches and racks, lifting belts, Olympic-style weights, lifting suits, and a multitude of other products. For a full price list write: Pat's Power Products, 124 E. State Street, West Lafayette, Indiana 47906.

**Weider Health and Fitness** is the equipment end of the vast Weider Enterprises, which includes the publication of *Muscle & Fitness, Shape,* and *Flex.* Weider offers a large selection of exercise and Olympic barbells, dumbbells, benches, and various lifting apparatus. Weider equipment is also on sale in many sporting-goods departments, or through mail order. Write Weider Health and Fitness, 21100 Erwin Street, Woodland Hills, California 91367, for full details.

**York Barbell Company** began selling weights and lifting equipment during the 1930s, and for years were the standard by which all other lifting equipment was compared. Both *Strength and Health* and *Muscular Development,* the York Barbell Company's magazines, contain numerous ads describing the Olympic weights, exercise sets, benches, and racks that are available. For further information write: York Barbell Company, York, Pennsylvania 17405.

There are many, many other barbell and equipment companies throughout the United States who also manufacture first-rate equipment. We have chosen to list these six companies simply because of our familiarity with their products.

# Suggestions for Further Reading

**American Health: Fitness of Body and Mind,** American Health Partners, 80 Fifth Avenue, Suite 302, New York, New York 10011. (American Health is editorially aimed more at the dispersal of health information than at exercise news, but we include it since we both always seem to learn a lot when the new issue arrives. We especially like the way they present the latest research findings so pleasantly.)

**Fit.** Runner's World Publishing Company, 1400 Stierlin Road, Mountain View, California 94043. (*Fit* started out along the lines of *Shape*, but since the birth of *Strength Training for Beauty*, the emphasis has switched from barbells to various forms of aerobic exercise. Besides the exercise information, each issue contains lots of good nutritional and health-related articles.)

**Flex,** 21100 Erwin Street, Woodland Hills, California 91367. (*Flex* is an offshoot of the enormously popular *Muscle & Fitness* magazine. Aimed at hard-core bodybuilders, the exercise routines and training advice are aimed at those with a desire to compete.)

**Iron Man,** P.O. Box 10, Alliance, Nebraska 69301. (*Iron Man* covers weightlifting, bodybuilding, powerlifting, nutrition, and also contains a good bit of information about weight training for fitness. *Iron Man*'s reputation for consistent integrity is unsurpassed in the field.)

**Muscle & Fitness,** 21100 Erwin Street, Woodland Hills, California 91367. (*Muscle & Fitness* is without a doubt the most sophisticated of the bodybuilding magazines now on the market. Gorgeous full-cover photography, skimpy swimsuits, and what is, for the most part, first-rate advice, have made this the biggest seller in the "muscle mag" section of most newsstands.)

**Muscular Development,** York Barbell Company, York, Pennsylvania, 17405. (In the mid-sixties the York people decided to split their coverage of the iron game into two separate publications. So, powerlifting and bodybuilding are now, for the most part, covered by *Muscular Development*, which is edited by John Grimek. *MD* and *Strength and Health* comes out in alternate months.)

**The National Strength and Conditioning Association Journal,** P.O. Box 81410, Lincoln, Nebraska 68501. (It's hard to say whether or not any of you will feel the need to subscribe to the *NSCA Journal*, but if you're at all interested in the real nuts and bolts of weight-training research, this would be a good place to start. Though the *Journal* is designed to meet the need of coaches and those involved with the hands-on training of athletes, many of the articles — as you can see in our bibliography — go far beyond how to be stronger for football.)

**Shape,** 21100 Erwin Street, Woodland Hills, California 91367. (Like *Flex*, *Shape* is the stepchild of *Muscle & Fitness*, although here, publisher Joe Weider has attempted to satisfy the needs of women. Each issue contains exercise routines, nutritional information, fashion and makeup tips, and more. Shape's emphasis is on fitness and weight reduction — not competitive bodybuilding.)

**Strength and Health,** York Barbell Company, York, Pennsylvania 17405. (*Strength and Health*, now published bi-monthly, contains information on Olympic weight lifting, health and physical culture. It is the oldest continuously published lifting magazine in the United States.)

**Strength Training for Beauty,** Runner's World Publishing Company, 1400 Stierlin Road, Mountain View, California 94043. (Like *Shape* and *Fit*, *STFB* is a woman's magazine that includes information on exercise, nutrition, beauty, fashion, and health, but unlike them, it is perhaps aimed a bit more at women who are seriously interested in training with weights. It includes lots of good bodybuilding information as well as the latet research findings.)

If you check your newsstands, you'll see that there are a number of other publications that also cover weight training and fitness. We don't intend this to be a complete list, only a list of some of the magazines we've found, through the years, to be helpful.

**Books**

Anderson, Bob. *Stretching*. Bolinas, CA: Shelter Publications, 1980.

Barrilleaux, Doris. *Forever Fit*. Southbend, IN: Icarus Press, 1983.

Darden, Ellington. *The Nautilus Book*. Chicago: Contemporary Books, 1982.

————. *The Nautilus Advanced Bodybuilding Book*. New York: Simon and Schuster, 1984.

Dominguez, Richard H., and Robert Gajda. *Total Body Training*. New York: Charles Scribner's Sons, 1982.

Goldman, Bob. *Death in the Locker Room — Steroids and Sports*. South Bend, IN: Icarus Press, 1984.

Mann, John A. *Secrets of Life Extenion*. New York: Bantam Books, 1980.

Mentzer, Mike, and Ardy Friedberg. *The Mentzer Method to Fitness*. New York: William Morrow and Co., 1980.

Pearl, Bill. *Keys to the Inner Universe*. Pasadena: Physical Fitness Architects, 1982.

Pearon, Durk and Sandy Shaw. *Life Extension*. New York: Warner Books, 1982.

Reeves, Steve. *Powerwalking*. New York: Bobb-Merrill Co., 1982.

Root, Allen W. *Human Pituitary Growth Hormone*. Springfield, IL: Charles C. Thomas Publishers, 1972.

Rosenzweig, Sandra. *Sportsfitness for Women*. New York: Harper & Row, 1982.

Sharkey, Brian. *Physiology of Fitness*. Champagne, IL: Human Kinetics Publishing, 1979.

Todd, Terry. *Inside Powerlifting*. Chicago: Contemporary Books, 1978.

Todd, Terry, and Dick Hoover. *Fitness for Athletes*. Chicago: Contemporary Books, 1977.

U.S. Department of Agriculture, Handbook #8, *Composition of Foods*. Washington, D.C.: U.S. Government Printing Office, 1975.

Walford, Roy L., M.D. *Maximum Lifespan*. New York: Avon Books, 1983.

Zane, Frank, and Christine Zane. *The Zane Way to a Beautiful Body*. New York: Simon & Schuster, 1979.

As with the magazines — even more so — there are many informative books not listed here. Our own library, in fact, includes over a thousand such books, but to list them all seems excessive. The ones we did list simply happen to be the ones we used most as we wrote our own.

# Bibliography

Abraham, William M. "Factors in Delayed Muscle Soreness." *Medicine and Science in Sports* 9, no. 1 (1977): 11–20.

Aloia, J. F., S. H. Cohn, J. A. Ostuni, R. Crane, and K. Ellis. "Prevention of Involutional Bone Loss by Exercise." *Annals of Internal Medicine* 89 (1978): 3.

Amatruda, J. M., S. M. Harman, G. Pourmotabbed, and D. H. Lockwood. "Depressed Plasma Testosterone and Functional Binding of Testosterone in Obese Males." *Journal of Clinical Endocrinology and Metabolism* 47 (1978): 268–271.

Anderson, Bob. *Stretching.* Bolinas, CA: Shelter Publications, 1980.

Archer, Patricia Ann. "The Relationship of Serum Testosterone Level to Strength, Percent Body Fat and $VO_2$ Max in Females." Master's thesis, Arizona State University, 1976. Published by Microform Publications, Physical Education and Recreation, University of Oregon, 1978.

Astrand, Per-Olaf, and Kaare Rodahl. *Textbook of Work Physiology.* New York: McGraw-Hill Book Co., 1977.

Barry, A., J. Steinmetz, H. Page, and K. Rodahl. "The Effects of Physical Conditioning on Older Individuals — Motor Performance and Cognitive Function." *Journal of Gerontology* 21 (1966): 182–191.

Berg, Kris. "Anaerobic Conditioning — Training the Three Energy Systems." *National Strength and Conditioning Association Journal* 4, no. 1 (1982): 48–52.

Clarke, D. H. "Adaptations in Strength and Muscular Endurance Resulting from Exercise." *Exercise and Sport Sciences Reviews* 1. J. H. Wilmore, ed. New York: Academic Press (1973): 74–98.

Cooper, K. H. *Aerobics.* New York: Evans Publishing Co., 1968.

————. *The New Aerobics.* New York: Evans Publishing Co., 1970.

Costill, David L., George E. Branam, Jack C. Moore, Kenneth Sparks, and Craig Turner. "Effects of Physical Training in Men with Coronary Heart Disease." *Medicine and Science in Sports* 6. no. 4 (1974): 95–100.

Cumming, Gordon R., and Lawrence M. Borysyk. "Criteria for Maximum Oxygen Uptake in Men over 40 in a Population Survey." *Medicine and Science in Sports* 4, no. 1 (1972): 18–22.

Cureton, Thomas K., ed. *Encyclopedia of Physical Education, Fitness and Sports — Training, Environment, Nutrition and Fitness.* Salt Lake City: Brighton Publishing Co., 1980.

Darden, Ellington. *The Nautilus Book.* Chicago: Contemporary Books, 1982.

————. *The Nautilus Bodybuilding Book.* Chicago: Contemporary Books, 1982.

De Kruif, Paul. *The Male Hormone.* Garden City, NJ: Garden City Publishing, 1945.

Desleypere, J. P., and A. Vermulen. "Aging and Tissue Androgens." *Journal of Clinical Endocrinology and Metabolism* 53 (1981): 430–434.

DeVries, Herbert A. *Fitness After Fifty.* New York: Charles Scribner's Sons, 1982.

————. *Physiology of Exercise for Physical Education and Athletics.* Dubuque: W. C. Brown Co., 1966.

————. "Physiological Effects of an Exercise Training Regimen upon Men Aged 52–88." *Journal of Gerontology* 25, no. 4 (1970): 325–336.

Dominguez, Richard H., and Robert Gajda. *Total Body Training.* New York: Charles Scribner's Sons, 1982.

Dunn, Bill, and Sue Halstead. "Strength Training for Women — Issues and Answers." *National Strength and Conditioning Coaches Association Journal* 4, no. 3 (1982): 32–36.

Elder, H. P. "The Effects of Training on Middle-aged Men." *Exercise and Fitness.* D. P. Franks, ed. Chicago: Athletic Institute, 1969.

Engle, Earl, and Gregory Pincus, eds. *Hormones and the Aging Process.* New York: Academic Press, 1956.

Fahey, Thomas, Richard Rolph, Pratoom Moungmee, James Nagel, and Stephen Mortara. "Serum Testosterone, Body Composition and Strength of Young Adults." *Medicine and Science in Sports* 8, no. 1 (1976): 31–34.

Ferris, S., F. Crook, G. Sathananthan, and S. Gershan. "Reaction Time as a Diagnostic Measure in Senility." *Journal of American Geriatric Society* 24 (1976): 529–533.

Flint, Marilyn, Barbara Drinkwater, and Steven Horvath. "Effects of Training on Women's Response to Submaximal Exercise." *Medicine and Science in Sports* 6, no. 2 (1974): 89–94.

Francis P. R., and C. M. Tipton. "Influence of a Weight Training Program on Quadriceps Reflex Time." *Medicine and Science in Sports* 1 (1969): 91–94.

Garhammer, John. "Power Production by Olympic Weightlifters." *Medicine and Science in Sports and Exercise* 12, no. 1 (1980): 54–60.

Gettman, L. R., M. L. Pollock, J. L. Durstine, A. Ward, J. Ayres, and A. C. Linnerud. "Physiological Responses of Men to 1, 3, and 5 Day per Week Training Programs." *Research Quarterly* 47 (1976): 638–646.

Gettman, Larry R., Paul Ward, and R. D. Hagan. "A Comparison of Combined Running and Weight Training with Circuit Weight Training." *Medicine and Science in Sports and Exercise* 14, no. 3 (1982): 229–234.

Gordon, G. A. "Proprioceptive Neuromuscular Facilitation — The Super Stretch." *National Strength and Conditioning Association Journal* 4, no. 2 (1982): 26–29.

Groves, Phil, Carol Lissance, and Mele Olsen. *The Natural Foods Calorie Counter.* New York: Bantam Books, 1982.

Guyton, Arthur C., M.D. *Textbook of Medical Physiology.* Philadelphia: W. B. Saunders Co., 1976.

Hilyer, James C., and William Mitchell. "Effect of Systematic Physical Fitness Training Combined with Counseling on the Self-Concept of College Students." *Journal of Counseling Psychology* 26, no. 5 (1979): 427–436.

Howley, Edward T., and Mary Edna Glover. "The Caloric Costs of Running and Walking One Mile for Men and Women." *Medicine and Science in Sports* 6, no. 4 (1974): 235–237.

Jankowski, Louis W., and Merle E. Foss. "The Energy Intake of Sedentary Men after Moderate Exercise." *Medicine and Science in Sports* 4, no. 1 (1972): 11–13.

Jezova, Daniela, and Milan Vigas. "Testosterone Response to Exercise during Blockade and Stimulation of Androgenic Receptors in Man." *Hormone Research* 15 (1981): 141–147.

Keizer, H. A. "Influence of Physical Exercise on Sex-Hormone Metabolism." *Journal of Applied Physiology* 48 (May 1980): 765–769.

Kent, Saul. "The Biologic Aging Clock." *Geriatrics* 37, no. 7 (1982): 95–99.

Kinsey, A. C., W. C. Pomeroy, and C. E. Martin. *Sexual Behavior in the Human Male*. Philadelphia: W. B. Saunders Co., 1948.

Kraus, Barbara. *Calorie Guide to Brand Names and Basic Foods*. New York: New American Library, 1981.

Lamb, David R. *Physiology of Exercise: Responses and Adaptations*. New York:MacMillan Co., 1978.

————. "Androgens and Exercise." *Medicine and Science in Sports* 7, no. 1 (1975): 1–5.

Liemohn, Wendell A. *Strength of Aging: An Exploratory Study." Journal of Aging and Human Development* 6, no. 4 (1975): 347–357.

Mann, John A. *Secrets of Life Extension*. New York: Bantam Books, 1980.

Maple, Terry L., and Michael Hoff. *Gorilla Behavior*. New York: Van Nostrand Reinhold Co., 1982.

Martin, L. G., J. W. Clarke, and T. B. Conner. "Growth Hormone Secretion Enhanced by Androgens." *Journal of Clinical Endocrinology* 38 (1968): 425–428.

Massie, J. F., and Roy J. Shephard. "Physiological and Psychological Effects of Training." *Medicine and Science in Sports* 3, no. 2 (1971): 110–117.

Masters, W. H., and V. Johnson. *Human Sexual Inadequacy*. Boston: Little, Brown and Co., 1970.

McFarland, R. "Experimental Evidence of the Relationship between Aging and Oxygen Want: In Search of a Theory of Aging." *Ergonomics* 6 (1975): 339–366.

McKerns, Kenneth W. *Steroids, Hormones and Metabolism*. New York: Appleton-Century-Crofts, 1969.

Metivier, G., R. Gauthier, J. De La Chevrotiere, and D. Grymala. "The Effect of Acute Exercise on the Serum Levels of Testosterone and Leuteinizing Hormone in Human Male Athletes." *Journal of Sports Medicine and Physical Fitness* 20, no. 3 (September 1980): 235–238.

Michael, R. P., and D. Zumpe. "Potency in Male Rhesus Monkeys: Effect of Continually Receptive Females." *Science* 200 (1978): 451–453.

O'Shea, John Patrick. *Scientific Principles and Methods of Strength Fitness*. Reading, MA: Addison-Wesley Publishing Co., 1976.

O'Shea, Pat. "The Endocrine System and Physical Activity — An Overview." *National Strength and Conditioning Association Journal* 6, no. 1 (1984): 31–36.

Padus, Emrika. *The Women's Encyclopedia of Health and Natural Healing*. Emmaus, PA: Rodale Press, 1982.

Pearl, Bill. *Keys to the Inner Universe*. Pasadena: Physical Fitness Architects, 1982.

Palmari, Gerard A. "The Principles of Muscle Fiber Recruitment Applied to Strength Training." *National Strength and Conditioning Association Journal* 5, no. 5 (1983): 22–26.

Pearson, Durk and Sandy Shaw. *Life Extension*. New York: Warner Books, 1982.

Pedemonte, Jimmy. "Periodization of Strength Training." *National Strength and Conditioning Association Journal* 4, no. 2 (1982): 10–11.

Pollock, Michael L., Jeffrey Broida, Zebulon Kendrick, Henry S. Miller, Richard Janeway, and A. C. Linnerud. "Effects of Training Two Days per Week at Different Intensities on Middle-aged Men." *Medicine and Science in Sports* 4, no. 4 (1972): 192–197.

Pollock, Michael L., Henry S. Miller, and Paul M. Ribsi. "Effect of Fitness of Aging." *The Physician and Sportsmedicine* 6, no. 8 (1978): 45–48.

Pollock, Michael, Jack Wilmore, and Samuel M. Fox. *Health and Fitness Through Physical Activity.* New York: Wiley, 1978.

Reeves, Steve. *Powerwalking.* New York: Bobbs-Merrill Co., 1982.

Richardson, John R. "A Comparison of Two Drugs on Strength Increase in Monkeys." *The Journal of Sports Medicine and Physical Fitness* 17, no. 3 (1977): 251–254.

Root, Allen W. *Human Pituitary Growth Hormone.* Springfield, IL: Charles C. Thomas Publishers, 1972.

Rosenzweig, Sandra. *SportsFitness for Women.* New York: Harper & Row, 1982.

Sale, D. G., A. R. M. Upton, A. J. McComas, and J. D. MacDougall. "Neuromuscular Function in Weight Trainers." *Experimental Neurology* 82 (1983): 521–531.

Selim, Robert D. *Muscles: The Magic of Motion.* Washington, D.C.: U.S. News Books, 1982.

Sharkey, Brian. *Physiology of Fitness.* Champagne, IL: Human Kinetics Publishing, 1979.

Sherwood, David E. and Dennis Selder. "Cardiorespiratory Health, Reaction Time and Aging." *Medicine and Science in Sports* 11, no. 2 (1979): 186–189.

Smith, Everett, William Reddan, and Patricia Smithy. "Physical Activity and Calcium Modalities for Bone Mineral Increase in Aged Women." *Medicine and Science in Sports and Exercise* 13, no. 1 (1981): 60–64.

Spirduso, Waneen W. "Exercise and the Aging Brain." The AAPHERD Research Consortium Third Annual C. H. McCloy Research Lecture. *Research Quarterly for Exercise Sciences* (1982).

————. "Physical Fitness in Relation to Motor Aging." *The Aging Motor System.* James A. Mortimer, Francis J. Pirozzolo, and Gabe J. Maletta, eds. New York: Praeger, 1982.

————. "Physical Fitness, Aging and Psychomotor Speed: A Review." *Journal of Gerontology* 35, no. 6 (1980): 850–865.

Stone, J. L. and A. H. Norris. "Activities and Attitudes of Participants in the Baltimore Longitudinal Study." *Journal of Gerontology* 21 (1966): 575–580.

Stone, Michael, Ron Byrd, Doug Boatwright, and John Tew. "Physiological Effects of a Short Term Resistive Training Program on Middle-age Sedentary Men." *National Strength and Conditioning Association Journal* 4 (October/November 1982): 16–20.

Stone, Michael, Dennis Wilson, Danny Blessing, and Ralph Rozenek. "Cardiovascular Response to Short Term Olympic-style Weight Training in Young Men." *Canadian Journal of Applied Sport Science* 8 (September 1983): 134–135.

Stone, Michael and John Garhammer. "Some Thoughts on Strength and Power." *National Strength and Conditioning Coaches Association Journal* 3, no. 5 (1981): 24–28, 30–32.

Stone, Michael, Ronald Byrd, and Cathy Johnson. "Observations on Serum Androgen Response to Short Term Resistive Training in Middle-age Sedentary Males." *National Strength and Conditioning Association Journal* 5, no. 6 (1984): 30–31.

Stone, Michael, and Harry Lipner. "Responses to Intensive Training and Methandrostenelone Administration: Part 1, Contractile and Performance Variables." *Pfluger Archiv* 375 (1978).

Stone, Michael, and Harry Lipner, and Michael Rush. "Responses to Intensive Training and Methandrostenelone Administration: Part 2, Hormonal, Organ Weights, Muscle Weights, and Body Composition." *Pfluger Archiv* 375 (1978: 147–151.

Sutton, J. R., M. J. Coleman, J. Casy, and L. Lazarus. "Androgen Responses during Physical Exercise." *British Medical Journal* 163 (1973): 520–522.

Tierney, John. "The Aging Body." *Esquire* (May 1982): 45–57.

Thorstensson, Alf, Lars Larson, Per Tesch, and Jan Karlsson. "Muscle Strength and Fiber Composition in Athletes and Sedentary Men." *Medicine and Science in Sports* 9, no. 1 (1977): 26–30.

Tsitouras, Panayiotis, Clyde E. Martin, and S. Mitchell Harman. "Relationship of Serum Testosterone to Sexual Activity in Healthy Elderly Men." *Journal of Gerontology* 37, no. 3 (1982): 288–293.

United States Department of Agriculture. Handbook #8, *Composition of Foods.* U.S. Government Printing Office, Washington, D.C.: 1975.

Wilmore, Jack H. *Athletic Training and Physical Fitness: Physiological Principles and Practices of the Conditioning Process.* Boston: Allyn and Bacon, 1976.

————. "Alterations in Strength, Body Composition and Anthropometric Measurements Consequent to a 10-Week Training Program." *Medicine and Science in Sports* 6, no. 2 (1974): 133–138.

Yessis, Michael. "Trends in Soviet Strength and Conditioning — The Soviet Sports Training System: The Yearly Cycle." *National Strength and Conditioning Association Journal* 3, no. 6 (1982): 42–45.

# Index

Calories: average daily expenditure, 72; average daily needs of men and women, 71; calculating requirements, 71–72; recording caloric intake, 72–73; reducing intake, 72–79
Cancer, STH and, 45
Calves, exercises for, 141, 154, 156, 159, 160, 257
Cardiovascular fitness, 29, 30; 52–54; aerobic exercise for, 124–25, 260–64; circuit training for, 283
Cardiovascular disease and memory and intelligence, 53, 67. *See also* Heart disease
Carrel, Alexis, 310–11
Cartilage and exercise, 56
"Cell therapy," 310–11
Cellular Theory of Aging, 312
Central Clock Theory of Aging, 312, 315–17
Central nervous system: aging of, 65–68; high-intensity training and, 113–14; "training," 33, 34
Checkup, physical, 124
Chest laterals: high-pulley, 243; single-arm, 243
Chin, the, 249, 269
Chinning bar, 186, 233, 249, 259
Cholesterol, 53, 54, 319; and response times, 67
Circuit training, 282–83; at home, 283
Circulation of blood, 52–54. *See also* Blood-flow
Clean, dumbbell, 196
Close-Grip Bench Press, 166; with curl bar, 195
Clothes, training, 129–31
Collagen, 5, 56, 314; cross-links in, 314
*Composition of Foods* (U.S. Department of Agriculture), 73, 79
Concentration Curl, 206
Cooper, Kenneth: *Aerobics,* 290
Cornell University Medical College, 29
Creatine phosphate, 36, 38
"Cross-links," 313–14; and immune system failure, 318

Crunch, 95, 180
Cunningham, L. H., 286
Curl, 172; reverse, 172
Curl, wrist, 173; with curl bar, 251; dumbbell, 252; reverse curl with dumbbells, 252; reverse wrist curl with curl bar, 251
Curl bar, 188, 233, 248; close-grip bench with, 195; curl, 193; wrist curl with, 251
Curls: cable, 198; concentration, 206; curl-bar, 193; dumbbell, 205; leg, 214; preacher bench, 248
Curry: Bill, 131, 286–87, 288, 289–92; Bill (son), 292–96; Eleanor, 131, 262, 264, 290, 299–301; Linda, 296, 298–99
Cycle training, 110, 111
Cycling, 35, 37, 189; as aerobic exercise, 124–25, 261, 263–64; as warm-up, 50, 134. *See also* Bicycle, exercise

Darden, Ellington: *The Nautilus Book,* 232, 258
Davis, Carol, 88, 90
Deadlift, 12, 153, 269; partial deadlift in power rack, 256, 269; stiff-legged, 157; women's world-record, 23
De Anza College, 43
Debris Theory of Aging, 318–19
Decline Bench Press, 239; Dumbbell Decline Press, 239
Decline Dumbbell Fly, 240
DECO (decreasing consumption of oxygen), 315–16
Deltoid Raises: low pulley, 247; rear deltoid raise, 204
Deltoids, exercises for, 150, 161, 162, 165, 166, 168, 170, 195, 196, 199, 200, 201, 202, 204, 207, 208, 212, 239, 240, 244, 246, 247
Denckla, W. Donner, 316
DeVries, Herbert, 68
Dieting, 71–73, 75–79. *See* Calories; Diets
Dietrich, Dr. John E., 29–30
Diets: calorie-counting, 75–76, 77–78;

Front Raise with Dumbbells, 207; alternating, 207; single dumbbell, 207
Front Squat, 216

Gant, Lamar, 59
Gastrocnemius muscle, exercises for, 159, 257
Gedney, Judy, 97–103, 112
General Adaptation Syndrome, 111
Genetic theories of aging, 312–17
Gerontology, 309
Gettman, Larry, 283
Glasser, William, 23
Gluteus maximus. *See* Buttocks
Glycogen, 37, 40
Glycolysis, 37–38
Goal-setting for weight poundages, 113, 116–18, 269
Gonyea, Dr. W. J., 34
Good Morning, the, 158
Grimek, John, 7, 8
*Guinness Book of World Records,* 18, 34
Gyms, 230–31
Gyms, commercial, 225–59; choosing, 226–29; "classes" at, 234–35; equipment, 231–32, 233; exercises for, 239–59; gym etiquette, 235–37; memberships in, 234; pitfalls at, 234–37; starting training, 237–38; types, 226, 229–31

Hack Squat, 254
Hagan, R. D., 283
Hamstrings, exercises for, 138, 139, 149, 153, 154, 156, 157, 160, 213, 214
Hand straps, 152
Hanging Knee-up, 259
Hanging Leg Raise, 259
Hayflick, Leonard, 312
Head strap or harness, 250
Health clubs. *See* Health spas
Health spas, 226, 227, 230, 234–35; visiting, 228–29
Heart disease, 44, 124–25. *See also* Cardiovascular disease

High blood pressure. *See* Hypertension
High Pull, 154–55, 269, 273
High repetition work, 110, 111, 115
"High volume-low intensity" training, 111, 113
Hilyer, Dr. James, 68, 95
Hips, exercises for, 137, 176
Home, training at, 107, 143–44; basic equipment for, 144–45; basic program for, 145–52; circuit training, 283; other exercises for, 153–82. *See also* Home gym
Home gym: equipment for, 183–91; exercises for, 193–224; training with, 191–92
Hormones, 40–47, 315–17; "death," 316; human growth, 45–46; synthetic, 41, 44; in women, 40, 46–47; "youth hormones," 316
Hydrostatic weighing, 69, 70, 76, 88, 89
Hyperextension machine, 233
Hyperextension, 242; twisting, 242; weighted, 242
"Hyperplasia," 34
Hypertension, 53–54, 67, 79, 124–25
Hypertrophy, 34, 39, 43, 112
Hypertrophy phase of periodization, 113, 115, 117, 118–20, 123; basic program for, 147; circuit training and, 283
Hypothalamus, 315

Immune system, 317–18
Incline benches, 144, 186, 233
Incline boards, 233
Incline Dumbbell Fly, 240
Incline Press, 199, 269; Dumbbell Incline Press, 199
Injury prevention, 124, 127, 238, 261, 264
Intercostal muscles, exercises for, 203
Intermediate sets, 113, 118, 123
International Powerlifting Federation, 23
*Iron Man* (magazine), 191
Isometric contraction, 110

Western Illinois Powerlifting Club, 100
Wide ("Sumo") Squat, 217
Wilcox, Dr. Richard, 66
Wilson, Dennis, 81
Wistar Institute, 312
Women: aging process in, 4–5, 47, 58; average daily caloric requirement, 71; bodybuilders, 60–64; exercises for, 208, 213, 214, 217, 223, 239, 272–73; facilities for in gyms, 228; hormones and, 40, 46–47; metabolic rate of, 71; in powerlifting competition, 19–21, 100–103; strength of, 31–32, 39. *See also* Sedentary middle-aged women

"Working in," 236–37
Workouts. *See* Routines; Training programs
Wrist Curl, 173; with curl bar, 251; dumbbell, 252; reverse with curl bar, 251; reverse with dumbbell, 252
Wrist weights, 262, 263

YMCA/YWCA, 229
York, Carol, 96
York Barbell Club, 12; 300-Pound Club, 286
York Barbell Company, 191, 286

Zane, Frank, 180